Optum

AF809011

Evaluation and Management Coding Advisor

Advanced guidance on E/M code selection for traditional documentation systems

2025

optumcoding.com

Optum Notice

Our Commitment to Accuracy

Optum is committed to producing accurate and reliable materials.

To report corrections, please email customerassistance@optum.com. You can also reach customer service by calling 1.800.464.3649, option 1.

American Medical Association Notice

Copyright

Made in the USA
ISBN 978-1-62254-976-4

Acknowledgments

Marianne Randall, *Product Manager*
Stacy Perry, *Manager, Desktop Publishing*
Leanne Patterson, CPC, *Subject Matter Expert*
Tara Rose, CPC, CPC-I, CPMA, RHIA, CCS-P, *Subject Matter Expert*
Tracy Betzler, *Senior Desktop Publishing Specialist*
Hope M. Dunn, *Senior Desktop Publishing Specialist*
Katie Russell, *Desktop Publishing Specialist*
Kimberli Turner, *Editor*

Subject Matter Experts

Leanne Patterson, CPC

Ms. Patterson has more than 20 years of experience in the health care profession. She has an extensive background in professional component coding, with proven expertise in assignment of E/M codes, general surgery coding, medical record documentation improvement, and HIPAA compliance. Her experience includes serving as Director of Compliance, conducting chart-to-claim audits, and physician education. She has been responsible for coding and denial management in large multi-specialty physician practices, and most recently has been part of a team developing content for products related to ICD-10-CM. Ms. Patterson is credentialed by and is a member of the AAPC.

Tara Rose, CPC, CPC-I, CPMA, RHIA, CCS-P

Ms. Rose has more than 15 years of experience in the health care profession. She has extensive experience in auditing, physician billing, and multi-specialty coding with assignment of CPT, HCPCS, and ICD-10-CM codes. She has served in roles as a coding consultant, trainer, clinical investigator, community college instructor, and coding lead. She has experience providing education to physicians and both new and experienced coders. Ms. Rose is a member of her local AAPC chapter and holds credentials from the American Health Information Management Association (AHIMA).

Product Updates

Significant updates to this manual will also be provided on our product updates page at Optumcoding.com, which can be accessed at the following:
https://www.optumcoding.com/ProductUpdates/
Password: EM25

Contents

Chapter 1. Introduction

About This Book

Evaluation and Management Coding Advisor is a reference guide to help providers select the correct code based on work, and to assist staff and compliance personnel in efforts to ensure that their medical record documentation substantiates the level of evaluation and management (E/M) service code selected. The guide can also be used as a training tool to help staff educate providers regarding the type and detail of documentation that is necessary.

The guide will provide:

- The American Medical Association's (AMA) guidelines for accurate E/M code selection and the documentation criteria necessary to support each E/M code. This text will familiarize readers with the basics.
- An analysis of the difference between correct coding and supporting documentation. This includes in-depth discussion of the medical decision making component and should result in an increase in E/M coding accuracy. This will include both AMA revisions and current CMS guidelines.
- A section prior to each range of E/M codes that will outline real-world issues with particular code types.
- Samples of proper medical documentation for both the level of service and the medical necessity for the service. Optum editors will endeavor to provide realistic samples as well as "perfect" notes.
- The potential for decreased audit liability by presenting guidelines for appropriate medical record documentation, including an explanation of the Subjective Objective Assessment Plan (SOAP) format, and examples of supporting documentation and standard abbreviations.

In addition to being a resource for solving day-to-day coding and documentation problems, the *Evaluation and Management Coding Advisor* can be used as a teaching tool for in-service education and as a source book for seminars, E/M coding and documentation training programs, and college and university courses.

Evaluation and Management Coding Advisor does not replace the Current Procedural Terminology (CPT®) code book, nor does it contain all the E/M coding guidelines created by the AMA. Rather, it is to be used to understand proper code selection and the linkage to medical record documentation.

Physician or Other Qualified Health Care Professional

The AMA's CPT book advises coders that the procedures and services listed throughout the book are for use by any qualified physician or other qualified health care professional or entity (e.g., hospitals, laboratories, or home health agencies).

The use of the phrase "physician or other qualified health care professional" was adopted to identify a health care provider other than a physician. This type of provider is further described in the CPT book as an individual "qualified by education, training, licensure/regulation (when applicable), and facility privileging (when applicable)" who performs a professional service within his/her scope of practice and independently reports that professional service." The professionals within this definition are separate from "clinical staff." The CPT book defines clinical staff as "a person who works under the supervision of a physician or other qualified health care professional and who is allowed, by law, regulation, and facility policy to perform or assist in the performance of a specified professional service, but who does not individually report that professional service." Keep in mind that there may be other policies, guidance, or payer policies that can affect who may report a specific service.

Contents

Organization

Evaluation and Management Coding Advisor is a resource for physicians and their staff with helpful sections to assist physicians in validating medical documentation and enable staff to verify support of the selected E/M code.

An Introduction and Overview of E/M Coding

This section gives a brief overview of the history and origin of evaluation and management (E/M) services, including the development of E/M documentation and coding. Coverage criteria and reimbursement issues for telehealth services are discussed, including information regarding the temporary expansion of telehealth services during the COVID-19 public health emergency (PHE).

The Building Blocks of Evaluation and Management Coding

This section details the categories and subcategories that must be considered when selecting the appropriate E/M code. Medical decision making (MDM) and time are covered in depth including definitions and descriptions of each element used in accurate code selection, as defined by the AMA and federal guidelines.

Modifiers that may be used with an E/M code are provided in this section, as well as the steps for selecting an E/M code. In addition, this section contains a list of terms commonly used in defining the E/M codes.

Quick Tip

Misuse of modifiers with E/M services has been, and continues to be, carefully reviewed by CMS and other payers as well as the OIG.

The Elements of Medical Documentation

Documentation principles are presented in this section, as well as information on how to evaluate medical chart documentation. This information is the result of a collaborative effort by representatives from national health information, medical societies, and insurance industry associations.

This section also explains components of the SOAP format, a method of medical chart documentation. It does not provide comprehensive instruction in using the SOAP format; it merely introduces the concept and states what is required for each component.

Adjudication of Claims by Third-Party Payers

This section outlines what third-party payers expect to find documented in the medical chart for a particular E/M service. The guidelines presented are not comprehensive, nor specific to a particular third-party payer. This section includes general information regarding teaching physician documentation requirements and incident-to protocols. Review sheets are also included and can be used by auditors to evaluate a provider's documentation and correct code assignment.

EM Code Types: Coding, Common Issues, and Documentation

This section is organized by E/M code type into 14 chapters numbered 6 through 19, with chapter 19 covering HCPCS Level II G codes applicable to evaluation and management coding. Each chapter contains general guidance on code selection, a discussion of issues that may surround particular codes (when applicable), a summary of individual code requirements, and sample documentation. When possible, Optum will provide both a complete note—samples of medical documentation taken from real-life clinical vignettes and patient presentations, with all elements clearly specified—and the more common "economical version" that many physicians currently provide. Each may be compliant but the difference in detail will illustrate varying approaches to documentation.

The information in these sections may be used to compare whether the E/M code documented in similar clinical scenarios in the typical physician practice resembles the documentation samples provided, or whether another code would be more appropriate for billing based on documentation deficiencies or surpluses. In addition, ICD-10-CM guidance as it relates to E/M coding including examples of details necessary in the E/M documentation for appropriate code selection has been provided.

Chapter 20, "Coding and Compliance," evaluates a variety of E/M compliance issues, both new and ongoing, that have been or currently are being investigated or scrutinized by different authoritative agencies including the OIG and recovery audit contractors (RAC). Issues discussed contain the investigating agency, details of the investigation, and applicable guidelines related to the E/M codes under investigation, as well as suggested strategies medical practices may employ to ensure compliance when reporting these specific E/M codes

Quick Tip

Providers should check with the hospitals with which they are affiliated or privileged for a listing of the acceptable abbreviations.

Knowledge Assessments

Chapter 21 provides the answers to and rationales for the knowledge assessments found in chapters 2 through 20.

Appendixes

Two appendixes are included in this publication. Each appendix provides valuable information for applying the E/M documentation guidelines and offers insight into potential areas of concern, such as fraud and abuse. Appendixes included in the book are:

- Appendix A: Physician E/M Code Self Audit Forms, as well as the documentation worksheets from Medicare contractor Novitas Solutions
- Appendix B: Evaluation and Management (E/M) Services Guidelines
- Glossary

Commonly used terms are found throughout the chapters and in a glossary at the back of this book.

How to Use *Evaluation and Management Coding Advisor*

To identify a particular E/M code, select an E/M level of service code from the CPT book. Next, locate this code in the E/M code types section of *Evaluation and Management Coding Advisor*.

The subsections within E/M code types are in numeric order according to the CPT book, and most subsections contain the following information:

- Quick comparison
  - at-a-glance chart for a quick review of all of the codes in that particular CPT code series and associated decision making, history, and exam requirements
- General guidelines
  - instructional notes for correct E/M code assignment within subset
- Common issue
  - outlines questions frequently associated with a code range or single code
- Documentation requirements
  - medically appropriate history
  - medically appropriate physical examination
  - medical decision making (MDM)
    - number and complexity of problems
    - amount and/or complexity of data reviewed and analyzed
    - risk of complications/morbidity or mortality
  - total time spent on the date of the encounter
    Note: For total time, counseling and coordination of care dominating more than 50 percent of the encounter is no longer a requirement. Time for these services includes total face-to-face and non-face-to-face time spent by the provider on the date of the encounter.
- Sample documentation
  - real-life clinical vignettes to assist in verifying the level of service and medical necessity for each CPT code in the series.
  - textbook- style notes, as well as samples, when practical, that provide a more real-life style of documentation

Review the coding and documentation requirements for the code selected. If the medical decision making documented in a chart being reviewed does not match the levels required for that particular code, locate a more appropriate code by reviewing the quick comparison chart or the code detail of the next code, higher or lower.

Note: Some sections may also contain additional information or instruction from a Medicare contractor, CMS, or other agency titled under the header "Special Instructions" or "Special Notice."

Follow these steps to validate medical documentation in a chart being reviewed

1. **Identify the MDM components in the medical record documentation (see the following example).**
2. **Select an E/M code from the CPT code book based on the MDM components, place and/or type of service, and/or time.**
3. **Review in the E/M code types section the documentation requirements and samples of documentation for the code selected.**

If the documentation does not include all of the necessary components to support the level of E/M code that has been chosen, it may be necessary for the physician/qualified health care professional to complete the chart note with correct details of the patient encounter, if appropriate, or select the documented E/M code for billing purposes.

Correcting documentation in "real time" is generally accepted; late entries for the purpose of filling documentation gaps to support billing a particular code level is not. If it takes a few charts being billed at a lower code level based on missing or insufficient documentation to get a provider's attention, this may prove a good lesson in the long run. The goal should be to teach the provider to recognize the key elements of services as they are provided and be certain that they are documented in the normal course of documentation.

Quick Tip

Review the practices policy for correcting documentation or creating an addendum.

Check for additional instructions under "General Guidelines," or situations that may be relevant in the common issues section. Such instructions include whether a modifier is necessary or what information may need to be reported separately. Consult the provider if chart documentation may not support medical necessity for services. While medical necessity is based on the judgment of the clinician, the chart documentation must clearly support the need for services provided.

The following medical documentation represents physician care consistent with a level IV ED service (99284):

Sample Documentation

History: the patient is a 19-year-old female who presents to the emergency department with a chief complaint of abdominal pain. The pain started approximately two days prior to her evaluation and has persisted. The pain increased in severity the morning of admission to the emergency department. The patient describes the pain as bilateral and lower in the abdominal area. The patient also experienced nausea and two episodes of vomiting. She denies other GI problems. She has recently noted abnormal menstrual periods over the last two or three months. She also noted an occasional or intermittent vaginal discharge.

Physical examination: the patient is a slender young female, well developed and well nourished. Her temperature is 100.5 degrees, blood pressure is 122/76, pulse is 64, respiratory rate is 26. Patient is somewhat anxious. Abdominal exam revealed a soft abdomen with decreased bowel sounds, and bilateral lower abdominal pain to deep palpation. The pain was greater in the right lower quadrant and there were signs of local rebound tenderness. No masses or hepatosplenomegaly were noted. Pelvic exam revealed a tender but normal cervix with minimal vaginal discharge. No bleeding was noted. There was right adnexal pain but no masses were noted.

Laboratory and procedures: Routine CBC, electrolytes, amylase and UA, as well as serum pregnancy tests were performed. The results of these tests revealed a white blood count of 11,500 and a negative b-HCG. Other tests were unremarkable. In view of the patient's condition, she underwent a routine ultrasound study of her lower abdominal and pelvic regions. The ultrasound revealed a right side ovarian cyst and was otherwise unremarkable.

Impression: abdominal pain secondary to ovarian cyst.

Treatment: The patient was treated in the emergency department with intravenous fluids and pain medications. Her course improved in the department and her pain resolved. Her vital signs remained stable. She was discharged after a total stay in the emergency department of two and one half hours. The patient was referred to her gynecologist for immediate follow-up.

Medical decision making (MDM) is classified as being of moderate complexity because the physician evaluated an undiagnosed new problem with an uncertain prognosis and ordered and reviewed laboratory tests (urinalysis, pregnancy test, U/S), and because the risk associated with intravenous pain medication is considered moderate.

Level of MDM is based on two out of three elements of MDM. In this example all three elements qualify as moderate complexity.

Quick Tip

Emergency department E/M services are reported with codes 99281–99285.

Quick Tip

When determining the amount and/or complexity of data reviewed and analyzed, each unique test ordered is counted once; the review of that test is included within the order.

Key Point

Tests that are results only and are analyzed as part of MDM do not count as an independent interpretation but may count as one item when determining the amount/complexity of data reviewed and analyzed (e.g., dipstick UA, CBC, quick strep test).

Summary of Recent Changes to the E/M Codes

New E/M Telemedicine Services Section

For the CY2025 update, the CPT Editorial Panel has added a new Telemedicine Services section within the Evaluation and Management (E/M) section of the CPT codebook.

Telemedicine services are synchronous, real-time, interactive encounters between a physician or other qualified health care professional (QHP) and a patient utilizing either combined audio-video or audio-only telecommunication.

Seventeen new telehealth codes have been added for reporting synchronous audio-video visits and synchronous audio-only visits for new or established patients. These include:

Synchronous Audio-Video E/M Services

- New Patient—98000-98003
- Established Patient—98004-98007

Synchronous Audio-Only E/M Services

- New Patient—98008-98011
- Established Patient—98012-98015

Brief Synchronous Communication Technology-Based Service

- Established Patient—98016

Chapter 2. Overview of E/M Coding

The evaluation and management (E/M) service codes, although some of the most commonly used codes by physicians of all specialties, are among the least understood. These codes, introduced in the 1992 CPT® book, were designed to increase accuracy and consistency of use in the reporting of levels of cognitive encounters. This was accomplished by defining the E/M codes based on the degree that certain elements common to cognitive services are addressed or performed and reflected in the medical record documentation. E/M codes have specific elements identified that must be documented to meet the level of care reported.

At the same time the E/M codes were introduced, the American Medical Association (AMA), in conjunction with other organizations, released general documentation guidelines. Over time the link between good patient care and good documentation has been realized. Documentation has gained importance not only for substantiating the services rendered for reimbursement but also for continuity of care with so many providers choosing specialty medicine, an increase in the use of electronic health record systems, the greater specificity found in ICD-10-CM coding, and even litigation support.

Objectives

This chapter discusses:

- **General overview of coding and documentation of evaluation and management (E/M) services**
- **The history and origin of E/M coding**
- **Telehealth and E/M coding**

Origin and Development of Evaluation and Management Codes

The AMA and the Centers for Medicare and Medicaid Services (CMS) developed the evaluation and management service codes in an effort to provide a more objective framework to represent services provided to patients and more clearly define work performed by the provider. These E/M codes were developed to replace codes that described brief, intermediate, and comprehensive visits in order to classify medical visits not only on the basis of time but also by the site of service, type of patient, and patient status.

Medicare physician payment was originally based on a calculation of the customary, prevailing, and reasonable cost.

In 1985, Congress authorized the development of a Medicare physician fee schedule (MFPS) based on the physician resources expended while rendering a medical service (e.g., skill, knowledge, specialty training, and time). Medicare's resource based relative value scale (RBRVS) measures the resources (i.e., physician work, practice expense, and malpractice expense) expended when physicians perform services and procedures. The resource costs of evaluation and management services were analyzed extensively as part of Medicare's RBRVS study.

Because studies determined that the duration of the face-to-face encounter with the patient was directly linked to the total amount of work, which did not increase proportionately with encounter time, CMS set the relative value units (RVU) for the work involved in E/M services by using "intraservice" time as the basis for each code.

E/M codes became an integral part of the AMA's CPT book and have constituted the first section of the book since 1992. Because these codes represent the services most frequently performed by providers (e.g., office, emergency department, inpatient visits), they are placed, for convenience, at the beginning of the book. The E/M section contains the codes applicable to all services commonly referred to as "visits." The following categories comprise the Evaluation and Management section of the CPT book as shown in the table below.

CPT Section	Code Range
Office or Other Outpatient Services	99202–99215
Telemedicine Services	98000-98016
Hospital Inpatient or Observation Services	99221–99223, 99231–99239
Consultations	99242–99255
Emergency Department Services	99281–99288
Critical Care Services	99291–99292
Nursing Facility Services	99304–99316
Home or Residence Services	99341–99350
Prolonged Services	99358–99360, 99415–99418
Case Management Services	99366–99368
Care Plan Oversight Services	99374–99380
Preventive Medicine Services	99381–99429

CPT Section	Code Range
Non-Face-to-Face Services	99421–99423, 99446–99458
Digitally Stored Data Services/Remote Physiologic Monitoring and Physiologic Monitoring Treatment Services	99453–99454, 99091, 99457–99458, 99473–99474
Special E/M Services	99450–99456
Newborn Care Services	99460–99463
Delivery/Birthing Room Attendance and Resuscitation Services	99464–99465
Inpatient Neonatal Intensive Care Services and Pediatric and Neonatal Critical Care Services	99466–99486
Cognitive Assessment and Care Plan Services	99483
Care Management Services	99424-99427, 99437, 99439, 99487–99491
Psychiatric Collaborative Care Management Services	99492–99494
Transitional Care Management Services	99495–99496
Advance Care Planning	99497–99498
General Behavioral Health Integration Care Management	99484
Other E/M Services	99459, 99499

General E/M guidelines precede the Evaluation and Management section of the CPT book. Guidelines specific to a particular subsection within the E/M section are also provided for additional clarification. The information contained in the guidelines provides definitions, explanations of terms, time-based instruction as applicable, and any other information unique to that set of codes necessary for appropriate E/M code assignment.

E/M codes were designed to increase accuracy and consistency when reporting the various levels of patient encounters and were jointly developed by the AMA and CMS. The AMA and CMS have, over time, developed guidelines for the use of evaluation and management codes to supplement the information found in the CPT book. The level of visit is based on the extent of the clinical history taken, the level of physical examination performed, and the complexity of medical decision making. In 1995, CMS published guidelines on how to appropriately document and quantify the provider's evaluation and plan of care for patients. These guidelines were expanded in 1997 to recognize that certain specialists like ophthalmologists, would not need to perform a cardiovascular or gastrointestinal exam, but, instead would need to perform a focused, complex, single-system examination. Both sets of guidelines are valid for services prior to 2023, and providers may choose either set to assist them in their documentation.

For More Info

A copy of the complete 1995 and 1997 Evaluation and Management Coding Guidelines can be found at https://www.cms.gov/outreach-and-education/medicare-learning-network-mln/mlnedwebguide/downloads/97docguidelines.pdf; https://www.cms.gov/outreach-and-education/medicare-learning-network-mln/mlnedwebguide/downloads/95docguidelines.pdf.

Effective January 1, 2021, CMS and the AMA adopted changes to coding and guidelines for codes 99202-99215 to ease the administrative burden on providers and decrease unnecessary documentation not required to achieve appropriate patient care. Effective January 1, 2023, CMS and the AMA adopted changes to code descriptions and guidelines for codes 99221–99223, 99231–99239, 99242–99245, 99252–99255, 99281–99285, 99304–99310, 99315–99316, 99341–99345, and 99347–99350 to ease the administrative burden on providers and decrease unnecessary documentation not required to achieve appropriate patient care.

Although the number of E/M codes is a relatively small percentage of the total Physicians' Current Procedural Terminology (CPT®) codes, they represent some of the most frequently reported services by physicians of all specialties and other qualified health care providers.

E/M services represent such a significant percentage of all billed services that every year, the Office of Inspector General (OIG) includes some evaluation and management services in the agency's annual work plan as an area of continued investigative review.

The OIG continually reviews the accuracy of E/M coding with emphasis on documentation. Documentation has always been an area of concern for the OIG. The key to making the determination of accuracy will be the medical record documentation. Although these statements link correct coding of E/M and attendant documentation, there is enough separation of these two concepts, correct coding and documentation, to illustrate an important point that this guide will repeatedly reference, that documentation should support the level of service assigned, but does not always dictate the correct code in terms of work performed. Any federal review will likely focus on documentation as the determinant of correct coding, but in fact the level of documentation merely supports, or does not support, the correctly assigned level of work performed.

Reimbursement for E/M services, and passing an audit of these services, is ultimately dependent on supporting documentation in the patient's medical chart and upon a determination that the services rendered were medically necessary. The latter aspect of medical necessity is linked to both the diagnosis code assigned and a determination of whether the documented elements are consistent with the problems addressed.

Telehealth Services

As technology and health care changes, the way that providers render care has also changed. Telemedicine continues to grow as a way to deliver appropriate health care to patients who might have difficulty being able to see a doctor in the traditional manner and is helping to facilitate greater access to health care for patients in medically underserved communities as well as to patients who desire traditional care delivered in a more modern, timely manner.

For the CY2025 update, the CPT Editorial Panel has added a new Telemedicine Services section within the Evaluation and Management section of the CPT codebook. Seventeen new telehealth codes have been added for reporting synchronous audio-video visits and synchronous audio-only visits for new or established patients. For details on the new codes, refer to chapter 7 of this book.

Telehealth services are largely evaluation and management services including, but not limited to teleconsultations via telecommunication systems for patients. The teleconsultations most often involve a primary care practitioner with a patient at a remote site and a consulting medical specialist at an urban or referral facility. The primary care practitioner is usually requesting advice from the consulting physician about the patient's conditions or treatment.

Billing and Coding Rules

An originating site is the location of the eligible Medicare beneficiary at the time the service is being furnished via a telecommunications system. All providers who are eligible to bill Medicare for professional services may provide distant-site telehealth through December 31, 2024.

Key Point

The Consolidated Appropriations Act of 2023 allows patients to receive telehealth services wherever they are located and not at an originating site, through December 31, 2024.

To be eligible for payment, interactive real-time audio and video telecommunications must be used and the patient must be present and participating in the conference. The entirety of the interaction between the physician and patient during a real-time telehealth service must be commensurate with the amount of time and nature sufficient to meet the key components or requirements of the service if performed face to face.

In the CY 2025 physician fee schedule proposed rule, CMS proposes to allow two-way, real-time, audio-only telehealth services when a patient is at home. The rule clarifies that this only applies when the provider can use an interactive telecommunications system, and the patient is not able to, or does not consent to, the use of video during the encounter. A list of allowed telehealth services can be found on the CMS List of Telehealth Services. See https://www.cms.gov/medicare/coverage/telehealth/list-services.

The CY 2025 proposed rule also addresses direct supervision by a physician or other supervising practitioner to allow the supervision to be provided through real-time audio and visual interactive telecommunications. Immediate availability requirements include virtual supervision through December 31, 2025. For teaching physicians, this includes virtual supervision of a resident when the service is furnished through telehealth.

Telehealth services guidelines, as well as the list of covered services, are continuing to evolve. For the most current changes, refer to https://www.cms.gov/Medicare/Medicare-General-Information/Telehealth/Telehealth-Codes. For more detailed information, refer to the 2025 final rule at https://www.cms.gov/medicare/payment/fee-schedules/physician/federal-regulation-notices.

Telehealth services are reimbursed when the technology is designated as a real-time interactive audio and video telecommunications system; to attest that the telehealth services furnished have been provided with this specific technology, CMS established two HCPCS modifiers to be used with the appropriate CPT code. These include modifier GT if the conference is via interactive audio and video telecommunications system or modifier GQ if via an asynchronous telecommunications system.

Asynchronous telecommunication and, therefore, the use of modifier GQ is restricted only to demonstration programs in Alaska and Hawaii. Providers, physicians, and practitioners who are affiliated with these demonstration programs may receive payment when using an asynchronous telecommunication system.

For payers that do not recognize these HCPCS modifiers, CPT modifier 95 was established to be used with certain CPT codes defined as synchronous telemedicine services rendered via a real-time interactive audio and video telecommunications system. Modifier 93 represents synchronous telemedicine services rendered via real-time interactive audio only. A list of codes associated with modifier 93 is found in CPT Appendix T while Appendix P lists those associated with modifier 95.

Beginning January 1, 2024, in lieu of modifier 95, CMS requires the use of place of service (POS) 02 or 10.

- POS 02 Telehealth to indicate you provided the billed service as a professional telehealth service when the originating site is other than the patient's home.
- POS 10 Telehealth for services when the patient is in their home.

Reimbursement Issues

The payment for the professional service from a distant site will be equal to what would have been paid without the use of telemedicine.

As a condition of Medicare payment for telehealth services, the physician or practitioner at the distant site must be licensed to provide the service. Medicare practitioners eligible to bill for covered telehealth services include:

- Physicians
- Nurse practitioners
- Physician assistants
- Nurse midwives
- Clinical nurse specialists
- Certified registered nurse anesthetists
- Clinical psychologists
- Clinical social workers
- Registered dietician or nutrition professional

Two place of service codes (POS) are available to report telehealth services.

POS	POS Name	POS Description
02	Telehealth Provided Other than in Patient's Home	The location where health services and health related services are provided or received, through telecommunication technology. Patient is not located in their home when receiving health services or health-related services through telecommunication technology. (Effective 1/1/17)
10	Telehealth Provided in Patient's Home	The location where health services and health related services are provided or received, through telecommunication technology. Patient is located in their home (which is a location other than a hospital or other facility where the patient received care in a private residence) when receiving health services or health-related services through telecommunication technology (Effective 1/1/22)

Code Examples

Payer does not accept modifier GT for telehealth services:
For 60 minutes of psychotherapy delivered via telemedicine, append CPT code 90837 with modifier 93 or 95 and use the originating place of service code 02.

MACs that have been accepting modifier GT for telehealth services:
For 60 minutes of psychotherapy delivered via telemedicine, report CPT code 90837 and use the originating place of service code 02.

Originating sites, those sites where the telehealth service is being provided to the patient, are paid an originating site facility fee for telehealth services. HCPCS Level II code Q3014 Telehealth originating site facility fee, describes this fee and should be submitted to the MAC as a separately billable Part B payment.

In November 2018, CMS announced via the 2019 Medicare Physician Fee Schedule Final Rule (MPFS) that CMS will be paying for more telehealth services. The agency established two new codes that will cover prolonged preventive services for Medicare beneficiaries. CMS is continuing efforts to ensure access, particularly for patients in rural areas, to access Medicare telehealth services by adding more codes for telehealth coverage, reimbursing for more services, and facilitating easier billing requirements for clinicians through the creation of new codes. In doing so, CMS has an ongoing focus committed to patient-centered, innovative quality, and efficient care.

For More Information

Information pertaining to reporting telehealth services may be found at:

https://telehealth.hhs.gov/providers/telehealth-policy/policy-changes-after-the-covid-19-public-health-emergency.

Temporary Expansion of Telehealth Services Due to COVID-19 Public Health Emergency

Although the COVID-19 PHE ended on May 11, 2023, section 4113 of the Consolidated Appropriations Act, 2023 has extended many of the telehealth flexibilities through December 31, 2024, and has made some of the changes and applicable services permanent.

For More Information

For more information, refer to COVID-19 Frequently Asked Questions (FAQs) on telehealth and other Medicare Fee-for-Service (FFS) Billing, see https://www.cms.gov/files/document/03092020-covid-19-faqs-508.pdf.

All health care practitioners who are authorized to bill Medicare for their services may continue to furnish and bill for telehealth services during this time, including physical therapists, occupational therapists, speech language pathologists, licensed clinical social workers, and clinical psychologists. Telehealth services should include the same level of documentation that would ordinarily be provided if the services were furnished in person.

The following areas were revised because of the PHE and remain in effect through December 31, 2024:

- Originating site
  - telehealth services can be provided to patients wherever they are located, including their home.
- Distant site
  - all providers who are eligible to bill Medicare for professional services may provide distant site telehealth

Telehealth technology requirements:

- "Interactive telecommunications system" is defined as multimedia communications equipment that includes, at a minimum, audio and video equipment permitting two-way, real-time interactive communication between the patient and distant-site physician or practitioner, including video-enabled phones.
- CMS is allowing some telehealth services to be provided using audio-only communications technology (telephones or other audio-only devices). These include telephone E/M services, certain counseling behavioral health care, and educational services, to name a few.

Effective January 1, 2024, for reporting telehealth services to CMS use POS 02 Telehealth to indicate you provided the billed service as a professional telehealth service when the originating site is other than the patient's home, or POS 10 Telehealth for services when the patient is in their home.

Additional information on POS, originating site, etc. can be found in the telehealth MLN Fact Sheet: https://www.cms.gov/files/document/mln901705-telehealth-services.pdf.

CMS continues to evaluate and make appropriate additions of services to the Medicare telehealth list. This current and evolving list of services is available at https://www.cms.gov/Medicare/Medicare-General-Information/Telehealth/Telehealth-Codes.

Knowledge Assessment Chapter 2

See chapter 21 for answers and rationale.

1. How is using a documentation method beneficial?
   a. Using a standardized documentation format expedites the revenue cycle process
   b. Using a standardized documentation format ensures a lower medical malpractice premium
   c. Using a standardized documentation format can help decrease audit liability
   d. Using a standardized documentation format has not been proven to be beneficial
2. Why are E/M services considered the dominant source of revenue for most providers?
   a. They are among the most frequently billed services
   b. They have high reimbursement values
   c. Providers can bill all high levels of care
   d. These services are not monitored
3. What can providers use to assess overall coding patterns?
   a. Reimbursement rates from payers
   b. Coder productivity
   c. Payer requests for documentation
   d. Benchmark data
4. Which modifier should be reported to indicate to a payer that service was provided via synchronous telemedicine?
   a. 25
   b. 57
   c. 95
   d. 97

Chapter 3. The Building Blocks of E/M Coding

The levels of evaluation and management (E/M) services define the wide variations in skill, effort, time, and medical knowledge required for preventing or diagnosing and treating illness or injury, and promoting optimal health. These codes are intended to represent provider work—mostly cognitive work. Because much of this work revolves around the thought process, and involves the amount of training, experience, expertise, and knowledge that a provider may bring to bear on a given patient presentation, the true indications of the level of this work may be difficult to recognize without some explanation.

At first glance, selecting an E/M code appears to be complex, but the system of coding medical visits is actually fairly simple once the requirements for code selection are learned and used.

Objectives

This chapter discusses:

- **Determining levels of evaluation and management (E/M) services using MDM or time**
- **Definitions of E/M services and the current E/M documentation guidelines**
- **Modifiers used with E/M codes**

Classification of Evaluation and Management (E/M) Services

The E/M section is divided into broad categories such as office visits, hospital inpatient or observation care visits, and consultations. Most of the categories are further divided into two or more subcategories of E/M services. For example, there are two subcategories of office visits (new patient and established patient) and there are two subcategories of hospital inpatient and observation care visits (initial and subsequent). The subcategories of E/M services are further classified into levels of E/M services that are identified by specific codes.

The basic format of codes with levels of E/M services based on medical decision making (MDM) or time is the same. First, a unique code number is listed. Second, the place and/or type of service is specified (eg, office or other outpatient visit). Third, the content of the service is defined. Fourth, time is specified.

The place of service and service type is defined by the location where the face-to-face encounter with the patient and/or family/caregiver occurs. For example, service provided to a nursing facility resident brought to the office is reported with an office or other outpatient code.

Categories of E/M Services

Codes for E/M services are categorized by the place of service (e.g., office or hospital) or type of service (e.g., critical care, preventive medicine services). Many of the categories are further divided by the status of the medical visit (e.g., new vs. established patient or initial vs. subsequent care).

New and Established Patients

A **new patient** is defined by the American Medical Association (AMA) and Centers for Medicare and Medicaid Services (CMS) as one who has *not* received any professional services from a provider or other qualified health care professional (OQHP) of the exact same specialty and subspecialty from the same group practice within the last three years. An **established patient** is defined as one who *has* received a professional service from a provider or OQHP of the exact same specialty and subspecialty from the same group practice within the last three years. If the patient is seen by a physician or OQHP who is covering for another physician or OQHP, the patient will be considered the same as if seen by the physician or OQHP who is unavailable.

Initial and Subsequent Services

An **initial** service is defined by the AMA as one who has *not* received professional services from a provider or OQHP of the exact same specialty and subspecialty from the same group practice during an inpatient, observation, or nursing facility admission. A **subsequent** service is defined as one who *has* received professional services from a provider or OQHP of the exact same specialty and subspecialty from the same group practice, during an inpatient, observation, or nursing facility admission. If the patient is seen by a physician or OQHP who is covering for another physician or OQHP, the patient will be considered the same as if seen by the physician or OQHP who is unavailable.

Note: Per the CY2023 Physician Fee Schedule Final Rule, CMS adopted these definitions with one exception. CMS does not recognize subspecialties and has left "subspecialty" out of their definitions.

Multiple Evaluation and Management Services on the Same Date

These guidelines apply when a patient in hospital inpatient care, observation care, or nursing facility care receives E/M services in more than one setting or multiple E/M services in the same setting on the same calendar date. These guidelines address multiple E/M services on the same date in which the patient has received multiple visits or services from the same physician or other QHP or another physician or other QHP of the exact same specialty and subspecialty who belongs to the same group practice.

- **Per day:** The hospital inpatient and observation care services and the nursing facility services are "per day" services. When multiple visits occur over the course of a single calendar date in the same setting, a single service is reported. When using MDM for code level selection, use the aggregated MDM over the course of the calendar date. When using time for code level selection, sum the time over the course of the day using the guidelines for reporting time.
- **Multiple encounters in different settings or facilities:** A patient may be seen and treated in different facilities (e.g., a hospital-to-hospital transfer). When more than one primary E/M service is reported and time is used to select the code level for either service, only the time spent providing that individual service may be allocated to the code level selected for reporting that service.

  No time may be counted twice when reporting more than one E/M service. Prolonged services are also based on the same allocation and their relationship to the primary service. The designation of the facility may be defined by licensure or regulation. Transfer from a hospital bed to a nursing facility bed in a hospital with nursing facility beds is considered as two services in two facilities because there is a discharge from one type of designation to another. An intra-facility transfer for a different level of care (e.g., from a routine unit to a critical care unit) does not constitute a new stay, nor does it constitute a transfer to a different facility.
- **Emergency department (ED) and services in other settings (same or different facilities):** Time spent in an ED by a physician or other QHP who provides subsequent E/M services may be included in calculating total time on the date of the encounter when ED services are not reported and another E/M service is reported (e.g., hospital inpatient and observation care services).
- **Discharge services and services in other facilities:** Each service may be reported separately as long as any time spent on the discharge service is not counted toward the total time of a subsequent service in which code level selection for the subsequent service is based on time. This includes any hospital inpatient or observation care services (including admission and discharge services) time (99234, 99235, 99236) because these services may be selected based on MDM or time. When these services are reported with another E/M service on the same calendar date, time related to the hospital inpatient or observation care service (including admission and discharge services) may not be used for code selection of the subsequent service.
- **Discharge services and services in the same facility:** If the patient is discharged and readmitted to the same facility on the same calendar date, report a subsequent care service instead of a discharge or initial service. For E/M reporting, this is considered a single stay.
- **Discharge services and services in a different facility:** If the patient is admitted to another facility, for the purpose of E/M reporting this is considered a different stay. Discharge and initial services may be reported if time spent on the discharge service is not counted toward the total time of the subsequent service reported when code level selection is based on time.
- **Critical care services (including neonatal intensive care services and pediatric and neonatal critical care):** Reporting guidelines for intensive and critical care services that are performed on the same calendar date as another E/M service are described in the service specific section guidelines.
- **Transitions between office or other outpatient, home or residence, or emergency department and hospital inpatient or observation or nursing facility:** See the guidelines for Hospital Inpatient and Observation Care Services or Nursing Facility Services. If the patient is seen in two settings and only one service is reported, the total time on the date of the encounter or the aggregated MDM is used for determining the level of the single reported service. If prolonged services are reported, use the prolonged services code that is appropriate for the primary service reported, regardless of where the patient was located when the prolonged services time threshold was met. The choice of the primary service is at the discretion of the reporting physician or other QHP.

Services Reported Separately

Any specifically identifiable procedure or service (i.e., identified with a specific CPT® code) performed on the date of E/M services may be reported separately.

The ordering and actual performance and/or interpretation of diagnostic tests/studies during a patient encounter are not included in determining the levels of E/M services when the professional interpretation of those tests/studies is reported separately by the physician or other qualified health care professional reporting the E/M service. Tests that do not require separate interpretation (e.g., tests that are results only) and are analyzed as part of MDM do not count as an independent interpretation, but may be counted as ordered or reviewed for selecting an MDM level.

Determining the Level of E/M Service

The levels of E/M services define the wide variations in skill, effort, time, and medical knowledge required for preventing or diagnosing and treating illness or injury. They also include services promoting optimal health and prevention of health conditions. These codes are intended to denote provider work, including cognitive work. Because much of this work revolves around the thought process of the provider, and involves a large amount of provider training, experience, expertise, and knowledge, the true indications of the level of work may be difficult to recognize without some explanation.

Key Point

Effective January 1, 2023, the 1995 and 1997 guidelines are no longer applicable to current E/M coding. The 1995 and 1997 have been removed from the Appendix of this book but may still be referenced for E/M coding prior to January 1, 2023, at https://www.cms.gov/outreach-and-education/medicare-learning-network-mln/mlnedwebguide/downloads/97docguidelines.pdf; https://www.cms.gov/outreach-and-education/medicare-learning-network-mln/mlnedwebguide/downloads/95docguidelines.pdf.

E/M services are divided into broad categories and subcategories. The following guidelines apply to categories:

- Office or Other Outpatient Services
- Telemedicine Services
- Hospital Inpatient and Observation Care Services
- Consultations
- Emergency Department Services
- Nursing Facility Services
- Home or Residence Services
- Prolonged Service With or Without Direct Patient Contact on the Date of an Evaluation and Management Service

Per CMS CY2020 Physician Fee Schedule (PFS) Final Rule and CPT guidelines, the history and examination are no longer used to select the code level for these services. These services, including a medically appropriate history and/or physical examination and the number of body systems/areas examined or reviewed as part of the history and examination are not used for code level selection. The history and examination are still required and should be documented, but the nature and extent of the history and/or physical examination will be determined by the treating clinician based on clinical judgement and what is deemed as reasonable, necessary, and clinically appropriate.

Selecting the level of service for these E/M categories should be based on the levels of medical decision making (MDM) or total time spent by the clinician on the day of the encounter, including face-to-face and non-face-to-face activities. Keep in mind that medical necessity is still the overarching criterion for selecting a level of service in addition to the individual requirements of the E/M code.

Key Point

Level one established visit (99211, 99281) describes and includes visits performed by clinical staff; the concept of MDM does not apply.

Medical Decision Making

MDM is used to establish diagnoses, assess the status of a condition, and select a management option(s). MDM for these services is defined by three elements detailed in the MDM table published in the CPT E/M guidelines. Note, new and established patient levels are scored the same and new and established codes require two out of three elements for any given code.

The MDM is defined by three elements:

- Number and complexity of problems addressed during the encounter
- Amount and/or complexity of data to be reviewed and analyzed
- Risk of complications and/or morbidity or mortality of patient management

Number and Complexity of Problems Addressed During the Encounter

The first element used in selecting these levels of E/M services is the number and complexity of problems addressed during the encounter. Several new or established problems may be addressed at the same time and may affect MDM.

Symptoms may cluster around a specific diagnosis and each symptom is not necessarily a unique condition. Comorbidities/underlying diseases, in and of themselves, are not considered in selecting a level of E/M service unless they are addressed and their presence increases the amount and/or complexity of data to be reviewed and analyzed or the risk of complications and/or morbidity or mortality of patient management.

The final diagnosis for a condition does not, in and of itself, determine the complexity or risk, as extensive evaluation may be required to reach the conclusion that the signs or symptoms do not represent a highly morbid condition. Therefore, presenting symptoms that are likely to represent a highly morbid condition may drive MDM even when the ultimate diagnosis is not highly morbid. The evaluation and/or treatment should be consistent with the likely nature of the condition. Multiple problems of a lower severity may, in the aggregate, create higher risk due to interaction.

Note: The AMA defines a problem as being addressed or managed once the problem has been evaluated and/or treated at the encounter by the physician or OQHP reporting the service. This service(s) includes consideration of additional testing and/or treatment that may not be provided due to risk vs. benefit analysis or patient/guardian/parent choice. Referring a patient without evaluation or consideration of treatment does not qualify as being addressed. For hospital inpatient or observation care services, the problem being addressed or managed may be different from the reason for the admission or extended stay.

CPT now includes definitions to assist in the selection of the different levels of problems listed in the MDM table.

- **Minimal problem:** A problem that may not require the presence of the physician or other qualified health care professional, but the service is provided under the physician's or other qualified health care professional's supervision (see 99211, 99281).
- **Self-limited or minor problem:** A problem that runs a definite and prescribed course, is transient in nature, and is not likely to permanently alter health status.
- **Stable, chronic illness:** A problem with an expected duration of at least one year or until the death of the patient. When it comes to defining chronicity, any variation in stage or severity (e.g., uncontrolled diabetes and controlled diabetes) is irrelevant, and the condition is considered chronic. Furthermore, when evaluating MDM, stability is determined by the patient's specific treatment goals. Therefore, if a patient is not meeting their treatment goals, they are considered unstable, even if their condition has not changed and there is no imminent threat to their life or health.

Key Point

Conditions are treated as chronic whether stage or severity changes (e.g., uncontrolled and controlled diabetes are single chronic conditions). "Stable" for the purposes of categorizing MDM is defined by the specific treatment goals for an individual patient. A patient not at his or her treatment goal is not considered stable.

- **Acute, uncomplicated illness or injury:** Recent or new short-term problem with low risk of morbidity for which treatment is considered. There is little to no risk of mortality with treatment, and full recovery without functional impairment is expected. A self-limited or minor problem that does not resolve consistent with a definite and prescribed plan of care.
- **Acute, uncomplicated illness or injury requiring hospital inpatient or observation level care:** A recent or new short-term problem with low risk of morbidity for which treatment is required. There is little to no risk of mortality with treatment, and full recovery without functional impairment is expected. The treatment required is provided in a hospital inpatient or observation setting.
- **Stable, acute illness:** A problem that is new or recent for which treatment has been initiated. The patient is improved and, while resolution may not be complete, is stable with respect to this condition.
- **Chronic illness with exacerbation, progression, or side effects of treatment:** A chronic illness that is acutely worsening, poorly controlled, or progressing with an intent to control progression and requiring additional supportive care or requiring attention to treatment for side effects.
- **Acute illness with systemic symptoms:** An illness that causes systemic symptoms and has a high risk of morbidity without treatment.
- **Acute, complicated injury:** An injury that requires treatment that includes evaluation of body systems that are not directly part of the injured organ, extensive injuries, or the treatment options are multiple and/or associated with risk of morbidity.
- **Chronic illness with severe exacerbation, progression, or side effects of treatment:** The severe exacerbation or progression of a chronic illness or severe side effects of treatment that have significant risk of morbidity and may require escalation in level of care.
- **Acute or chronic illness or injury that poses a threat to life or bodily function:** An acute illness with systemic symptoms, an acute complicated injury, or a chronic illness or injury with exacerbation and/or progression or side effects of treatment that poses a threat to life or bodily function in the near term without treatment.
- **Undiagnosed new problem with uncertain prognosis:** A problem in the differential diagnosis that represents a condition likely to result in a high risk of morbidity without treatment.

Level Low: Number and Complexity of Problems Addressed

Level of MDM	Number and Complexity of Problems Addressed at the Encounter
Low	**Low** • Two or more self-limited or minor problems *or* • One stable, chronic illness *or* • One acute, uncomplicated illness or injury • One stable, acute illness • One acute, uncomplicated illness or injury requiring hospital inpatient or observation level of care

Note: Each level has the same requirements for new or established patients.

Amount and/or Complexity of Data to be Reviewed and Analyzed

Each level of service has the same requirements for new or established patients. The four levels for this category are minimal, limited, moderate, and extensive.

Key Point

When determining the amount and/or complexity of data reviewed and analyzed, each unique test ordered is counted once; the review of that test is included within the order.

This MDM element includes medical records, tests, and other information that must be obtained, reviewed, ordered, and/or analyzed for the visit, including information obtained from multiple sources or interprofessional correspondence and interpretation of tests that aren't reported separately. Ordering and subsequently reviewing test results are considered part of the current encounter, not a subsequent encounter. Ordering a test may include those considered but not selected following the shared decision making process. For example, a patient requests diagnostic imaging that may not be necessary based on their condition and discussion of the lack of benefit may be necessary. Alternatively, a test that is normally ordered for a specific condition is not ordered because of risk to a specific patient. These considerations should be documented. Data elements are divided into three categories:

1. Tests, documents, orders, or independent historian(s). (Each unique test, order, or document is counted to meet a threshold number.)
2. Independent interpretation of tests (not separately reported).
3. Discussion of management or test interpretation with external physician or other qualified health care professional or appropriate source (not separately reported).

CPT now includes definitions of certain elements used within the data category of the MDM table to help with the interpretation of these elements.

- **Analyzed:** Each specific data element may not be subject to analysis (e.g., glucose), but it is instead included in the thought process for diagnosis, evaluation, or treatment. Tests ordered are typically analyzed when the results are reported. Consequently, when ordered during a specific encounter, tests are counted in that encounter. Tests ordered outside of an encounter may be counted in the encounter in which they are analyzed. For recurring orders, each new result may be counted in the encounter in which it is analyzed. Services for which the professional component is separately reported by the provider reporting the E/M service should not count as a data element ordered, reviewed, analyzed, or independently interpreted for the purposes of determining the level of MDM.
- **Unique:** A unique test is defined by the CPT code, not section/category (e.g., laboratory, 80000 series). When multiple results of the same unique test (e.g., serial blood glucose values) are compared during an encounter, this counts as one unique test. Test elements that overlap are not unique, even if they are identified with distinct CPT codes. For example, a CBC with differential would incorporate the set of hemoglobin, CBC without differential, and platelet count. A unique source is defined as a physician or qualified heath care professional in a separate group or different specialty or subspecialty, or a unique entity. Review of materials from any unique source counts as one data element toward MDM.
- **Combination of data elements:** A combination of different data elements, for example, a combination of notes reviewed, tests ordered, tests reviewed/analyzed, or independent historian, allows these elements to be summed. It does not require each item type or category to be represented. A unique test ordered, a note reviewed, and an independent historian counts as three data elements.
- **Test:** Imaging, laboratory, psychometric, or physiologic data. A clinical laboratory panel (e.g., basic metabolic panel [80047]) is a single test. The differentiation between single or multiple tests is defined in accordance with the CPT code set. Pulse oximetry is not counted toward data reviewed and analyzed.
- **External:** Records, communications, and/or test results from an external physician, other qualified health care professional, facility, or health care organization.
- **External physician or other qualified health care professional:** An external physician or other qualified health care professional who is not in the same group practice or is of a different specialty or subspecialty. This includes licensed

professionals who are practicing independently. The individual may also be a facility or organizational provider such as from a hospital, nursing facility, or home health care agency.

- **Discussion:** Discussion requires a direct interactive exchange. The exchange cannot be through intermediaries (e.g., clinical staff or trainees) to be counted. Sending chart notes or written exchanges that are in the medical record does not qualify as an interactive exchange. The discussion does not have to be on the date of the encounter, but it is counted only once and only when it is used in the decision making of the encounter. It may be asynchronous (i.e., does not need to be in person), but it must be initiated and completed within a short time (e.g., within a day or two).
- **Independent historian(s):** Individual (e.g., parent, guardian, surrogate, spouse, witness) who provides a history in addition to a history provided by the patient who is unable to provide a complete or reliable history (e.g., due to developmental stage, dementia, or psychosis) or because a confirmatory history is judged to be necessary. In the case where there may be conflict or poor communication between multiple historians and more than one historian is needed, the independent historian requirement is met. It does not include translation services. The independent history does not need to be obtained in person but does need to be obtained directly from the historian providing the independent information.
- **Independent interpretation:** Interpretation of a test for which there is a CPT code and an interpretation or report is customary. This does not apply when the physician or other qualified health care professional who reports the E/M service is reporting or has previously reported the test. A form of interpretation should be documented but need not conform to the usual standards of a complete report for the test. A test that is ordered and independently interpreted may count both as a test ordered and interpreted.
- **Appropriate source:** Professionals who are not health care professionals but may be involved in the management of the patient (e.g., lawyer, parole officer, case manager, teacher). It does not include discussion with family or informal caregivers. For the purpose of documents reviewed, documents from an appropriate source may be counted.

Low Level: Amount and/or Complexity of Data Reviewed and Analyzed

Level of MDM	**Amount and/or Complexity of Data to be Reviewed and Analyzed** ***Each unique test, order, or document contributes to the combination of two or combination of three in Category 1 below.***
Low	**Limited** *(Must meet the requirements of at least one of the two categories.)* **Category 1: Tests and documents** • Any combination of two from the following: – review of prior external note(s) from each unique source* – review of the result(s) of each unique test* – ordering of each unique test* *or* **Category 2: Assessment requiring an independent historian(s)** *(For the categories of independent interpretation of tests and discussion of management or test interpretation, see moderate or high)*

Note: Each level has the same requirements for new or established patients.

Key Point

Tests that are results only and are analyzed as part of MDM do not count as an independent interpretation but may count as one item when determining the amount/complexity of data reviewed and analyzed (e.g., dipstick UA, CBC, quick strep test).

Risk of Complications and/or Morbidity or Mortality of Patient Management

The third element listed for determining the level of service includes decisions made during the encounter associated with the patient's problems, diagnostic procedures, and treatments. This includes potential management options selected, and those considered but not selected, after shared MDM with the patient and/or family. Shared MDM involves eliciting patient and/or family preferences, patient and/or family education, and explaining risks and benefits of management options.

The four levels for this category are minimal, low, moderate, and high.

CPT now includes definitions of certain elements used within the data category of the MDM table to help with the interpretation of these elements.

- **Risk:** The probability and/or consequences of an event. The assessment of the level of risk is affected by the nature of the event under consideration. Definitions of risk are based upon the usual behavior and thought processes of a physician or other qualified health care professional in the same specialty. Trained clinicians apply common language usage meanings to terms such as high, medium, low, or minimal risk and do not require quantification for these definitions (though quantification may be provided when evidence-based medicine has established probabilities). For the purposes of MDM, level of risk is based upon consequences of the problem(s) addressed at the encounter when appropriately treated. Risk also includes MDM related to the need to initiate or forego further testing, treatment, and/or hospitalization.

- **Morbidity:** A state of illness or functional impairment that is expected to be of substantial duration during which function is limited, quality of life is impaired, or there is organ damage that may not be transient despite treatment.
- **Social determinants of health:** Economic and social conditions that influence the health of people and communities. Examples may include food or housing insecurity.
- **Drug therapy requiring intensive monitoring for toxicity:** A drug that requires intensive monitoring and is a therapeutic agent that has the potential to cause serious morbidity or death. The monitoring is performed for assessment of these adverse effects and not primarily for assessment of therapeutic efficacy. The monitoring should be that which is generally accepted practice for the agent but may be patient-specific in some cases. Intensive monitoring may be long-term or short-term. Long-term intensive monitoring is not performed less than quarterly. The monitoring may be performed with a laboratory test, a physiologic test, or imaging. Monitoring by history or examination does not qualify. The monitoring affects the level of MDM in an encounter in which it is considered in the management of the patient.
- **Surgery:** *Minor or major*—These are not defined by a surgical package classification. The classification is based on the common meaning of such terms when used by trained clinicians.

  Elective or emergency—These describe the timing of a procedure when the timing is directly related to a patient's condition. Elective procedures are usually planned in advance. Emergent procedures are usually performed immediately or with minimal delay. Both types of procedures may be considered minor or major.

  Risk factors—Evidence based risk calculators may be used but are not required when assessing patient/procedure risk. Risk factors are those that are relevant to the patient and procedure.
- **Parenteral controlled substances:** The level of risk is based on the common behavior and thought process of a provider in the same specialty and subspecialty, it is not simply based on the presence of an order for parenteral controlled substances.

Low Level to Moderate: Risk of Complications and/or Morbidity or Mortality of Patient Management

Level of MDM	Risk of Complications and/or Morbidity or Mortality of Patient Management
Low	**Low risk of morbidity from additional diagnostic testing or treatment**
Moderate	**Moderate risk of morbidity from additional diagnostic testing or treatment** *Examples only:* • Prescription drug management • Decision regarding minor surgery with identified patient or procedure risk factors • Decision regarding elective major surgery without identified patient or procedure risk factors • Diagnosis or treatment significantly limited by social determinants of health

Note: Each level has the same requirements for new or established patients.

The Levels of Medical Decision Making (MDM) is a guide to help select the appropriate level of MDM for reporting an E/M code. The table includes the four levels of MDM (i.e., straightforward, low, moderate, high) and the three elements of MDM (i.e., number and complexity of problems addressed at the encounter, amount and/or complexity of data reviewed and analyzed, and risk of complications and/or morbidity or mortality of patient management). To qualify for a specific level of MDM, two out of three elements for that level of MDM must be met or exceeded.

When the physician or other qualified health care professional (OQHP) performs and reports additional procedures that include interpretation and/or report, the interpretation and/or report is not counted toward the level of MDM. When the physician or OQHP is reporting a separate service for discussion of management with a physician or OQHP, the discussion is not counted toward the level of MDM when selecting a level of E/M services.

Examples in the table may be applicable to specific settings of care. For example, the decision to hospitalize applies to the outpatient or nursing facility encounters, whereas the decision to escalate hospital level of care (e.g., transfer to ICU) applies to the hospitalized or observation care patient.

2025 Medical Decision Making Table

Level of MDM (Based on 2 out of 3 Elements of MDM)	Number and Complexity of Problems Addressed at the Encounter	Amount and/or Complexity of Data to Be Reviewed and Analyzed **Each unique test, order, or document contributes to the combination of 2 or combination of 3 in Category 1 below.*	Risk of Complications and/or Morbidity or Mortality of Patient Management
Straightforward	**Minimal** • **1** self-limited or minor problem	**Minimal or none**	**Minimal risk of morbidity from additional diagnostic testing or treatment**
Low	**Low** • **2** or more self-limited or minor problems; **or** • **1** stable, chronic illness; **or** • **1** acute, uncomplicated illness or injury; **or** • **1** stable, acute illness; **or** • **1** acute, uncomplicated illness or injury requiring hospital inpatient or observation level of care	**Limited** *(Must meet the requirements of at least 1 out of 2 categories)* **Category 1: Tests and documents** • Any combination of 2 from the following: – Review of prior external note(s) from each unique source*; – Review of the result(s) of each unique test*; – Ordering of each unique test* **or** **Category 2: Assessment requiring an independent historian(s)** *(For the categories of independent interpretation of tests and discussion of management or test interpretation, see moderate or high)*	**Low risk of morbidity from additional diagnostic testing or treatment**
Moderate	**Moderate** • **1** or more chronic illnesses with exacerbation, progression, or side effects of treatment; **or** • **2** or more stable, chronic illnesses; **or** • **1** undiagnosed new problem with uncertain prognosis; **or** • **1** acute illness with systemic symptoms; **or** • **1** acute, complicated injury	**Moderate** *(Must meet the requirements of at least 1 out of 3 categories)* **Category 1: Tests, documents, or independent historian(s)** • Any combination of 3 from the following: – Review of prior external note(s) from each unique source*; – Review of the result(s) of each unique test*; – Ordering of each unique test*; – Assessment requiring an independent historian(s) **or** **Category 2: Independent interpretation of tests** • Independent interpretation of a test performed by another physician/other qualified health care professional (not separately reported); **or** **Category 3: Discussion of management or test interpretation** • Discussion of management or test interpretation with external physician/other qualified health care professional/appropriate source (not separately reported)	**Moderate risk of morbidity from additional diagnostic testing or treatment** *Examples only:* • Prescription drug management • Decision regarding minor surgery with identified patient or procedure risk factors • Decision regarding elective major surgery without identified patient or procedure risk factors • Diagnosis or treatment significantly limited by social determinants of health
High	**High** • **1** or more chronic illnesses with severe exacerbation, progression, or side effects of treatment; **or** • **1** acute or chronic illness or injury that poses a threat to life or bodily function	**Extensive** *(Must meet the requirements of at least 2 out of 3 categories)* **Category 1: Tests, documents, or independent historian(s)** • Any combination of 3 from the following: – Review of prior external note(s) from each unique source*; – Review of the result(s) of each unique test*; – Ordering of each unique test*; – Assessment requiring an independent historian(s) **or** **Category 2: Independent interpretation of tests** • Independent interpretation of a test performed by another physician/other qualified health care professional (not separately reported); **or** **Category 3: Discussion of management or test interpretation** • Discussion of management or test interpretation with external physician/other qualified health care professional/appropriate source (not separately reported)	**High risk of morbidity from additional diagnostic testing or treatment** *Examples only:* • Drug therapy requiring intensive monitoring for toxicity • Decision regarding elective major surgery with identified patient or procedure risk factors • Decision regarding emergency major surgery • Decision regarding hospitalization or escalation of hospital-level care • Decision not to resuscitate or to de-escalate care because of poor prognosis • Decision regarding parenteral controlled substances

Time as the Basis for Code Selection

Certain categories of time-based E/M codes do not have levels of services based on MDM (e.g., Critical Care Services). It is important to review the instructions for each category.

Time is not a descriptive component for the emergency department levels of E/M services because emergency department services are typically provided on a variable intensity basis, often involving multiple encounters with several patients over an extended period of time.

When time is used for reporting E/M services codes, the time defined in the service descriptors is used for selecting the appropriate level of services.

Time alone may be used to select the appropriate code level for 99202–99205, 99212–99215, 98000-98007, 98008-98015, 98016, 99221–99239, 99242–99255, 99304–99316, 99341–99350, 99358–99359, and 99415–99418. Time includes face-to-face and non-face-to-face time personally spent by the provider or OQHP on the date of the encounter count toward the total reported time.

Key Point

Per CMS, medical necessity is still the overarching criterion for selecting a level of service in addition to the individual requirements of the E/M code.

The time defined in the code descriptor is used for selecting the appropriate level of service. Applicable time spent on the date of the encounter should be documented in the medical record when it is used as the basis for code selection.

Time includes time spent in activities that require the physician or other qualified health care professional (OQHP) and does not include time in activities normally performed by clinical staff. It includes time regardless of the location of the physician or OQHP (e.g., whether on or off the inpatient unit or in or out of the outpatient office).

For services that allow for time-based selection of code levels, a time threshold must be met. The concept of reaching a mid-point between levels does not apply. For example, to report 99417 and 99418 both require at least 15 minutes of prolonged service.

The total time personally spent by the physician(s) and other qualified health care professional(s) on the date of the patient encounter should be summed to determine total time when selecting the applicable code level. This time includes time spent assessing and managing the patient, as well as time spent counseling, educating, and communicating results. If two or more individuals meet or discuss the patient together, only the time of one individual should be included.

Key Point

Third-party payer reporting guidelines may differ from CPT coding guidelines. Coverage and payment policies are determined by individual insurers and third-party payers. Check with the specific payer for specific guidelines and to determine coverage.

The following activities may be counted toward total time on the date of the encounter.

- Preparing to see the patient
- Obtaining/reviewing a separately obtained history
- Performing a medically appropriate physical examination
- Counseling and education (patient, family, caregiver)
- Ordering tests, procedures and/or medications
- Referring and communicating with other clinicians (not reported separately)
- Documenting in the electronic or other medical record
- Independently interpreting results (not reported separately) and communicating results with the patient, family and/or caregiver
- Care coordination (not reported separately)

The following should not be counted when using time as the basis for code selection:

- Performance of services that are reported separately
- Travel
- Teaching that is general and not limited to discussion required for management of the patient

The time defined in the code descriptor is used for selecting the appropriate level of service. Applicable time spent on the date of the encounter should be documented in the medical record when it is used as the basis for code selection.

Modifiers Used with E/M Codes

The following modifiers apply to E/M codes; other modifiers may apply in some situations.

24 Unrelated Evaluation and Management Service by the Same Physician or Other Qualified Health Care Professional During a Postoperative Period
The physician or other qualified health care professional may need to indicate that an evaluation and management service was performed during a postoperative period for a reason(s) unrelated to the original procedure. This circumstance may be reported by adding modifier 24 to the appropriate level of E/M service.

25 Significant, Separately Identifiable Evaluation and Management Service by the Same Physician or Other Qualified Health Care Professional on the Same Day of a Procedure or Other Service
It may be necessary to indicate that on the day a procedure or service identified by a CPT code was performed, the patient's condition required a significant, separately identifiable E/M service above and beyond the other service provided or beyond the usual preoperative and postoperative care associated with the procedure that was performed. A significant, separately identifiable E/M service is defined or substantiated by documentation that satisfies the relevant criteria for the respective E/M service to be reported (see **Evaluation and Management Services Guidelines** for instructions on determining level of E/M service). The E/M service may be prompted by the symptom or condition for which the procedure and/or service was provided. As such, different diagnoses are not required for reporting of the E/M services on the same date. This circumstance may be reported by adding modifier 25 to the appropriate level of E/M service. **Note:** This modifier is not used to report an E/M service that resulted in a decision to perform surgery. See modifier 57. For significant, separately identifiable non-E/M services, see modifier 59.

Optum Note: This modifier is used to identify the E/M service when provided with another service reported with a CPT or HCPCS code.

Key Point

Modifier 25 is appended to the E/M code and not to codes for other procedures or services performed.

27 Multiple Outpatient Hospital E/M Encounters on the Same Date
For hospital outpatient reporting purposes, utilization of hospital resources related to separate and distinct E/M encounters performed in multiple outpatient hospital settings on the same date may be reported by adding modifier 27 to each appropriate level outpatient and/or emergency department E/M code(s). This modifier provides a means of reporting circumstances involving evaluation and management services provided by physician(s) in more than one (multiple) outpatient hospital setting(s) (eg, hospital emergency department, clinic). **Note:** This modifier is not to be used for physician reporting of multiple E/M services performed by the same physician on the same date. For physician reporting of all outpatient evaluation and management services provided by the same physician on the same date and performed in multiple outpatient setting(s) (eg, hospital emergency department, clinic), see **Evaluation and Management, Emergency Department, or Preventive Medicine Services** codes.

32 Mandated Services
Services related to mandated consultation and/or related services (eg, third-party payer, governmental, legislative, or regulatory requirement) may be identified by adding modifier 32 to the basic procedure.

52 Reduced Services
Under certain circumstances a service or procedure is partially reduced or eliminated at the discretion of the physician or other qualified health care professional. Under these circumstances the service provided can be identified by its usual procedure number and the addition of modifier 52, signifying that the service is reduced. This provides a means of reporting reduced services without disturbing the identification of the basic service. **Note:** For hospital outpatient reporting of a previously scheduled procedure/service that is partially reduced or cancelled as a result of extenuating circumstances or those that threaten the well-being of the patient prior to or after administration of anesthesia, see modifiers 73 and 74 (see modifiers approved for ASC hospital outpatient use).

Optum Note: This modifier cannot be appended to an E/M code for Medicare.

Quick Tip

Do not use modifier 52 to report a reduced fee. It is specific to a service that was less than that described by the CPT code but not described by another available code.

57 Decision for Surgery
An evaluation and management service that resulted in the initial decision to perform the surgery may be identified by adding modifier 57 to the appropriate level of E/M service.

Optum Note: Medicare recognizes modifier 57 only for major procedures, those with 90 follow-up days.

95 Synchronous Telemedicine Service Rendered Via a Real-Time Interactive Audio and Video Telecommunications System
Synchronous telemedicine service is defined as a real-time interaction between a physician or other qualified health care professional and a patient who is located at a distant site from the physician or other qualified health care professional.

The totality of the communication of information exchanged between the physician or other qualified health care professional and the patient during the course of the synchronous telemedicine service must be of an amount and nature that would be sufficient to meet the key components and/or requirements of the same service when rendered via a face-to-face interaction. Modifier 95 may only be appended to the services listed in Appendix P of the AMA's official CPT codebook. Appendix P is the list of CPT codes for services that are typically performed face-to-face, but may be rendered via a real-time (synchronous) interactive audio and video telecommunications system.

AI Principle Physician of Record
Modifier AI identifies the principal physician of record—that is, the admitting or attending physician who is overseeing the patient's care while in an inpatient or nursing facility setting. Only the admitting physician should report this modifier. The use of this modifier is subject to individual commercial payers' policies regarding inpatient admissions and consultative services; therefore, it is advised to always check with individual payers for specific guidelines regarding the use of this modifier.

Selecting an E/M Code

To select the appropriate level of service, one should take the following steps:

- Identify the place of service (e.g., office, inpatient hospital, emergency room visit) or type of service (e.g., consultation) provided, and select the appropriate category and subcategory from the CPT book.
- Read the guidelines at the beginning of the category and subcategory to determine what special instructions, if any, apply to that subcategory of E/M codes.
- Determine the complexity of the medical decision making from the medical record documentation.
- Review the code narratives in the appropriate category and subcategory. Each narrative includes the specific criteria that must be met or exceeded if the code is to be assigned correctly.
- For billing purposes, select the code that matches the levels of medical decision making or total time.
- Apply appropriate E/M modifiers, as needed.

Knowledge Assessment Chapter 3

See chapter 21 for answers and rationale.

1. Tests that are results only and are reviewed (e.g., quick strep test) do not count when determining the amount/complexity of data reviewed.
   a. True
   b. False
2. Using the MDM table included in the CPT E/M guidelines section, level of MDM is based on how many elements?
   a. One out of three
   b. Two out of three
   c. Three out of three
3. When using time to determine the level of E/M service, which of the following count toward total time?
   a. Reviewing a separately obtained history
   b. Documenting information regarding the patient in an electronic health record
   c. Ordering medication or tests
   d. All of the above
   e. None of the above
4. Which is an example of additional information to determine ICD-10-CM code selection for the chief complaint of "my foot hurts"?
   a. What caused the pain?
   b. Do other body parts hurt?
   c. Which foot?
   d. Is the injury weather related?
5. Of all the body areas/organ systems reviewed during an E/M encounter, which body system requires the greatest level of specificity in terms of documentation as it relates to ICD-10-CM?
   a. Neurological
   b. Respiratory
   c. Ears, nose, throat
   d. Musculoskeletal

Chapter 4. The Elements of Medical Documentation

Medical documentation furnishes the pertinent facts and observations about a patient's health, including past and present history, tests, treatment and medications, and outcomes. The primary purpose of the medical chart is continuity of patient care. An accurate and complete medical chart protects the patient by providing complete information about the patient's history, current health status, and the effectiveness of past and current therapy. An accurate and comprehensive medical chart can also protect the physician, when necessary, in liability actions.

Objectives

This chapter discusses:

- **The principles of documentation**
- **SOAP and SNOCAMP formats**
- **Common documentation deficiencies**
- **Electronic health records (EHR) and documentation**

The medical chart also provides the information that supports the ICD-10-CM and CPT®/HCPCS codes used to report the services provided and submitted to various payers for reimbursement. Therefore, it is absolutely essential that the medical record—whether office, emergency department, or hospital—is complete and concise and contains all information regarding the following:

- Reason for the encounter
- Complete details of the information provided by the patient and by the clinician's evaluation of the patient
- Results of diagnostic, consultative, and/or therapeutic services provided to the patient
- Assessment of the patient's conditions
- Plan of care for the patient, including advice from other physician specialists
- Other services, procedures, and supplies provided to the patient
- Total time personally spent by the provider or other qualified health care professional (OQPH) on the date of the encounter

The style and form of medical documentation depends on the provider, as demonstrated by the samples of documentation included in this book. However, it is important that any reader of the medical record be able to understand, from the documentation, the service rendered and medical necessity for the service.

In addition, the medical documentation must be legible and understandable for all providers who care for the patient. If the handwriting of the provider cannot be read, Medicare auditors, as well as other payers, consider the service to be unbillable.

Key Point

Authentication of documentation is the key to identifying the author, credential, and date of service. Addendums should be dated when written and refer to the date they are modifying.

Abbreviations or shorthand used in medical record documentation should be listed on an identification key accessible to all who read the documentation. Abbreviation lists should be specific to the facility or practice and identify abbreviations that have more than one applicable definition.

All entries should be dated and legibly signed according to the *Evaluation and Management Services Guide*, revised by CMS in August 2023. It is recommended that the signature also include credentials (e.g., MD, DO, DC, etc.). Moreover, medical documentation should be completed during or immediately following the services provided.

Note that the work involved in charting and dictation of medical records is included in all CPT codes.

Principles of Documentation

To provide a basis for maintaining adequate medical record information, follow the official medical record documentation standards listed below. The following principles were developed jointly by representatives of the American Health Information Management Association, the American Hospital Association, the American Managed Care and Review Association, the American Medical Association, American Health Quality Association, the Blue Cross and Blue Shield Association, and the Health Insurance Association of America:

- The medical record should be complete and legible
- The documentation of each patient encounter should include; the reason for the encounter; appropriate history and physical examination; review of lab, x-ray data, and other ancillary services, where appropriate; assessment; and plan for care (including discharge plan, if appropriate)
- Past and present diagnoses should be accessible to the treating and/or consulting provider
- The reasons for and results of x-rays, lab tests, and other ancillary services should be documented or included in the medical record; CMS documentation guidelines state that the reason for tests and procedures should be indicated in the documentation or "easily inferred."
- Relevant health risk factors should be identified
- The patient's progress, including response to treatment, change in treatment, change in diagnosis, and patient noncompliance, should be documented
- The written plan for care should include, when appropriate, treatments and medications, specifying frequency and dosage; any referrals and consultations; patient/family education; and specific instructions for follow-up
- The documentation should support the intensity of the patient's evaluation and/or treatment, including thought processes and the complexity of medical decision making
- All entries to the medical record should be dated and authenticated

Documentation guidelines in the *Evaluation and Management Services Guide* also indicate that the documentation should be able to validate where the services were rendered and that the services were medically necessary and appropriate.

The CPT/ICD-10-CM codes reported on the health insurance electronic or paper claim form or billing statement should be supported by the documentation in the medical record.

Evaluating Your Documentation

If you answer "yes" to all of the following questions, your documentation contains the information necessary to correctly assign and/or support evaluation and management codes.

- Is the reason for the patient encounter documented in the medical record?
- Are all services that were provided correctly documented?
- Does the medical record clearly explain the medical necessity of the level of E/M service, diagnostic and therapeutic procedures, support services and supplies provided?
- Is the assessment of the patient's condition apparent in the medical record?
- Does the medical record contain information about the patient's progress, as well as the results of treatment?
- Does the medical record include the patient's plan for care?
- Does the information in the medical record describing the patient's condition provide reasonable medical rationale for the services and the choice of setting in which the services were provided?
- Does the information in the medical record support the care given, especially when another health care professional must assume care or perform medical review?
- Is the medical record legible and comprehensible to the other health care personnel?

The SOAP Format

Many medical school and residency programs advocate a method of problem-oriented medical record (POMR) documentation. In this system, known by its acronym SOAP, the provider's notes concerning a patient's health and treatment are divided into four parts (the bolded and italicized terms identify where the components of the E/M levels of service can be found in the SOAP format):

- **(S)ubjective:** This component summarizes the patient's complaints, generally using the patient's own words or a synopsis (e.g., chest pain or sore throat). It should include the nature and duration of the patient's symptoms, the time the patient first noticed the symptoms, the patient's opinion as to the possible causes of the illness or condition, any remedies that the patient may have tried, or other medical treatment previously received for the same illness or condition, any contributory factors that may influence the patient's health or response to treatment.

  In the SOAP format, the subjective (S) component documents the ***chief complaint*** and the ***history of the present illness, review of systems***, and relevant ***past, family, and or social history***.
- **(O)bjective:** This section gives the measurable, pertinent findings of the provider's actual examination, as well as the results of diagnostic tests (e.g., laboratory tests or x-rays), which are recorded or referenced in this portion of the medical documentation.

  In the SOAP format, the objective (O) component documents the ***physical examination*** and the ***diagnostic evaluation***.
- **(A)ssessment:** This component of the documentation defines the provider's determination of the cause of the patient's condition, based on the information recorded in the subjective and objective components, and includes the provider's differential diagnoses, diagnostic and therapeutic options, and potential for complications.
- **(P)lan:** This part of the medical record documentation states the agreed-upon treatment plans for the patient.

  In the SOAP format, the assessment (A) and plan (P) document the ***complexity of medical decision making.***

Quick Tip

The SOAP format is the most commonly used documentation tool used by providers and ancillary staff.

The POMR generally incorporates a baseline database of information that includes the patient's past, family, and social history, as well as a chronological problem list. In this format, the provider identifies each problem being addressed from the patient's problem list and then documents each individual problem addressed during an encounter within the SOAP note. Past, family, and social history database information should be updated at appropriate intervals, annually in most cases.

As we reviewed in the previous chapter, this approach is a sequential record of how information was obtained, analyzed, and acted upon in the order in which it appeared. But remember, that for ease of identifying the general level of decision making, much of the nature of the encounter can be determined very early on. If the reason for the visit is follow-up of hypertension, diabetes, hyperlipidemia, and obesity there is a reasonable certainty that this encounter may be a level four established patient visit.

The reason we continue to make this point is that when the provider recognizes early on what the general tenor of the encounter is, he/she can be certain to *document* those ROS or exam elements that may be performed but not turn out to be particularly relevant. Remember that the nature of the presenting problem is not just a contributing component; it will most often drive the breadth and depth of the components within the SOAP format.

Over-Documenting the Encounter

Providers who are unfamiliar with EHR templates or are not fully trained may consider the template to be a "mandatory" list of check boxes that all must be completed. The documentation templates need to be completed so that the higher level of E/M service can be captured and documented. However, providers should perform only as much history, exam, and decision making as is necessary for appropriate treatment of the presenting problem. Over-documenting on a template uses provider time performing and documenting unnecessary components.

This is reiterated by CMS in the *Medicare Claims Processing Manual,* Pub. 100-04, chapter 12, section 30.6:

- Medical necessity of a service is the "overarching criterion" for payment in addition to the individual requirements as defined by the CPT code nomenclature
- It is not medically necessary or appropriate to bill a higher level of evaluation and management service when a lower level of service is warranted
- Sheer volume of documentation is not a factor for selecting a specific level of service

Under the 1995 and 1997 E/M guidelines, the sheer volume of documentation was often felt to support a higher level of E/M code. With the changes to E/M codes in 2021 and 2023, the emphasis is not on the volume of documentation but content.

Providers must still document appropriate history and exam, but focus is no longer on counting specific elements of the history and exam. Rather than completing a template, many providers will revert back to free-form text to report the encounter. The documentation must still reflect the services rendered and provide a record for continuity of care and support of the medical decision making. Detail of the history and exam performed is more beneficial than simply stating the patient returns for follow-up. Although the detailed template may not be used, details such as chief complaint, changes to history, and exam are still useful elements in treating the patient and supporting the medical decision making.

Key Point

The E/M guidelines state: The extent of history and/or physical examinations performed and documented is dependent upon clinical judgment and the nature of the presenting problem(s)."

The medical decision making documentation should identify the three elements and support a final level of complexity. Identification of problems addressed includes signs and symptoms where a final diagnosis may not be made, as well as other coexisting conditions and possible complications. The data reviewed should be documented including laboratory results, pathology reports, radiology exams, patient monitoring, and all other data pertinent to diagnosing and treating the patient. The patient risk, including monitoring of medications and treatment, possible complications, or other factors should also be noted.

Documentation should still present a "snapshot" of the encounter that supports the testing and treatment, level of care, and provides information for other providers who may participate in the patient care.

Signatures

Complying with payers' signature guidelines is vital, especially when a practice is audited. CMS has modified its signature guidelines several times over the years. These guidelines not only apply to providers, but they serve as a reference for medical reviewers when reviewing medical records and claim documentation.

If a signature is illegible, practices may choose to use a signature log (a list of the typed or printed name of the author associated with initials or illegible signatures) or an attestation statement to determine the identity of the author of a medical record entry.

If a signature is missing from the medical record, an attestation statement may be completed. Below is an example of a CMS approved attestation statement:

"I, ____________________**[print full name of the physician/practitioner**], hereby attest that the medical record entry for _________**[date of service]** accurately reflects signatures/notations that I made in my capacity as _________**[insert provider credentials, e.g., M.D.]** when I treated/diagnosed the above-listed Medicare beneficiary. I do hereby attest that this information is true, accurate, and complete to the best of my knowledge and that I understand that any falsification, omission, or concealment of material fact may subject me to administrative, civil, or criminal liability."

Providers should avoid adding late signatures to the medical record (beyond the short delay that occurs during transcription) but instead use the signature attestation. The signature attestation can also be used for illegible signatures.

Medical Documentation Elements

Electronic Health Records

With the adoption of electronic health records (EHR) in both the hospital and outpatient clinical settings. Some of the obvious benefits include legibility, portability within a clinic or facility, and improved quality of care.

The EHR should be a compilation of patient-centered records that can be securely accessed by the appropriate care providers. It is hoped that eventually the health-related information of the patient from "cradle to grave" will be available to assist in the care of current conditions and managing long-term conditions. It is hoped that the longitudinal record will also aid in the concept of patient wellness by monitoring change over time and appropriate health counseling. A good way of thinking about an EHR is that it functions as the portal to manage and control patient information and appropriate access. These systems typically feature organized patient documents that can be readily accessed and searched for pertinent information. Providers may enter encounter or procedural information by keyboard, voice recognition software, or by conventional dictation that is converted into the system. However, whenever using EHR documentation, careful attention must be paid to include only those elements that occur during the encounter. Populating a note with outdated, conflicting, incomplete, or inaccurate information can result from many of the copy functions available in an EHR.

The EHR will also aid in the promotion of telehealth applications such as remote monitoring of devices. Telehealth encounters can be documented and recordings of vital signs, monitoring, and testing can be immediately available.

EHR Documentation of Encounters

One benefit to adopting an EHR is the increase in legibility of provider documentation. When determining which EHR system to adopt, the ability to create and define documentation templates is an important consideration.

When professionals use templates, many mistakenly use the template as a mandatory checklist of history and exam elements that must be completed regardless of medical necessity. Professionals should instead use the template as a prompter to document the necessary elements performed.

Quick Tip

Each encounter should be a snapshot of that visit documenting the unique nature of the patient and service provided.

Because of the misunderstanding of how to effectively use EHR templates, there is often a significant increase in the levels of codes reported without an increase in the severity of patients seen. This may trigger a payer audit to determine why there is such a shift in billing practices. For this reason, it is suggested that internal audits be performed to verify understanding and completion of templates with consideration of medical necessity.

Other common errors associated with the adoption of an EHR include the copy function. Instead of considering each encounter with the patient as a separate item, there is a commonly adopted habit of copying over history and exam elements. This has resulted in incorrect reporting of services, especially when compared to the patient's account of the encounter. This is often identified by auditors and payers when every chart note appears to be exactly the same.

What is important, with regard to the use of templates, is that only the elements of the exam *actually* performed are documented on the template. This is important not only from a coding and billing compliance standpoint but also from a legal and liability standpoint. It is easy to start clicking and select elements that a provider did not actually perform.

Providers must remember that each encounter is a unique document. Just as there is variation from patient to patient, there should be variances, even with templates, in the documentation of the patient encounter. Even when treating the same patient for chronic conditions there are variations in the necessity of exam elements or review of history. This type of documentation is often called cloning and is a common problem with EHR systems.

Key Point

Beginning January 1, 2019, providers are not required to redocument elements of a physical examination, for an established Medicare patient, that haven't changed since the previous encounter when seen for an office/other outpatient E/M encounter (99212-99215). Providers need only to indicate in the medical record that the information was reviewed and updated as necessary.

Lack of narration is another problem often seen when using an EHR. Many of the templates are very good at identifying the history and exam elements and providing fill-in-the-blank areas for the decision making or pick lists to select diagnostic tests and procedures. These same templates may also lack appropriate places to provide additional narration. For example the chief complaint should be a descriptive statement taken from the patient account of the illness or injury that occasioned the encounter. Choosing a chief complaint from a pick list is inappropriate.

Another example of narration is elaboration of negative or unexpected results of the physical exam. For example, a skin lesion should include documentation of the size, color, shape, and location. A heart murmur should describe the quality, loudness, and nature of the murmur. It is appropriate to include a check box for tympanic membrane's red, but bleeding, abrasions, and other abnormalities may need to be elaborated in a narrative manner.

By learning how to use an EHR template, the routine portions of history and exam can be completed quickly leaving time for the provider to document meaningful narrative regarding the patient and his or her condition.

Electronic Health Record Templates

Another key benefit of an EHR is that documenting a patient encounter can be standardized. While almost all EHR systems have parts that require manual entry of text, there are other portions that can be streamlined through the use of templates to help expedite documentation.

In order for documentation to serve its designated purpose, it should summarize the provider's thought sequence that led to the specific orders as well as function as clear communication to other providers involved with the patient's care and convey the diagnosis and plan of treatment.

Accurate templates designed in an intuitive manner will also help to increase provider productivity, reduce denials, and help to increase the accuracy of documentation and ultimately code selection. Workflow can be evaluated, streamlined, and coordinated between providers.

Customized templates with prompts can help to achieve consistent care opportunities for all patients. Templates enable consistent documentation. Information can be captured and relayed to other care providers and printed for patient use. Templates can also remind the provider to check for health maintenance milestones.

Quality in health care is increasing in importance and more and more carriers are moving towards proactive preventive and wellness medicine to treat conditions and injuries before they become more serious and chronic. The emphasis is now on helping patients to be more actively involved in managing their own health and wellness. Templates can serve as reminders to the provider of age- and sex-appropriate screenings for patients. It may also be tied to the results of the last screening or even vaccinations. Additionally, templates help ensure documentation contains important and necessary information such as a problem list or reconciling the patient's medication list. Lastly, templates aid in providing complete data regarding the patient encounter.

Examples of the different types of templates, include, but are not limited to:

- Chart documentation of encounter procedures, phone calls, medication lists, and problem lists
- Prescriptions and refills, including e-prescribing
- Referral to other provider forms
- Requests for ancillary services such as x-rays, lab services, or physical therapy
- Patient instruction sheets

Templates can be customized to the specialty of the practice; for example, a pediatric practice would have age–appropriate, well-child visit templates as well as common pediatric condition templates such as those for an ear ache (otitis media), sore throat (e.g., strep throat), and respiratory issues (e.g., croup, RSV, asthma) as well as injury templates.

A number of methods are available for help in determining template types for a practice. The use of a frequency report of the diagnosis codes reported offers guidance to determine what type of preventive, injury or illnesses are most common to the practice and can serve as the basis for a solid, general all-purpose template that can be modified as needed.

EHR Encoders

Many EHR systems offer an encoder option. In the truest sense an encoder is a set of algorithms and computer code that takes the documented medical record and selects codes for the encounter. Some encoders will select the E/M codes based upon the completed check marks in a template. Other encoders will provide guidance and the provider determines the final code selection.

Definitions

encoder. Computer application that assists in the assignment of a diagnosis or procedure code and may also assign reimbursement categories and values.

On the surface it is appealing to use an encoder to select the codes to be reported on a claim. However, providers should carefully consider certain issues prior to selecting and using an encoder system. The auto selection program is most often the defining feature of an encoder. An auto selection encoder does not consider medical necessity. These systems consider that if the documentation is in the chart, the level of history, exam, or decision making was necessary. When compared to the presenting problem or final diagnosis, this may not hold true.

A provider should also be able to override the auto selection recommendation of an encoder system. The trained provider can determine the code selection for those cases where the documentation may overstate complexity of the visit.

Coder Verification

Although the provider may select the E/M or other codes to be reported or may use an auto-selection system to provide an initial recommendation, some practices choose to have the codes verified by a coder. This practice prevents over and under reporting of services. The coder can also detect errors in correlation between the procedure codes and diagnosis codes. However, final code assignment should be made by the clinician.

Even when using an auto-selection encoder, the coder should verify any questionable code assignments. The practice may choose, for example, to have all high-level E/M codes verified before the bills are submitted. The coder could review all codes selected based on moderate or high MDM. The coder could also verify any diagnosis codes that are not on the template. Lastly, the coder could verify the documentation for a code selected based upon time to ensure that the time components were adequately documented.

Once an EHR system has been implemented and providers and staff have become comfortable with the system, it is imperative that billing patterns be evaluated and monitored by performing a month-by-month comparison of codes billed over the prior year. In doing so, practices will be able to determine any potential shift in coding patterns, such as changes in levels of E/M encounters reported or frequency of services reported.

Knowledge Assessment Chapter 4

See chapter 21 for answers and rationale.

1. Abbreviations can have multiple meanings and can confuse those who need to review the medical record documentation.
   a. True
   b. False
2. Why is legibility a key requirement of documentation?
   a. Patient care and treatment may be delayed and/or compromised
   b. If the handwriting of the provider cannot be read, Medicare auditors, as well as other payers, consider the service as not billable or reimbursable
   c. Legibility is not a key requirement of documentation at the present time
   d. None of the above
3. The benefits of the SOAP formats of documentation are that the SOAP format is a sequential record of how information is obtained, analyzed, and acted upon during the encounter .
   a. True
   b. False
4. What is a common reason a provider might over-document an encounter?
   a. Using a template as a documentation mandate and completing all fields regardless of the presenting problem and misinterpretation of the Table of Risk
   b. Using a template as a prompter to record the history and exam completed
   c. Using nursing and ancillary staff as scribes
   d. Using the Table of Risk for the final level of E/M service
5. What is an advantage to using templates with an electronic health record?
   a. Templates are used to document all necessary elements for a specific level of E/M service
   b Templates help provide consistent format and tools for electronic documentation
   c. Templates allow other staff to fill in blank data
   d. Templates are mandated by the EHR legislation
6. Why should billing patterns be evaluated after implementing an EHR?
   a. To penalize providers not using an EHR
   b. To verify any shift in coding patterns
   c. To keep the coders busy
   d. Both a and b

Chapter 5. Adjudication of Claims by Third-Party Payers and Medicare

The following are medical documentation guidelines many third-party payers use when reviewing claims for accuracy of payment or when performing an audit. Many commercial reviews are geared more towards medical necessity than evaluation and management (E/M) documentation guidelines, as many of the third-party payers have not formally adopted federal documentation guidelines. If they have done so, this should be clear in any contracting language relative to chart or service audit activity. Also, be sure you thoroughly examine your provider's manual, as provided by your third-party payers. Your contract with that payer typically binds your practice to follow the rules as set forth in the provider's manual.

Although the specific federal guidelines may not be required by any given payer, it is a prudent policy to have providers document to the level of the highest requirements. Some facilities and practices bill E/M codes based on payer type, and have lesser documentation standards for nongovernmental payers. Though legal at this time, because contractual arrangement supersedes general conventions, this may not be the wisest course. Providers should likely be taught one set of coding and documentation requirements for all patients for at least two reasons: 1) Does the practice truly always know what coverage is in effect on a given day, and who secondary payers might be? and 2) It is hard enough for providers to remember one set of rules much less different rules for different payers. Following a single set of coding and documentation requirements is much safer for practices from a compliance perspective.

Objectives

This chapter discusses:

- **Documentation guidelines that payers use**
- **How documentation supports medical necessity**
- **Documentation aids**

Medically Necessary Services

Appropriate documentation is important to substantiate services as medically necessary. For a service to be deemed medically necessary, most third-party payers expect the service to be medically required and appropriate for diagnosing and treating the patient's condition and consistent with professionally recognized standards of medical care.

Claims reviewed for medical necessity are usually reimbursed based on the medical documentation supporting the level of service selected. If the documentation does not verify the level of service code reported, the third-party payer, upon review of the documentation, may assign a lesser level of service code and pay accordingly.

Many payers may also use background edits that will evaluate the reported diagnoses with the level of E/M service reported. This is not an invitation to over-diagnose the patient as manual review of the documentation will not support a higher level of care.

Key Point

The level of MDM is determined based on the patient's current conditions at this encounter. A stable patient with a long-term illness that may eventually result in death is not an automatic high level of MDM.

The following sections outline the contents of the medical record documentation that are necessary to substantiate and validate the medical necessity of services provided to patients. Various types of services (e.g., office visit, consultation) and medical settings (e.g., medical office, inpatient hospital) are illustrated.

Key Point

The E/M guidelines state: The extent of history and/or physical examinations performed and documented is dependent upon clinical judgment and the nature of the presenting problem(s).

Office or Other Outpatient Services

For the initial E/M visit, the medical record should include specific documentation for the level of E/M services provided.

- Medically appropriate history, as well as the reason the patient sought medical care
- Medically appropriate physical/psychological examination
- Results of diagnostic tests
- Elements of medical decision making
- Allergy status
- Diagnostic assessment
- Treatment plan and rationale
- Immunization record (for pediatric patients)
- Total time on the date of the encounter, if time is used for code selection

For subsequent visits, the medical record should include specific documentation for the level of E/M of ongoing medical care provided.

- Interval history, including current symptoms and the patient's response to therapy
- Results of any further diagnostic testing
- Elements of medical decision making
- Clinical findings on reexamination
- Diagnostic assessment
- Therapy plan and rationale (including specific documentation of any treatment or procedure performed or prescribed)
- Total time on the date of the encounter, if time is used for code selection

Key Point

Effective January 1, 2021, providers may base the level of office/other outpatient visits (99202–99205 and 99212–99215) solely on the level of medical decision making. For these specific services, revisions were made to the three elements of MDM, as well as utilization of a new MDM table developed by the CPT Editorial Panel and adopted by CMS.

Effective January 1, 2023, these same guidelines, including additional code description changes, apply to the following E/M services 99221–99239, 99242–99255, 99281–99285, 99304–99316, and 99341–99350.

Initial Inpatient Hospital or Observation Care

For initial hospital or observation care, the medical record should include specific documentation for the level of E/M services provided.

- Medically appropriate history, as well as the reason the patient sought medical care
- Medically appropriate physical/psychological examination
- Clinical findings
- Results of diagnostic tests
- Elements of medical decision making
- Diagnostic assessment
- Therapy plan and rationale
- Total time on the date of the encounter if time is used for code selection

According to the hospital's conditions of participation, a complete history and physical (H&P) should be dictated or written within 48 hours of admission, including comprehensive documentation of the elements outlined above.

If the current hospitalization is a readmission within 30 days for the same or related problems, an interval H&P documenting any changes in the patient's condition may substitute for a new H&P as long as a legible copy of the original H&P is included with the interval H&P in the medical record for the current hospitalization.

For subsequent inpatient hospital or observation care, the medical record should include specific documentation for the level of E/M services provided.

- Interval history, including current symptoms and reference to patient's response to therapy
- Clinical findings on reexamination
- Interpretation of results of diagnostic tests
- Diagnostic assessment
- Medical decision making
- Changes in the therapy plan and rationale (including specific documentation of any treatment or procedure performed or prescribed)

Progress notes should be written daily, with time of the encounter noted. This includes the time spent establishing and reviewing the patient's chart, examining the patient, writing notes, and communicating with other professionals and the patient's family.

The patient's medical record should show that the provider's orders were acted on in a timely manner and that the physician's action was consistent with the working diagnoses and therapeutic rationale as documented in the progress notes. In addition, a physician's or other qualified health care professional's orders should be dated and signed and countersigned by the provider within 24 hours if given orally in person or by phone.

Subsequent hospital care is often one of the least well documented levels of care which may open it up for review. Decision making is often split between order sheets and documentation forms. Some electronic records are easier to review as they may "link" the components from a single encounter or day together.

Consultations

The medical documentation of consultations should contain complete information for the level of E/M services provided.

- Name of the requesting provider
- Reason for the consultation
- Date the consultant was notified
- Date and time the consultation was completed
- Medically appropriate history
- Medically appropriate physical examination including system review of the affected body areas or organ systems
- Consultant's findings, diagnostic impressions, and recommendations
- Signature of the consultant
- Copy of the letter or report sent by the consultant to the provider who requested the consultation detailing findings and recommendations (in outpatient records)
- A patient/family referral, not requested by a provider or other appropriate source, is not reported with consultation codes
- Subsequent care is reported using an established patient office, home or residence code; or subsequent inpatient or observation care, or subsequent nursing facility care codes
- Instructional notes clarify what an appropriate source is to request a consult. The guidelines indicate that an appropriate source includes:
  - another physician
  - physician assistant
  - nurse practitioner
  - doctor of chiropractic
  - physical therapist or occupational therapist
  - speech-language pathologist
  - psychologist or social worker
  - lawyer
  - insurance company

Quick Tip

Medicare does not cover consultations. The appropriate inpatient or outpatient service should be reported.

Teaching Physician Documentation

Medicare will cover professional services provided by attending physicians when they deliver personal direction to interns or residents participating in the care of their patients in teaching hospitals and in skilled nursing facilities with teaching programs. Payment is based on the physician fee schedule and is subject to strict guidelines.

Medicare guidelines for payment of physician services provided in a teaching setting require that the teaching physician be present during any services involving a resident for which payment will be sought under the Medicare program. Under Medicare's teaching physician reimbursement guidelines, the services provided by the teaching physician must be of the same character (in terms of responsibilities to the patient that are assumed and fulfilled) as the services rendered to other paying patients. These responsibilities by the teaching physician are demonstrated by:

- Reviewing the patient's history and conducting a physical examination
- Personally examining the patient within a reasonable period of time after admission
- Confirming or revising the diagnosis
- Determining the course of treatment to follow
- Assuring that any supervision needed by the interns and residents is furnished
- Making frequent review of the patient's progress

For More Information

For additional information regarding teaching physician documentation guidelines, refer to MLN006347 at https://www.cms.gov/files/document/guidelines-teaching-physicians-interns-and-residents.pdf

When a teaching physician reports an E/M service to Medicare, the medical record must show his or her participation in the management of the patient. This includes personally performing the service or being present during the critical or key portions when services are performed by a resident. The presence of the teaching physician can be shown through notes in the medical record created by physicians, residents, or nurses (IOM Pub. 100-04, Chapter 12, Section 100.1.1, a).

Students may document in the medical record. However, the teaching physician must verify all portions of the medical record, including history, physical examination, and medical decision making. The teaching physician must personally perform or re-perform the physical examination and medical decision making activities. However, these elements do not have to be re-documented by the teaching physician, verification of the students' documentation is sufficient.

When total time is used to decide the office or outpatient E/M visit level, only include teaching physician time when the physician is performing qualifying activities, including time present when the resident is performing qualifying activities.

Fellows and the Teaching Physician Guidelines

Since the term "fellow" can be applied to individuals for different reasons, understanding the relationship between services provided by fellows and the teaching physician guidelines can be confusing. This term may be used for either an individual who:

- Has completed a basic residency program and is now in a formally organized and approved subspecialty program, which may or may not be recognized as an approved residency program under Medicare
- Has completed all residency programs but is staying at the teaching hospital/medical school complex for a variety of reasons, such as a faculty appointment or the opportunity to develop or refine his or her skills outside the context of the residency program

Medicare law has clearly established direct graduate medical education (GME) payments as the payment mechanism for services provided in a hospital by individuals in an approved residency training program that leads to certification in a specialty or subspecialty. However, fees for some physicians who are designated as fellows may also be appropriately billed as physician services.

According to the CMS instructions for billing the services of supervising physicians in a teaching setting, Medicare will pay for physician services furnished in a teaching setting under the physician fee schedule only if:

- Services are provided personally by a physician who is not a resident
- The teaching physician was physically present during the critical or key portions of the service performed by the resident
- The teaching physician provides care under the exception for E/M services furnished in certain primary care centers

Under the circumstances listed above, the services rendered by the resident are paid by Medicare through the direct GME payment or on a reasonable cost basis.

Key Point

The notes recorded in a patient's medical record by the resident, teaching physician, or others regarding the service provided may be dictated and typed, hand-written, or computer generated. They must be dated and include a legible signature or identity. In the very least, they must describe the service rendered, the participation of the teaching physician, and whether the teaching physician was physically present.

Exception: E/M Services Furnished in Certain Primary Care Centers

Physician claims for services furnished by residents without the presence of the teaching physician may be paid when furnished in primary care centers that were granted the primary care exception. These centers must attest in writing that they meet specific criteria for a particular residency program. The E/M codes that may be billed in these cases are 99202–99203 (new patient) and 99211–99213 (established patient). Code G0402 Initial preventive physical examination; face-to-face visit, services limited to new beneficiary during the first 12 months of Medicare enrollment, as well as G0438 and G0439 are also included under the primary care exception.

For this exception to be applicable, the center must attest in writing that all of the following conditions are met:

- The services must be furnished in a center located in the outpatient department of a hospital or another ambulatory care entity in which the time spent by residents in patient care activities is included in determining direct GME payments to a teaching hospital. This requirement is not met when the resident is assigned to a physician's office away from the center or makes home visits.
- Any resident furnishing the service without the presence of a teaching physician must have completed more than six months of an approved residency program.
- The teaching physician must not supervise more than four residents at a given time and must direct the care from such proximity as to constitute immediate availability. The teaching physician must:
  - have no other responsibilities at the time of the service for which payment is sought
  - have the primary medical responsibility for those patients seen by the residents and ensure that the services furnished are appropriate
  - review with each resident during or immediately after each visit the patient's medical history, physical examination, diagnosis, and record of tests and therapies
  - document the extent of his or her own participation in the review and direction of the services furnished to each patient
  - ensure care is reasonable and medically necessary

- The patients seen must be an identifiable group of individuals who consider the center to be the continuing source of their health care and in which services are furnished by residents under the medical direction of teaching physicians. The residents must generally follow the same group of patients throughout the course of their residency program, but there is no requirement that the teaching physician remain the same over any period of time.
- The range of services furnished by residents includes all of the following:
  - acute care for undifferentiated problems or chronic care for ongoing conditions, including chronic mental illness
  - coordination of care furnished by other physicians and providers
  - comprehensive care not limited by organ system or diagnosis

Some state Medicaid programs also recognize the teaching physicians primary care exception guidelines. The state Medicaid programs also recognize the preventive medicine codes not recognized by Medicare. These include codes 99381–99397. It is important that you verify with your specific state whether they recognize these codes in addition to those recognized by CMS. As with other primary care exception guidelines, the supervising physician must be available to provide care if the resident encounters a problem requiring additional care or treatment during the provision of a preventive medicine service.

Outlined in the CY 2022 Medicare Physician Fee Schedule Final Rule, under the primary care exception, only MDM may be used to select office/outpatient E/M visit level. In the context of teaching hospital primary care centers that are staffed by residents and teaching physicians, CMS believes that MDM is a more accurate indicator of the complexity of the visit as opposed to time. Since residents are in training, they may need more time than is reflected in the code descriptor to furnish a visit that has a low-level of medical decision making. CMS determined that MDM is a more accurate indicator of the level of visit relative to time as it relates to the primary care exception.

Psychiatry

For psychiatry services furnished under an approved GME program, the requirement for the presence of the teaching physician during service may be met by concurrent observation of the service using one-way mirrors or video equipment. Audio-only equipment does not suffice, however. The Medicare teaching physician policy is not applicable to psychologists who supervise psychiatry residents in approved GME programs.

Although psychiatric intake evaluation and psychotherapy services are reported with codes 90785–90899, a psychiatrist may also report E/M services. It should be noted that physicians, NP's, and PA's may also report E/M services. However, other behavioral health providers are not licensed to provide diagnostic or prescriptive services not specific to psychiatric conditions and, therefore, may not report E/M services or psychotherapy with E/M codes such as 90832. Care should be taken when reporting codes from 90785–90838 that the licensure of the provider is also considered to appropriately report the service.

Time-Based Services

For procedures based on time, the teaching physician must be present for the period of time for which the claim is made. Time spent by the resident in the absence of the teaching physician cannot be added to the time spent by the resident and teaching physician or the teaching physician alone with the patient. For example, if a code specifically describes a service of from 20 to 30 minutes it should be billed only if the teaching physician is present for 20 to 30 minutes.

Examples of services in this category include the following:

- Individual medical psychotherapy
- Critical care services
- Office or outpatient E/M codes in which time is used to select a particular level of E/M service
- Prolonged services
- Care plan oversight services
- Hospital discharge day management

Services rendered by teaching physicians involving a resident in the care of their patients must be identified using one of the following modifiers. The modifiers are required only for teaching physicians in a teaching setting (a program receiving Part A graduate medical education funding). These modifiers were developed to assist CMS in its postpayment audits of Medicare Part B payments for services involving residents.

GC: This service has been performed in part by a resident under the direction of a teaching physician. This modifier is to be used with all services provided by a teaching physician except where modifier GE is applicable. It certifies that the physician was present during the key portion of the service and was immediately available during the other parts of the service.

GE: This service has been performed by a resident without the presence of a teaching physician under the primary care exception. This modifier is used to indicate that the teaching physician was not present during the E/M service being billed, but that the requirements for billing E/M services under the primary care exception have been met. Teaching physicians who seek to submit services with modifier GE must file an attestation with the carrier that their services meet the conditions for this exception.

Documenting Teaching E/M Services

For a given encounter, the selection of the appropriate level of E/M service should be based on the documentation guidelines for evaluation and management services developed by the AMA and CMS, and published by the AMA. When E/M services are billed by teaching physicians, the following must be personally documented:

- The teaching physician personally performed the service or was physically present during the key or critical portions of the service performed by the resident (resident documentation of the presence and participation of the teaching physician is inadequate)
- The teaching physician participated in the management of the patient

The documentation of these key elements may be satisfied by the combination of entries into the medical record made by the resident and the teaching physician.

Sample Documentation

Meets Expected Requirements:
Admitting note. "I performed a history and physical examination of the patient and discussed his management with the resident. I discussed the findings and plan of care with the resident and agree with the documented findings and plan of care."

Follow-up visit. "Hospital day 5. I saw and examined the patient. I agree with the resident's note except the heart murmur is louder, so I will obtain an echo to evaluate."

Does NOT Meet Expected Requirements:
Admitting or Follow-up visit.
A countersignature only or a countersignature with:

"Agree with above."

"Rounded, reviewed, agree."

"Discussed with resident. Agree."

"Seen and agree."

"Patient seen and evaluated."

All required elements are obtained by the resident in the presence of, or jointly with, the teaching physician and documented by the resident. In this situation, the teaching physician is required to document that he or she was present during the critical or key portions of the service and directly involved in the patient's management. In addition, the note of the teaching physician should reference the resident's note. For purposes of payment, the combination of the teaching physician's and the resident's documentation must reflect the medical necessity of the service provided as well as the level of service that is billed by the physician.

Sample Documentation

The teaching physician is required to document that he or she was present during the critical or key portions of the service and directly involved in the patient's management.

Meets Expected Requirements:
I was present with the resident during the history and examination. I discussed the case with the resident and agree with the findings and plan as documented in the resident's note."

Does NOT Meet Expected Requirements:
A countersignature only or countersignature with:

"Agree with above."

"Rounded, reviewed, agree."

"Seen and agree."

Sample Documentation

Meets Expected Requirements:
Initial visit. "I saw and evaluated the patient. I reviewed the resident's note and agree, except that the picture is more consistent with pericarditis than myocardial ischemia. Will begin NSAIDs."

Follow-up visit. "I saw and evaluated the patient. Discussed with resident and agree with resident's findings and plan as documented in the resident's note."

Does NOT Meet Expected Requirements:
A countersignature only or countersignature with:

"Discussed with resident. Agree."

"Patient seen and evaluated."

Documentation by Students

Any time a student participates in performing a billable service (other than the review of systems and/or past, family, or social history, which are part of an E/M service), it has to be performed in the physical presence of a physician. Students are allowed to document services in the medical record. If the medical student documents E/M services, the teaching physician is required to verify the patient's history and perform or re-perform the physical exam and medical decision making portions of the service. The teaching physician's personal note can refer to a student's documentation of physical exam findings or medical decision making rather than redocumenting the work. To meet requirements, the teaching physician should sign and date the medical student's entry in the medical record.

Incident-to Services

If the practice employs limited-licensed practitioners, it is advisable to periodically determine that the "incident-to" guidelines are being adhered to. Incident-to services are defined by CMS as "those services that are furnished incident to a physician professional services in the physician's office (whether located in a separate office suite or within an institution) or in a patient's home."

To qualify as incident-to, the services must be part of the patient's normal course of treatment, during which a physician personally performed an initial service and remains actively involved in the course of the patient's treatment. Auxiliary personnel performing these services must be employed by the physician or clinic and services must be performed under the direct supervision of the physician and billed by the physician. The physician does not have to be physically present in the treatment room while these services are provided but must be present in the office suite to render assistance, if necessary (direct supervision).

Definitions

auxiliary personnel. Individual acting under the supervision of a physician; may be an employee, leased employee, or independent contractor of the physician (or other practitioner) or of the same entity that employs or contracts with the physician (or other practitioner).

direct supervision. Physician must be present in the office suite and immediately available to provide assistance and direction throughout the procedure; however, the physician is not required to be present in the room when the procedure is performed.

independent contractor. Individual who performs full- or part-time work for which an IRS1099 form is required.

leased employee. Legal employment relationship established by a contract where an employer hires the services of an employee through another employer.

noninstitutional setting. All settings other than a hospital or skilled nursing facility.

practitioner. Physician or nonphysician practitioner authorized to receive payment for services or incident-to services he or she provides.

To be considered an employee, the nonphysician performing an incident-to service may be a part-time or full-time employee, independent contractor, or leased employee of the supervising physician, physician group, or the legal entity that employs the physician who provides the supervision.

To qualify as "incident to," services and supplies must be:

- An integral, although incidental, part of a physician professional service
- Commonly rendered without charge or included in the physician bill
- Commonly furnished in physician offices or clinics
- Furnished by the physician or by auxiliary personnel under the physician's direct supervision

"Incident to" services cannot be provided to a patient on the first visit, or for an established patient with a new problem or change to plan of care.

Documentation Requirements

Documentation must indicate that the patient is established. That is, the patient has seen the physician previously and is not considered a new patient to the practice.

Documentation must specify a physician was present to supervise the service. The physician does not have to be in the room with the NPP, but they must be present in the office suite. If the established patient has a new problem, the physician must see the patient face-to-face during the encounter and initiate a course of treatment for the new problem to meet "incident to" requirements.

The patient record should document the essential requirements for incident-to services. The medical records should document the following:

- The service was an integral part of the patient's treatment course.
- The service is commonly included in the physician's services.
- The service is furnished in a physician's office or clinic (not in an institutional setting).
- The service was an expense to the practice.

Commonly furnished services and supplies are those customarily considered incident-to physicians' personal services in the office or physician-directed clinic setting. The requirement could not be considered to be met where supplies are clearly of a type that a physician is not expected to have on hand in his or her office or where services are of a type not considered medically appropriate to provide in the office setting.

Services performed by the nonphysician practitioner (NPP) "incident to" a physician's professional services include not only services typically rendered by a nurse or medical assistant (i.e., blood pressure and temperature measurements, injections, and dressing changes) but also services reserved for the physician such as minor surgery, casting, treating simple fractures, reviewing x-rays, and other activities that involve evaluation or treatment of a patient's condition. However, only those services that are within the individual's legal scope of practice, and for which the individual is qualified, may be furnished.

Key Point

The incident-to provision requires that services and supplies must be:

- **Provided in a noninstitutional setting to noninstitutional patients**
- **An integral, although incidental, part of the service of a physician (or other practitioner) provided during the course of diagnosis or treatment of an injury or illness**
- **Commonly furnished without charge or included in the bill of a physician (or other practitioner)**
- **Commonly provided in the office or clinic of a physician (or other practitioner)**
- **Provided under the direct supervision of the physician (or other practitioner)**
- **Furnished by the physician, practitioner with an incident-to benefit, or by auxiliary personnel**

Sample Documentation

Meets Expected Requirements:
The patient presents for monthly blood pressure check; no new problems or complaints; BP: 145/85; Wt. 215 lbs, pulse 88, Resp. 20. Diet reviewed with patient. Scheduled an appointment with Dr. Jones next month; has enough meds to last until next appointment.

Dr. Jones (signature)

J. Smith, RN

Does NOT Meet Expected Requirements:
Monthly BP check; BP:145/85

J. Smith, RN

E/M services provided in the office or clinic setting by the physician must be billed using the physician's NPI. When the E/M service is provided by an NPP, such as a nurse practitioner (NP), physician assistant (PA), clinical nurse specialist (CNS), or a certified nurse midwife (CNM), it may be reported in one of two ways:

- If the service is provided to an established patient, and the incident-to requirements are met, the service is billed using the physician's NPI.
- If the incident-to provisions are not met, the service must be billed using the NPI of the NPP.

Key Point

For incidental services performed by a nonphysician practitioner, there must have been direct, personal, professional services furnished by the physician to initiate the course of treatment. There must also be documentation of subsequent services by the physician that reflects his/her continuing active participation in the management of the course of treatment.

Finally, medical records should be evaluated to validate the medical necessity of the codes assigned and reported.

To substantiate that the "incident to" guidelines were met, the medical record should contain at a minimum:

- Some indication of the supervising physician's involvement with the patient's care. This indication could be satisfied by:
  - notation of supervising physician's involvement (the degree of which must be consistent with clinical circumstances of the care) within the text of the associated medical record entry OR
  - documentation from other dates of service (e.g., initial visit, etc.) other than those requested, establishing the link between the two providers OR
  - cosignature or legible identity and credentials (i.e., MD, DO, NP, PA, etc.) of the practitioner who provided the service and the supervising physician

Split and Shared E/M Services Facility Setting

When the E/M service in a facility setting is shared or split between the physician and an NPP from the same group, the provider who performs the substantive portion of the service reports the E/M code under their own NPI.

The CPT book includes guidelines for split and shared visits to help determine who performed the substantive portion of the encounter. These include:

- When the physician or other qualified health care professionals (QHP) provide services to the patient as a team, only one may report the specific encounter.
- When time is used to select the level of care, the physician or QHP who provides the substantive portion (i.e., the majority of the face-to-face or non-face-to-face time) of the encounter reports the service.
- When medical decision making is used to determine the level of care, the provider who performs the substantive portion of the care reports the encounter. The reporting provider makes or approves and takes responsibility for the management plan, including inherent risk of complications, morbidity, or mortality and the number and complexity of problems addressed at the encounter. When the amount and/or complexity of data to be reviewed and analyzed is used for code selection, the reporting provider must personally perform any independent interpretation of tests and discussion of the management plan or test interpretation. However, the reporting provider does not have to personally order or review tests/documents or assess an independent historian's narrative because these elements are already considered when the provider formulates the management plan.

Split (or shared) visits may be reported for new and established patients, initial and subsequent visits, and prolonged services.

For shared/split E/M services, each provider should document his or her portion of the E/M service. The provider responsible for the substantive portion of the visit must sign and date the record.

Coding Axiom

For shared/split E/M services, each provider should document his or her portion of the E/M service. The documentation must support the face-to-face requirement and must clearly identify both providers involved in the service. Select the code for the level of E/M service based on the combined documentation.

In the 2024 MPFS final rule, CMS announced that it has adopted the CPT book definition of the substantive portion of a split or shared visit to allow code selection based on MDM or time. Note that critical care services do not use MDM, the substantive portion for critical care services is defined as more than half of the total time spent by the physician and NPP. In the context of critical care, split (or shared) visits occur when the total time of the critical care service provided by a physician and NPP in the same group on a specific date is summed, and the provider who furnishes the substantive portion of the cumulative critical care time reports the critical care service(s). Modifier FS Split (or shared) evaluation and management visit, should be appended to the appropriate E/M code when the E/M service is split between the physician and qualified health care professional.

For details on the updates to these sections go to: https://www.cms.gov/files/document/r11288CP.pdf.

Comprehensive Error Rate Testing (CERT) Program

The Comprehensive Error Rate Testing (CERT) program is one of the programs that CMS established to monitor and report the accuracy of Medicare fee-for-service payments.

Under this program, independent reviewers review random samples of claims as they are accepted into contractor and intermediary claims processing systems and follow them through the system. CERT medical reviewers strictly follow documentation standards as outlined in Medicare regulation, statute, and policy, including local coverage determinations (LCD), rather than allowing for clinical review judgment based on billing history and other available information.

As a result of CERT and its strict adherence to policy requirements, a significant number of errors have been identified, including:

- Missing or no documentation for services rendered
- Missing or illegible signature
- Documentation does not support medical necessity
- Documentation is not sufficient to substantiate a claim
- Incorrect coding

The CERT contractor requests medical records and supporting documentation from the provider. Once they are received, the contractor's medical review staff (i.e., nurses, physicians, and other qualified health care practitioners) perform a complete review, comparing the claims data to the medical record to verify the services billed were rendered and medically necessary. If the documentation supports the service and medical necessity, no further action is required. However, if the documentation fails to support the service billed, an error is determined and a refund requested.

E/M coding continues to be an ongoing issue for providers. Most incorrect payments for E/M services were due to lack of documentation in the medical record that failed to support the service reported or missing and inadequate documentation to substantiate the level of E/M service reported.

For More Information

Information regarding the CERT program can be found at: http://www.cms.gov/cert/.

Medical Necessity

Medical necessity is another factor used to determine if code assignment is appropriate. Medical necessity refers to services required to prevent harm to the patient or an adverse effect on the patient's quality of life. The term usually determines whether insurance will cover a procedure or service. It is important to remember that the most accurate method of supporting medical necessity is through good, clear, and complete documentation.

Medicare pays for services that are determined to be reasonable and necessary for the diagnosis and treatment of a specific illness or injury, or in the treatment of a malformed or missing body member.

Private payers often define medical necessity as:

- Services appropriate to prevent, diagnose, or treat the patient's condition, illness, or injury
- Consistent with standards of good medical practice in the United States
- Not primarily for personal comfort of the patient, the family, or the provider
- Not part of or associated with scholastic education or vocational training of the patient
- In the case of inpatient care, cannot be provided safely on an outpatient basis

For example, based on findings from a routine x-ray exam, a radiologist may feel additional studies are warranted. The record must clearly demonstrate the medical necessity for performing the additional studies. In such a situation, the radiologist is usually not required to check with the ordering provider before proceeding. However, the service may require prior authorization from the payer, depending upon that payer's guidelines.

Knowledge Assessment Chapter 5

See chapter 21 for answers and rationale.

1. Medical necessity is a critical element to medical record documentation because without it claims may be rejected or outright denied.
   a. True
   b. False
2. What is the description of "incident-to" services?
   a. Services provided by auxiliary personnel of a facility for a physician
   b. Services provided by a nurse practitioner using their own provider identification number
   c. Services provided by auxiliary personal under the supervision of and billed by the physician
   d. Services provided directly by the physician for secondary conditions
3. What are the disadvantages of using documentation templates?
   a. They can be abused by providing "stock" or comprehensive prerecorded histories or exams
   b. No disadvantages; they are designed to replace provider work
   c. May not be used solely as a prompt to document elements performed
   d. Both a and c
4. The teaching physician does not need to be present for the key portion of an encounter if the resident relays all pertinent information in chart notes.
   a. True
   b. False
5. Which of the following is acceptable teaching physician documentation?
   a. Seen and agreed
   b. No changes
   c. Patient evaluated, care plan reviewed with resident and agreed with findings, no additional changes
   d. Signature and date
6. What is the responsibility of the teaching physician in a primary care exception program?
   a. Supervise residents in providing all E/M services
   b. Supervise up to four residents providing primary responsibility for the patient's care and review each case with the resident during or immediately after the encounter
   c. Have a full schedule of patients concurrent with the residents
   d. Cosign all resident notes
7. What is conveyed with modifier GC?
   a. The teaching physician completed the service without resident participation
   b. The teaching physician and the resident provided the service
   c. The resident provided the service under the primary care exception
   d. The resident acted as scribe for the teaching physician
8. What special criteria must a teaching physician utilize for psychiatric services?
   a. The resident service is concurrently monitored using one-way mirrors or video equipment and audio transmission
   b. The teaching physician records the audio transmission for review
   c. The teaching physician is not required to participate in the service due to patient privacy
   d. The teaching physician is only required to review medication changes

Chapter 6. Office or Other Outpatient Services (99202–99215)

New Patient (99202–99205)

E/M Code	Medical Decision Making	History	Exam	Time Spent on Date of Encounter
99202	Straightforward	Medically appropriate	Medically appropriate	15 min.
99203	Low	Medically appropriate	Medically appropriate	30 min.
99204	Moderate	Medically appropriate	Medically appropriate	45 min.
99205	High	Medically appropriate	Medically appropriate	60 min.

General Guidelines

- Code selection is based on MDM or total time, including face-to-face and non-face-to-face time spent on the date of the encounter.
- History and physical examination elements are not required for code level selection for office and other outpatient services. However, a medically appropriate history and/or physical examination should still be documented. The nature and degree of the history and/or physical examination is determined by the treating physician or other qualified health care professional reporting the service.
- Clinical staff may collect information pertaining to the history and exam and the patient and/or caregiver may provide information directly (e.g., by electronic health record [EHR] portal or questionnaire) that is reviewed by the reporting provider.
- Total time for these services includes total face-to-face and non-face-to-face time personally spent by the physician or other qualified health care professional on the day of the encounter.

Quick Tip

Medical necessity is still the overarching criterion for selecting a level of service in addition to the individual requirements of the E/M code.

- Physician or other qualified health care professional time may include the following activities:
  - preparing to see the patient (e.g., review of tests)
  - obtaining and/or reviewing separately obtained history
  - performing a medically appropriate examination and/or evaluation
  - counseling and educating the patient/family/caregiver
  - ordering medications, tests, or procedures
  - referring and communicating with other health care professionals (when not separately reported)
  - documenting clinical information in the electronic or other health record
  - independently interpreting results (not separately reported) and communicating results to the patient/family/caregiver
  - care coordination (not separately reported)

Key Point

A "results" only test that does not require separate interpretation, but is analyzed as part of the MDM for the encounter, counts as one ordered/reviewed item under the Data element.

- Comorbidities or other underlying conditions should not be considered when selecting the level of service unless they are addressed during the encounter and their presence increases the amount and/or complexity of data to be reviewed and analyzed or the risk of complications and/or morbidity or mortality.
- Use these codes if the patient has not been seen or had a professional service provided by this physician/qualified health care professional or any other physician/qualified health care professional from the same practice and exact same specialty and subspecialty in the past three years.
- Consider using the appropriate critical care code instead of these codes if the physician/qualified health care professional provided constant care to a critically ill patient. Critical care codes are based on the patient's condition, not the site of service, and are selected according to time spent in attending the patient.
- Consider assigning the appropriate consultation code instead of these codes if the provider provided an opinion or advice about a specific problem at the request of another provider or other appropriate source.
- Report only the appropriate initial hospital or observation care or comprehensive nursing facility assessment code if the patient was admitted to the hospital or nursing facility on the same day as another visit.

- Do not include the time spent by any other staff (e.g.,nurse, nurse practitioner or physician assistant) toward the time thresholds. Face-to-face and non-face-to-face time is the time the treating provider spent on the date of the encounter.
- Use case management codes when coordination of care is provided on a date without a patient encounter. Case management codes are "bundled" according to Medicare and cannot be billed to the carrier. Other third-party payers may reimburse for these services.
- Report prolonged service code 99417 with 99205 when the service runs 15 minutes beyond the time specified in the CPT® code narrative. The time must be clearly documented in the medical record. For Medicare, report prolonged services code G2212 with 99205 when the service runs 15 or more minutes beyond the total time indicated in the E/M code description. See Chapter 19 for more information on G2212.

Key Point

Modifiers 25 and 57 are to be appended to the E/M code and not to the codes for other procedures that may be performed.

- Append modifier 25 to report that a separately identifiable E/M service was performed by the same provider on the same date as a minor procedure or other service. Only the content of the note documenting the separate E/M service should be used to determine the level of an additional E/M service.
- Append modifier 57 to report that the decision to perform surgery was made during this visit. For Medicare patients, modifier 57 is used to report the fact that the decision was made to perform major surgery (a procedure with a 90-day postoperative period).
- Append modifier 95 to indicate that the E/M service was rendered to a patient at a distant site via a real-time interactive audio and video telecommunications system. The communication between the physician or other qualified health care professional and the patient should be commensurate with the same key components or requirements of those that would be required if the service had been rendered in a face-to-face setting.
- Performance of diagnostic tests or studies during an encounter that require separate interpretation are not included when determining the level of E/M service when reported separately. A separate code(s) for the diagnostic tests or studies performed in addition to the E/M codes may be reported.
- Simple tests, such as UA, CBC, and quick strep, that are results only tests and do not require separate interpretation can be counted as ordered or reviewed as part of the Data element for MDM even if the test is reported by the provider performing the office E/M visit.
- A test/study that is independently interpreted by the provider that is not separately reported but is part of the E/M service is considered part of MDM.

APC Note: Under the Medicare ambulatory payment classification (APC) system, the definition of a new patient is a patient who has not been registered as an inpatient or outpatient of the hospital within the three years prior to a visit.

Also, it is important to note that the use of the CPT evaluation and management codes in provider-based clinics and emergency departments for APC billing is not determined or reported the same as for a facility.

Issues in This Code Range

- When a patient has been seen or treated in the hospital within the last three years, as a consult or otherwise, he or she is no longer a new patient. Likewise, when moving to a new practice, and taking old patients along, they are best considered established.
- If a nonphysician practitioner is allowed to see new patients be certain the practitioner uses his or her own provider number.
- Codes for high-level E/M services have been targeted in the CERT program as being overutilized. Medical necessity and the level of medical decision making should be verified for all high-level E/M services.

99202

Documentation Requirements

Medical Decision Making: Straightforward
- Minimal number and complexity of problems addressed
- No or minimal amount and complexity of data reviewed and analyzed
- Minimal risk of complications and/or morbidity or mortality

History: Medically appropriate

Examination: Medically appropriate

Key Point

The nature and extent of the patient history and physical examination are determined by the treating provider reporting the service.

Code Indicators (from the MDM table)

Number and Complexity of Problem(s)
- One self-limited or minor problem

Amount and/or Complexity of Data
- Minimal or none

Risk of Complications/Morbidity or Mortality
Minimal risk of morbidity from additional diagnostic tests or treatment

Time Spent on Date of the Encounter
- 15 minutes

Quick Tip

CMS documentation guidelines indicate that documentation should include the reason for the encounter and relevant history and physical examination findings.

Sample Documentation—99202

Level II Initial Office Visit
S: This 20-year-old male patient, new to my practice, who presents with a three-day duration of painful right middle finger nail bed and surrounding area. Pt. denies trauma to the area. The fingernail discomfort has rapidly progressed to its present state. Pt. denies noticing suppuration/drainage. No self-treatment.

ROS: No arthralgias. All other joints without complaint.

O: Right hand—middle distal phalange with periungual induration. Skin with increased warmth and sensitivity. Joints WNL. Full ROM. Other right hand nail beds WNL. Remainder of upper extremity WNL. Neuro intact; sensory as stated.

A: Paronychia, right third digit.

P: Warm soaks q.4 to 6 hrs. Begin E-mycin 333 mg one every eight hours, #21. Protect digit. ASA/Tylenol PRN pain. Return as needed.

(General multisystem)

99203

Documentation Requirements

Medical Decision Making: Low

- Low number and complexity of problems addressed
- Limited amount and complexity of data reviewed and analyzed
- Low risk of complications and/or morbidity or mortality

History: Medically appropriate

Examination: Medically appropriate

> **Key Point**
>
> **The nature and extent of the patient history and physical examination are determined by the treating provider reporting the service.**

Code Indicators (from the MDM table)

Number and Complexity of Problem(s)

- Two or more self-limited or minor problems
- One stable, chronic illness
- One acute, uncomplicated illness or injury
- One stable, acute illness
- One acute, uncomplicated illness or injury requiring hospital inpatient or observation level of care

Amount and/or Complexity of Data

**Each unique test, order, or document contributes to the combination of two or combination of three in Category 1 below.*

- Limited

(Must meet the requirements of at least one of the two categories.)

Category 1: Tests and documents

- Any combination of two from the following:
  - review of prior external note(s) from each unique source*
  - review of the result(s) of each unique test*
  - ordering of each unique test*

  or

Category 2: Assessment requiring an independent historian(s)

(For the categories of independent interpretation of tests and discussion of management or test interpretation, see moderate or high)

Risk of Complications/Morbidity or Mortality

Low risk of morbidity from additional diagnostic tests or treatment

Time Spent on Date of the Encounter

- 30 minutes

Sample Documentation—99203

Level III Initial Office Visit
Reason for visit: "Something is really wrong"

HPI: This 18-year-old white female complains of vaginal itching, burning, and pain for three days, getting "worse and worse." She tried an OTC preparation, but it provided little relief. She has never had a GYN exam before and is apprehensive. She has been sexually active for three years, has had four partners and "always" uses condoms for protection. Past history unremarkable. She denies use of tobacco, drugs, or alcohol except for a "beer or two" on weekends. She is a university student, lives in the dorms, works part time at the university. No known allergies. Menses regular, lasting three to four days, normal flow; LMP 10 days ago. No history of STD or previous GU infections. Review of systems otherwise within normal limits.

Physical exam: Vital signs: T: 97.8, R: 18, P: 76, BP: 116/78. Abdomen: no organomegaly, no masses or tenderness. External genitalia, red and irritated with a foul-smelling creamy discharge oozing from the vagina; no lesions noted. No adnexal tenderness or ovarian masses. Uterus 8 cm. Cervix firm, pink no discharge from os. Rectal negative. Pap smear deferred. Gram stain of vaginal discharge negative for GC. Wet mount + clue cells. KOH prep revealed no yeast or hyphae.

Impression: Bacterial vaginitis.

Plan: The patient was reassured, and her condition was explained. She was given an RX for metronidazole gel intravaginally BID x five days, and was also instructed that her partner should be treated concurrently. GC culture and VDRL sent.

How This Level of E/M Service Was Assigned:

- **History:** Medically appropriate as deemed by the provider.
- **Physical Examination:** Medically appropriate as deemed by the provider.
- **Medical Decision Making:** Diagnosis made by the physician is "Bacterial vaginitis." Using the redefined MDM table published by the AMA and adopted by CMS, the note indicates that one acute, uncomplicated illness was addressed, which equates to low number and complexity of problems addressed. Two unique laboratory tests (GC culture and VDRL test) are ordered/reviewed, which equates to a limited amount and/or complexity of data reviewed and analyzed. The level of risk for this encounter is low. The level of MDM is based on two out of three elements; all three elements in this case equate to Low MDM and code 99203.

Level III Initial Office Visit
History: A 41-year-old male complaining of pain, stiffness, "clicking" and swelling of both knees that is of gradual onset but seems to be getting worse. He cannot pinpoint when he first noticed a problem, but it was several months before his move here six months ago. He first noted pain in his knees after exercise but notes that exercise also makes the stiffness better. He occasionally gets nonradiating backache, especially after lifting and doing yard work, but sometimes it happens for no apparent reason. Over-the-counter preparations such as Advil with rest and heat help his back and used to make his knees feel better, but lately they seem worse. He notes no paresthesias from his back. Past history is otherwise noncontributory. He notes no problems with gait or stability.

Physical Exam: Well-developed, somewhat obese white male. Height 5'10", weight 205 pounds. BP 130/92. Gait and station are normal. Back appears normal; no kyphosis or scoliosis; no tenderness upon palpation of the lumbar area. Flexes to 90 degrees. Leg lengths even and joints symmetrical. Knees are nontender and are not erythemic or warm. Full range of motion. No back pain on straight leg raising. McMurray's negative. There is moderate crepitation noted on movement of the knees. Hip movement is normal and the patient reports no pain. Muscle strength, pulses and reflexes are all within normal limits. Babinski is negative. Normal response to touch and pinprick.

Impression:

1. Osteoarthritis, bilateral knees.
2. History of lumbago without evidence of sciatic nerve involvement.

Plan: Discussion with the patient regarding osteoarthritis, treatment options and nature of the condition. Patient instructed in the importance of daily exercise including stretching exercises to avoid further damage to the joints. Importance of weight reduction in management of DJD was also strongly stressed. Patient was instructed to use aspirin to relieve knee and back pain, and was given a referral for physical therapy evaluation and instructions on exercises and activities to help manage his condition. The patient was instructed to return in four months for follow-up and to call sooner if there are any problems. The patient was advised to contact his PCP for hypertension follow up.

How This Level of E/M Service Was Assigned:

- **History:** Medically appropriate as deemed by the provider.
- **Physical Examination:** Medically appropriate as deemed by the provider.
- **Medical Decision Making:** Diagnosis made by the physician is "Osteoarthritis, bilateral knees." Using the redefined MDM table published by the AMA and adopted by CMS, the note indicates that one acute, uncomplicated illness was addressed, which equates to low number and complexity of problems addressed. There were no data elements reviewed or analyzed and the level of risk for this is encounter is low. The level of MDM is based on two out of three elements; two elements in this case equate to Low MDM and code 99203.

Office/Other Outpatient Services

99204

Documentation Requirements

Medical Decision Making: Moderate

- Moderate number and complexity of problems addressed
- Moderate amount and complexity of data reviewed and analyzed
- Moderate risk of complications and/or morbidity or mortality

History: Medically appropriate

Examination: Medically appropriate

> **Key Point**
>
> **The nature and extent of the patient history and physical examination are determined by the treating provider reporting the service.**

Code Indicators (from the MDM table)

Number and Complexity of Problem(s)

- One or more chronic illnesses with exacerbation, progression, or side effects of treatment
- Two or more stable chronic illnesses
- One undiagnosed new problem with uncertain prognosis
- One acute illness with systemic symptoms
- One acute, complicated injury

Amount and/or Complexity of Data

**Each unique test, order, or document contributes to the combination of two or combination of three in Category 1 below.*

- Moderate

(Must meet the requirements of at least one of the three categories.)

Category 1: Tests, documents, or independent historian(s)

- Any combination of three from the following:
  - review of prior external note(s) from each unique source*
  - review of the result(s) of each unique test*
  - ordering of each unique test*
  - assessment requiring an independent historian(s)

  or

Category 2: Independent interpretation of tests

- Independent interpretation of a test performed by another physician/other qualified health care professional (not separately reported)

  or

Category 3: Discussion of management or test interpretation

- Discussion of management or test interpretation with external physician/other qualified health care professional/appropriate source (not separately reported)

Risk of Complications/Morbidity or Mortality

Moderate risk of morbidity from additional diagnostic testing or treatment

Examples only:

- Prescription drug management
- Decision regarding minor surgery with identified patient or procedure risk factors
- Decision regarding elective major surgery without identified patient or procedure risk factors
- Diagnosis or treatment significantly limited by social determinants of health

Time Spent on Date of the Encounter

- 45 minutes

Sample Documentation—99204

Level IV Initial Office Visit

This is a 34-year-old female, who presents to my office today as a new patient to the clinic. She has had a three-day history of lower right back pain, which she believes is due to a muscle strain after shoveling snow. However, several hours prior to her presentation here, she developed rapid onset of fever, severe shaking chills, and nausea and vomiting. No diarrhea. She also has a headache currently. She denies dysuria, polyuria, and change in urine color or stool color/consistency. She denies any real injury to her back, except possibly straining it while shoveling snow. Positive history of frequent UTIs. Has not self-treated. No increase in fluid intake.

ROS: Feels well in general except for this episode. CV: Negative except for a heart murmur since childhood. Resp: No issues. Neg. GI or GU symptomatology, but frequent UTIs as noted. Skin: No complaints. Tends to scar easily. Has developed keloids on the earlobes, they have been removed twice now but she no longer wears pierced earrings. Musculoskeletal: No arthritis. Neuro: Without complaint. Allergic: Severely allergic to bee stings and is "deathly" afraid to have these insects around her.

PMH: Gravida 1, para 1 vaginal delivery three years ago. History of heart murmur present since a child.

SH: Taking BCPs now. Smokes 1/2 pack cigarettes/day. Drinks occasionally. Unmarried.

FH: Positive for CA of lungs, HTN in paternal grandfather, CAD in maternal grandmother, and DM in mother.

O: Vitals: T; 104.4; BP: 124/82; R: 22. General: Well-developed, well-nourished female appearing her stated age. HEENT: Unremarkable. Nasopharynx normal. Eyes WNL. Ears WNL. Throat WNL. Chest: Clear to P&A. Heart auscultation reveals grade II/VI holosystolic murmur along the left sternal border; otherwise WNL. GI: Sl. tenderness over epigastrium referred to the right flank region. No guarding or rebound. Negative psoas sign. No organomegaly. No mass. Right CVA tenderness. Unable to touch her chin to her chest. Negative Kernig's sign. Neuro: Unremarkable. Normal DTRs. Musculoskeletal exam: Entirely WNL. No muscle spasm. Lymph: Axillary/cervical/inguinal nodes negative. GU: Deferred.

Labs: CBC, UA with culture and sensitivity, and blood chemistries ordered. KUB ordered. (all STAT labs)

A: Right acute pyelonephritis.

P: Patient is well hydrated and tolerating oral agents well; therefore, begin Cipro 500 mg q.12h. for two weeks. An appointment will be scheduled in three to four days to recheck her condition. PRN sooner. Tylenol for temperature elevations. Encourage fluids.

How This Level of E/M Service Was Assigned:

- **History:** Medically appropriate as deemed by the provider.
- **Physical Examination:** Medically appropriate as deemed by the provider.
- **Medical Decision Making:** Diagnosis made by the physician is "Acute pyelonephritis." Using the redefined MDM table published by the AMA and adopted by CMS, the note indicates that one acute illness with systemic symptoms was addressed, which equates to moderate number and complexity of problems addressed. Three unique laboratory tests (CBC, UA, and blood chemistries) and a KUB test are ordered/reviewed for a total of four unique tests. The combination of four items under Category 1 equates to a moderate amount and/or complexity of data reviewed and analyzed. The level of risk for this encounter is moderate based on the prescription drug prescribed. The level of MDM is based on two out of three elements; all three elements in this case equate to Moderate MDM and code 99204.

(continued)

Sample Documentation—99204 (Continued)

Level IV Initial Office Visit
Reason for visit: "Mom and my school counselor say that I need to see you."

S: This 15-year-old white male high school tenth grader came in accompanied by his mother; she states that the counselor suggested an evaluation because he skipped school several times in the past three months, and they do not know why this has started. Prior to this time, the patient was a "model student" and an "all around good kid." His behavior and general attitude changed "for the worse—big time" about four months ago, and the mother is very concerned.

The patient was then interviewed privately, and initially stated that this interview is "a waste of time." He states that "people just don't understand" and he is "just being a normal kid," and that "everyone is overreacting all over the place." He also expressed concerns that if he talked with me, I would "tell everyone that he is depressed or nuts" and he'd have "even more problems" than he does now.

He is not currently dating, although he says he knows a girl he wants to ask out but she only goes out with "older guys." He tried to find part-time work but states that employers want him to wait till he is 16 so he won't need a work permit. He is not currently involved in any sports or school activities although he played football in middle school, and last year in ninth grade; he states that he "just didn't feel like doing it" this year. He states that he is just nervous all the time and that sometimes he thinks that "everyone is just trying to make me angry so I'll do something so really stupid that they can just lock me up and forget about me."

Past history, according to the form completed by his mother, is relatively unremarkable. Patient had a Colles fracture at age five, and otherwise has had no significant health problems. No hospitalizations, no other trauma and no surgery; no current medications. Family history is unremarkable. Patient denies use of alcohol, tobacco or drugs, although he does admit that he "smoked a joint" once. He states that he and his friend "borrowed" a joint from a third friend's older brother (apparently without the knowledge of either of the brothers) so they could "try it," but it "didn't do much."

Complete review of systems was generally within normal limits. The patient noted that his face "breaks out a lot" and that he gets "tension headaches" when his parents "bug" him, but otherwise no complaints.

Records from his family physician were unremarkable except for notations of "marked change in attitude, probably age-related" on his last visit three weeks ago.

O: BP 110/70, temperature 98.6, height 5'9", weight 150 lbs.; well-developed, well-nourished adolescent male, appropriate dress, defensive postures. Patient's speech was appropriate, a little reticent and flat initially but eventually became more animated and normal. Thought processes intact, well organized and logical; abstract reasoning and computative skills intact and normal, associations appropriate. Patient denies any suicidal ideation; says that he has "wondered what it would be like to be dead" but states that he certainly doesn't want to know about it "right now." Admits that he sometimes gets so "shaky" inside that he is afraid he will die. Patient's overall judgment and insight seem to be age appropriate. Patient is well oriented to time and place; attention span is age appropriate. The patient seems generally bewildered by what he is doing and by the reactions of his parents and school officials to his behavior.

I spent 50 minutes of face-to-face time with this young man today.

A: Depression.
P:
1. Administer the children's depression inventory; the children's depression scale and depression self-rating scale.
2. Psychotherapy twice weekly for now
3. Consider Desyrel or Prozac once testing is completed.

Quick Tip

It may also be appropriate to report a psychiatric diagnostic interview examination if this service was performed by a psychologist and not a psychiatrist.

99205

Documentation Requirements

Medical Decision Making: High
- High number and complexity of problems addressed
- Extensive amount and complexity of data reviewed and analyzed
- High risk of complications and/or morbidity or mortality

History: Medically appropriate

Examination: Medically appropriate

> **Key Point**
> **The nature and extent of the patient history and physical examination are determined by the treating provider reporting the service.**

Code Indicators (from the MDM table)

Number and Complexity of Problem(s)
- One or more chronic illnesses with severe exacerbation, progression, or side effects of treatment
- One acute or chronic illness or injury that poses a threat to life or bodily function

Amount and/or Complexity of Data
**Each unique test, order, or document contributes to the combination of two or combination of three in Category 1 below.*
- Extensive

(Must meet the requirements of at least two of the three categories.)

Category 1: Tests, documents, or independent historian(s)
- Any combination of three from the following:
  - review of prior external note(s) from each unique source*
  - review of the result(s) of each unique test*
  - ordering of each unique test*
  - assessment requiring an independent historian(s)

  or

Category 2: Independent interpretation of tests
- Independent interpretation of a test performed by another physician/other qualified health care professional (not separately reported)

  or

Category 3: Discussion of management or test interpretation
- Discussion of management or test interpretation with external physician/other qualified health care professional/appropriate source (not separately reported)

Risk of Complications/Morbidity or Mortality
High risk of morbidity from additional diagnostic testing or treatment

Examples only:
- Drug therapy requiring intensive monitoring for toxicity
- Decision regarding elective major surgery with identified patient or procedure risk factors
- Decision regarding emergency major surgery
- Decision regarding hospitalization or escalation of hospital-level care
- Decision not to resuscitate or to de-escalate care because of poor prognosis
- Parenteral controlled substances

Time Spent on Date of the Encounter
- 60 minutes

> **Key Point**
> **A "results" only test that does not require separate interpretation, but is analyzed as part of the MDM for the encounter, counts as one ordered/reviewed item under the Data element.**

Sample Documentation—99205

Level V Initial Office Visit
Reason for visit: "Need a new doctor."

History: This 47-year-old male states he "needs a new doctor" because he was discharged by his former physician about three months ago for noncompliance with hypertensive regimen. He has not seen anyone in the interim, and he takes his medications only sporadically when "it gets really bad." He uses a home BP monitor to check his blood pressure weekly. The patient sought treatment today following an episode of apparent amaurosis fugax last night, with vision returning to normal after about one hour. This was the first such episode for this patient who recognized the episode from his reading material. The patient also reports at least two episodes of probable TIA.

He was diagnosed with hypertension at age 38, and has been on a variety of hypertensive medications since then, with reportedly continual problems with various side effects of treatment. He has investigated a variety of alternative treatments for hypertension including various diets, herbs, and vitamins, acupuncture, various devices such as metal bracelets, prayer meetings, meditation, etc, in an attempt to control his disease without medications, with admitted limited success. He has not tried biofeedback training. He admits his blood pressure has not been well controlled.

Patient history is otherwise unremarkable. No surgery. Fractured ankle at age 24. No meds except antihypertensives and a variety of over-the-counter vitamins and herbal preparations.

His mother is alive and well at age 74, no known health problems except "her age." His father died of MI at the age of 57 and was hypertensive. He has one sister, age 50, who is overweight and hypertensive; he is divorced with two children ages 15 and 12 and apparently has little contact with the children but believes they are healthy. Grandparents apparently all died of "old age" at age 75 and older; his paternal grandfather died in an accident. Family history is otherwise unknown. He quit smoking about five years ago; was a one-pack a day smoker since age 16; drinks "four to five" beers three to four times a week; hard liquor rarely. Reports no illicit drug use; has lived with his girlfriend for the past four years; works as an executive for a manufacturing firm. Exercise includes walking "an hour or so" three to four times a week apparently depending on the weather. Otherwise the patient reports no other problems. Review of systems otherwise negative. See self-history form completed by patient.

Physical Examination:
BP supine 240/110 (left arm); P 80, BP (left leg) 254/118;
BP standing 226/112 (left); P 84; BP 222/110 (Right standing); R: 18, not labored; T: 98.8; weight 198 lbs.; Ht. 5'9"

Well-developed overweight white male in no acute distress.
Eyes—PERRL, EOMI, Fundi flat. + venous pulsations, arteriolar narrowing, copper wiring and A-V nicking. No hemorrhages or exudates.
ENT—good dentition, normal mucosa.
Neck supple, no masses or thyromegaly, no JVD
Respiratory—normal excursion, clear to percussion and auscultation.

Heart—regular rate and rhythm, S4 gallop and grade II non-radiating murmur at left sternal border. Normal carotid upstrokes with bruit on left.
Abdomen—rounded, soft, non tender, no masses or organomegaly. No aortic bruit or pulsation.
Rectal—normal tone, no masses, BPH Gr. I, heme neg.

Musculoskeletal back non tender, straight, motor + 4/4—all 4 extremities, no joint deformities.
Extremities—no clubbing, cyanosis, edema. Pulses +2 arms, +1 legs (no dorsalis pedis either foot).

Skin dry, normal turgor.
Neuro/Psychiatric—alert and oriented X3, normal gait and station, no focal defects. DTR's +2; affect defensive and anxious

Impression and plan:

1. Longstanding hypertension, uncontrolled, with probable end organ changes. Exam indicates no real emergency; therefore, will treat as outpatient. The patient indicates that lightheadedness and impotence are the most bothersome residuals.
2. Begin Moexipril 15 mgm qd
3. UA, full chemistry panel, EKG, cholesterol today.
4. Return in three weeks, recheck orthostatics, K, and creatinine. .
5. I had a discussion with this patient about his hypertension. The patient has a good understanding about the potential side effects of the various drugs used to treat his disease. I apprised the patient in detail of the potential side effects of not treating his condition. The patient expressed an understanding of the high risks of non-compliance, stating no one had "spelled it out before." I firmly explained to the patient that I would be willing to help him explore alternative therapy for hypertension, but only if he were to strictly adhere to a conventional regimen of therapy until his hypertension was well controlled and stable, and to explore the alternatives in addition to conventional therapy and not instead of it.

I spent 65 minutes with this patient today, including reviewing his previous records, examination, and a long discussion regarding the treatment of his uncontrolled hypertension.

Sample Documentation—99205 (Continued)

Level V Initial Office Visit

A 47 year-old white female presents to an OB/GYN on the advice of her primary care doctor. At her 'get established' visit there last week her hemoglobin was 6.3. He had wanted her to go to the hospital for transfusion. She refused and presents here today for evaluation.

This patient had a D/C four months ago in another state. Pathology was suggestive of perimenopause. She had been amenorrheic for the first two months following the D/C, then had a normal period menses last month. This month she has had an extremely heavy menses for 10 days. Her previous doctor started her on Climara .025 and Provera and she has not had a withdrawal period since. The plan was to have her stop her Provera, and expect a period, but he had doubled the dose up to 20 a day to try and keep her amenorrheic.

She has had some fatigue, occasional headache and dizziness. She states her heart feels like its beating fast. All other systems are negative by review with the patient.

Her past medical history is notable for the anemia, and her social history does not include alcohol, tobacco or social drug use. She has previously had three vaginal deliveries, G3, P3.

She is a well-developed, well-nourished pale white female in no acute distress. Her pulse is 92, BP 130/80 and weight is 190 lbs. A & O x 3, affect normal. Her neck and thyroid are normal. Her heart has regular rhythm with no murmur. Lungs clear. The abdomen is soft, non-tender, no masses, and the liver and spleen are non-palpable. No inguinal or axillary adenopathy. The vulva, vagina, periurethral, perirectal, periclitoral areas are normal. The cervix and uterus are normal and adnexa negative. Skin warm and dry.

Hurricane spray and a single-tooth tenaculum to the cervix result in its coming down moderately. Her uterus and vagina are well-supported.

Her diagnosis is menorrhagia with severe anemia. We discussed the complexity of the problem. She has tried a hormonal regimen in the past and it did not work. She tried a
D & C and it did not work. There has been no anatomical problem found. I suggest a hysterectomy as the only viable option. She understands this will make her infertile. We need to build up her hemoglobin and stop her period. The Hemocyte Plus bothers her stomach and she will be switched to a slow Iron. She is also taking Biaxin for upper respiratory problems and her chronic cough.

We need to keep her amenorrheic. We'll continue the Provera 20 mg per day. We'll give her Lupron 3.75 IM today. We discussed the risks and benefits of this. She will get a surge of estrogen in about 10–14 days. That is when she is likely to get a period. If the bleeding gets heavy, we can try switching her to Aygestin at that point. We will plan for surgery in about seven weeks. She should return in two weeks for a hemoglobin check. She will report any further bleeding in the meantime.

We also discussed Depo-Provera, but I am concerned that in about six weeks the lining may get too thin and she could bleed from that between the Depo-Provera and the Depo-Lupron. If there is any more significant bleeding she will need to be transfused. If this occurs in the next few days for any reason we will proceed with the hysterectomy much sooner to prevent another bleeding episode. One hour and 10 minutes was spent on the patient's case today, including review of records, documenting in the medical record, and face-to-face time with the patient.

Established Patient (99211–99215)

E/M Code	Medical Decision Making	History	Exam	Time Spent on Date of Encounter
99211	Does not apply	N/A	N/A	N/A
99212	Straightforward	Medically appropriate	Medically appropriate	10 min.
99213	Low	Medically appropriate	Medically appropriate	20 min.
99214	Moderate	Medically appropriate	Medically appropriate	30 min.
99215	High	Medically appropriate	Medically appropriate	40 min.

General Guidelines

The following guidelines apply to codes 99211–99215.

- Code selection is based on MDM or total time, including face-to-face and non-face-to-face time spent on the date of the encounter.
- History and physical examination elements are not required for code level selection for office and other outpatient services. However, a medically appropriate history and/or physical examination should still be documented. The nature and degree of the history and/or physical examination will be determined by the treating physician or other qualified health care professional reporting the service.
- Clinical staff may collect information pertaining to the history and exam and the patient and/or caregiver may provide information directly (e.g., by electronic health record [EHR] portal or questionnaire) that is reviewed by the reporting provider.
- Total time for these services includes total face-to-face and non-face-to-face time personally spent by the physician or other qualified health care professional on the day of the encounter.

Key Point

Medical necessity is still the overarching criterion for selecting a level of service in addition to the individual requirements of the E/M code.

- Physician or other qualified health care professional time may include the following activities:
  - preparing to see the patient (e.g., review of tests)
  - obtaining and/or reviewing separately obtained history
  - performing a medically appropriate examination and/or evaluation
  - counseling and educating the patient/family/caregiver
  - ordering medications, tests, or procedures
  - referring and communicating with other health care professionals (when not separately reported)
  - documenting clinical information in the electronic or other health record
  - independently interpreting results (not separately reported) and communicating results to the patient/family/caregiver
  - care coordination (not separately reported)
- Comorbidities or other underlying conditions should not be considered when selecting the level of service unless they are addressed during the encounter, their presence increases the amount and/or complexity of data to be reviewed and analyzed, or there is an increased risk of complications and/or morbidity or mortality.
- Use these codes if the patient has been seen by this physician/qualified health care professional or any other physician/qualified health care professional from the same practice and exact same specialty and subspecialty in the past three years.
- Consider using the appropriate critical care code instead of these codes if the physician provided constant care to a critically ill patient. Critical care codes are based on the patient's condition, not the site of service.
- Consider assigning the appropriate consultation code instead of these codes if the physician provided an opinion or advice about a specific problem at the request of another physician or other appropriate source.
- Report only the appropriate initial hospital care, hospital observation or comprehensive nursing facility assessment code if the patient was admitted to the hospital or nursing facility on the same day as another visit.
- Do not include the time spent by any other staff (nurse, nurse practitioner or physician assistant) towards the time threshold. Face-to-face and non-face-to-face time is the time the treating provider spent on the date of the encounter.
- Use case management codes when coordination of care is provided on a date without a patient encounter. Case management codes are "bundled" according to Medicare and cannot be billed to the carrier.

- Report prolonged services code 99417 with 99215, when the service runs 15 minutes beyond the time specified in the CPT® code narrative. The time must be clearly documented in the medical record. For Medicare, report prolonged services code G2212 with 99215 when the service runs 15 or more minutes beyond the total time indicated in the E/M code description. See Chapter 19 for more information on G2212.

Key Point

Modifiers 25 and 57 are to be appended to the E/M code and not to the codes for other procedures that may be performed.

- Append modifier 25 to report that a separately identifiable E/M service was performed by the same provider on the same date as a minor procedure or service. Only the content of the note documenting the separate E/M service should be used to determine the correct level of service code.
- Append modifier 57 to report that the decision to perform surgery was made during this visit. For Medicare patients, modifier 57 is used to report the fact that the decision was made to perform a major surgery (a procedure with a 90-day postoperative period).
- Append modifier 95 to indicate that the E/M service was rendered to a patient at a distant site via a real-time interactive audio and video telecommunications system. The communication between the physician or other qualified health care professional and the patient should be commensurate with the same key components or requirements of those that would be required if the service had been rendered in a face-to-face setting.
- Performance of diagnostic tests or studies during an encounter that require separate interpretation are not included when determining the level of E/M service when reported separately. A separate code(s) for the diagnostic tests or studies performed in addition to the E/M codes may be reported.
- Simple tests, such as UA, CBC, and quick strep, that are results only tests and do not require separate interpretation can be counted as ordered or reviewed as part of the Data element for MDM even if the test is reported by the provider performing the office E/M visit.
- A test/study that is independently interpreted by the provider that is not separately reported but is part of the E/M service is considered part of MDM.
- CPT code 99211 is a nonphysician service and is usually performed as part of an "incident to" service as defined in the code descriptor. For more information on "incident to", see Chapter 5: Adjudication of Claims by Third-Party Payers and Medicare.

APC Note: Under the Medicare ambulatory payment classification (APC) system, the definition of an established patient is a patient who has been registered as an inpatient or outpatient of the hospital within the 3 years prior to a visit would be considered to be an established patient for that visit.

Also, it is important to note that the use of the CPT E/M codes in provider-based clinics and emergency departments for APC billing is not determined or reported the same as for a facility.

Issues in This Code Range

- Do not assign 99211 for a Medicare patient presenting for periodic surveillance unless the labs are drawn in the office.
- Codes for high-level E/M services have been targeted in the CERT program as being overutilized. Medical necessity and the level of medical decision making should be verified for all high-level E/M services.
- CPT code 99211 cannot be submitted to Medicare with a drug administration service (e.g., a therapeutic or diagnostic injection code, chemotherapy, or nonchemotherapy drug infusion code). However, if a medically necessary, significant, and separately identifiable E/M service that meets a higher complexity level than CPT code 99211 is performed in addition to one of these drug administration services, the appropriate E/M CPT code should be reported with modifier 25. Documentation should support the level of E/M service billed; a different diagnosis is not required. See Pub.100-04, *Medicare Claims Processing Manual*, chapter 12, section 30.6 and 30.6.6-B.

Quick Tip

CPT Category II codes identify other health surveillance services considered part of the E/M service.

99211

Documentation Requirements

Problem Severity

- Problem not requiring the presence of the physician, but service provided under physician's supervision.

Special Coding and Documentation Considerations

- The concept of the level of MDM does not apply and time is not used in reporting this service.
- Report separately the codes for the diagnostic test or studies performed.
- Documentation of these nonphysician visits should be individualized to the patient, relevant to the problem present and include evidence of the evaluation and management of the patient and the presenting problem.
- The management documentation should clearly state the treatment or care plan related to the identified problem. It should also state who was involved in the development and initiation of the care plan and follow standard documentation guidelines, including date, patient name, and provider's signature with credentials. This documentation is to be part of the patient's permanent medical record.
- This code has been erroneously used to report nonphysician services that do not have an evaluation and/or a management component. Examples include:
  - taking of any or all of the routine vital signs (e.g., blood pressure check)
  - administering previously prescribed medication only
  - filling out forms
  - collecting blood or other specimens
  - dispensing educational material without further evaluation or management of the patient
- A blood pressure log alone is insufficient documentation. Appropriate documentation is important to substantiate services as medically necessary. For a service to be deemed medically necessary, most payers expect the service to be medically required and appropriate for diagnosing and treating the patient's condition and to be consistent with professionally recognized standards of medical care.
- Do not bill this code with any other E/M service provided on the same day.

Special Instructions for Code 99211

Wisconsin Physician Services (WPS), a Medicare contractor, released an updated article in September 2017 detailing findings from a CERT review indicating CPT code 99211 is an area of concern. As stated earlier in this section, the lack of supporting documentation continues to be an ongoing issue for providers. Oftentimes, an audit or medical records review will demonstrate documentation that simply indicates a lab service result or the type of service that was performed during the encounter such as "blood draw." However, reporting 99211-25 with a venipuncture code requires the documentation to demonstrate that a separately identifiable E/M service was performed. Clearly, noting "blood draw" does not substantiate a separate E/M service even if it is a low level encounter.

Any E/M service should be considered medically necessary; that is, reasonable and required in order to make a diagnosis and treat an illness or injury. WPS has stated that a face-to-face encounter with the patient that includes the elements of an E/M service is necessary. Furthermore, WPS defines the evaluation portion of the service to be that "clinically relevant and necessary exchange of information between provider and patient" and the management portion to be the components that influence patient care such as medical decision making or patient education.

Sample Documentation—99211
Level I Established Patient Office Visit The patient is here for monthly blood pressure check; no new problems or complaints; BP: 145/85; Wt. 215 lbs, pulse 88, Resp. 20. Scheduled an appointment with Dr. Jones next month; has enough meds to last until next appointment. Diet reviewed with patient. Dr. Jones (signature) J. Smith, RN
Level I Established Patient Office Visit The patient is here for periodic lipid surveillance. Labs drawn. Results discussed with Dr. Underwood. Continue present regimen. Dr. Underwood has updated flow sheet.
Level I Established Patient Office Visit Patient returns for blood pressure check after two weeks of current medication. Blood pressure remains at 160/98. Patient states compliance with medication and denies new or significant stress or other risk factors. Discussed the patient's response with the internist who requested the patient increase Vasotec from 10mg to 15mg daily and return to see him in one week. Patient to have blood pressure checked daily in the interim and bring log to appointment with internist.

99212

Documentation Requirements

Medical Decision Making: Straightforward

- Minimal number and complexity of problems addressed
- No or minimal amount and complexity of data reviewed and analyzed
- Minimal risk of complications and/or morbidity

History: Medically appropriate

Examination: Medically appropriate

> **Key Point**
>
> **The nature and extent of the patient history and physical examination are determined by the treating provider reporting the service.**

Code Indicators (from the MDM table)

Number and Complexity of Problem(s)

- One self-limited or minor problem

Amount and/or Complexity of Data

- Minimal or none

Risk of Complications/Morbidity or Mortality

Minimal risk of morbidity from additional diagnostic tests or treatment

Time Spent on Date of the Encounter

- 10 minutes

Sample Documentation—99212
Level II Established Patient Office Visit Patient comes in for suture removal; three sutures were placed in left index finger 10 days ago in the ED, following an accidental laceration from a broken glass. Tetanus booster given in ER. **Exam:** Digit healing well. No erythema, exudate or tenderness. **Plan:** All sutures removed without difficulty. Wound dressed. Patient given instructions on wound care; instructed to call with any problems.
Level II Established Office Visit **S:** This 6-year-old male pt. returns today for follow up of left otitis media. Finished antibiotics three days ago. **O:** Left TM clear, no signs of infection. Rest of ENT WNL. **A:** Otitis resolved. **P:** Return as needed.

99213

Documentation Requirements

Medical Decision Making: Low

- Low number and complexity of problems addressed
- Limited amount and complexity of data reviewed and analyzed
- Low risk of complications and/or morbidity

History: Medically appropriate

Examination: Medically appropriate

Key Point

The nature and extent of the patient history and physical examination are determined by the treating provider reporting the service.

Code Indicators (from the MDM table)

Number and Complexity of Problem(s)

- Two or more self-limited or minor problems
- One stable, chronic illness
- One acute, uncomplicated illness or injury
- One stable, acute illness
- One acute, uncomplicated illness or injury requiring hospital inpatient or observation level of care

Amount and/or Complexity of Data

**Each unique test, order, or document contributes to the combination of two or combination of three in Category 1 below.*

- Limited

(Must meet the requirements of at least one of the two categories.)

Category 1: Tests and documents

- Any combination of two from the following:
  - review of prior external note(s) from each unique source*
  - review of the result(s) of each unique test*
  - ordering of each unique test*

  or

Category 2: Assessment requiring an independent historian(s)

(For the categories of independent interpretation of tests and discussion of management or test interpretation, see moderate or high)

Risk of Complications/Morbidity or Mortality

Low risk of morbidity from additional diagnostic testing or treatment

Time Spent on Date of the Encounter

- 20 minutes

Sample Documentation—99213

S: A 59-year-old male patient returning for recheck of prostatic hypertrophy discovered six months ago; he says Proscar has reduced the urgency and frequency and improved the diminished urinary stream and nocturia; he says urinary function is "not perfect but a lot better" than before. No dysuria; no other complaints except for seasonal allergies treated by his ENT physician. Medications sheet reviewed as well as health questionnaire.

O: Abdomen soft, no organomegaly, no masses. Bladder not percussible. Genitalia normal circumcised male penis; testes normal size; no masses; rectal sphincter tone normal; prostate enlarged, firm consistency. Rectal exam otherwise normal.

Labs: Urinalysis shows a few white cells, otherwise clear.

A: 1: BPH, stable at this time with improved urinary function on Proscar.
2. No indications of infection.

P: 1. Continue Proscar.
2. Recheck in six months; sooner if any change in urinary status or other problems.
3. Urinalysis on next visit.

How This Level of E/M Service Was Assigned

- **History:** Medically appropriate as deemed by the provider.
- **Physical Examination** Medically appropriate as deemed by the provider.
- **Medical Decision Making:** Diagnosis made by the physician is "BPH, stable—with improved urinary function on Proscar." Using the redefined MDM table published by the AMA and adopted by CMS, the note indicates that one stable but chronic condition was addressed, which equates to low number and complexity of problems addressed. A laboratory test (UA) is reviewed, and a UA is ordered for the next visit. The AMA's definition for "Analyzed" as it pertains to the Amount and/or complexity of data element states, "Tests ordered are presumed to be analyzed when the results are reported. Therefore, when they are ordered during an encounter, they are counted in that encounter." In this case, the encounter included review of a UA ordered during a previous encounter and an order (UA) for a future visit. Only the UA analyzed as part of MDM counts towards data reviewed and analyzed. The data element for this visit is minimal. The level of risk for this encounter is low. Level of MDM is based on two out of three elements; these two elements equate to Low MDM and code 99213.
- **Final E/M Level of Service:** CPT code 99213 is assigned.

Level III Established Patient Office Visit

A 48-year-old woman presents to her primary care physician complaining of a nine-day history of weakness, aching joints, cough and a sore throat. OTC meds provide temporary relief she reports on questioning. Fever to 102 on/off for five days, cough productive of thick green sputum.

Weight 290 lbs, Temp. 99.6, BP sitting 162/100. Obese WF in obvious discomfort. OP clear, no nodes, lungs clear w/upper airway mucus, CV RRR.

Imp. Bronchitis. Ceftin 25 mg, Muco-Fen 800.

99214

Documentation Requirements

Medical Decision Making: Moderate

- Moderate number and complexity of problems addressed
- Moderate amount and complexity of data reviewed and analyzed
- Moderate risk of complications and/or morbidity

History: Medically appropriate

Examination: Medically appropriate

Key Point

The nature and extent of the patient history and physical examination are determined by the treating provider reporting the service.

Code Indicators (from the MDM table)

Number and Complexity of Problem(s)

- One or more chronic illnesses with exacerbation, progression, or side effects of treatment
- Two or more stable, chronic illnesses
- One undiagnosed new problem with uncertain prognosis
- One acute illness with systemic symptoms
- One acute, complicated injury

Amount and/or Complexity of Data

**Each unique test, order, or document contributes to the combination of two or combination of three in Category 1 below.*

- Moderate

(Must meet the requirements of at least one of the three categories.)

Category 1: Tests, documents, or independent historian(s)

- Any combination of three from the following:
  - review of prior external note(s) from each unique source*
  - review of the result(s) of each unique test*
  - ordering of each unique test*
  - assessment requiring an independent historian(s)

  or

Category 2: Independent interpretation of tests

- Independent interpretation of a test performed by another physician/other qualified health care professional (not separately reported)

  or

Category 3: Discussion of management or test interpretation

- Discussion of management or test interpretation with external physician/other qualified health care professional/appropriate source (not separately reported)

Risk of Complications/Morbidity or Mortality

Moderate risk of morbidity from additional diagnostic testing or treatment.

Examples only:

- Prescription drug management
- Decision regarding minor surgery with identified patient or procedure risk factors
- Decision regarding elective major surgery without identified patient or procedure risk factors
- Diagnosis or treatment significantly limited by social determinants of health

Time Spent on Date of the Encounter

- 30 minutes

Sample Documentation—99214

Level IV Established Patient Office Visit
Chief complaint: One day history of left ear pain and discharge.

This 5-year-old female presents with left ear pain and discharge from the left ear canal. The mother reports the child awakened during the night complaining of pain in the left ear. The mother noted purulent discharge coming from the left ear canal which she states was increased this morning. The mother reports that the child was swimming in a lake at a family picnic two days prior to this visit. The child says she cannot hear well and appears to have difficulty in hearing questions. The mother says the child had a fever of 100 degrees this morning. The child indicates that her throat is sore; no G.I. complaints or other symptoms. She slept poorly last evening and refused to eat or drink. Immunizations are up to date. The child has had four prior episodes of serous otitis media associated with tonsillitis and pharyngitis; no prior episodes of otitis externa. She had chickenpox at age 16 months. No other pertinent history; no medications, no known allergies. Developmental milestones are within normal limits. No other family members are ill or have been within the past few weeks.

PE: Pulse 94 and regular, respirations 20 and unlabored, temperature 101.7; wt. 42. Well-developed, well-nourished child, appearing somewhat flushed, cranky and tired. HEENT normocephalic, no tenderness over the sinuses. Eyes clear, conjunctivae pink; nose, clear. Pharynx shows red, infected tonsils, +2 enlarged, no Koplik's spots on palate. Mouth otherwise normal. Left ear canal red, swollen with purulent material filling the canal and tenderness of the external ear. Right canal is clear—the TM is erythematous and slightly bulging. Fluid level noted retro-tympanically. The left TM was not visualized. Neck supple, minimal cervical lymphadenopathy present. Exam of the nose revealed yellow discharge. Chest is clear to P&A with no wheezes, rales or rhonchi. Heart regular rate and rhythm, no murmurs. Abdomen soft non-tender. No organomegaly. Skin: no rash, turgor good.

Impression:
1. Left otitis externa with possible tympanitis
2. Right otitis media
3. Acute tonsillopharyngitis

Plan:
1. 4 drops of Pedi-Otic were placed in the left canal, and the mother was given a prescription for same, three drops, TID x one week, both ears.
2. Amoxicillin Suspension 250 mgm TID x 10 days.
3. Recheck 10–14 days.
4. Consider ENT referral if no improvement.

Level IV Established Patient Office Visit
Chief Complaint:A 55-year-old male patient presents for evaluation of mandibular jaw pain.

The patient has experienced a dull, aching pain in the left lower jaw for approximately three weeks that occasionally radiates to his neck or upper shoulder. I have reviewed dental records from his recent dental exam, which revealed no causal pathology. Dental x-rays revealed no abnormalities of the temporomandibular joint (TMJ). Family history is positive for cardiovascular disease, resulting in the early demise of the patient's father at the age of 52. Patient is otherwise healthy.

Physical Examination: Patient is a mildly obese, middle-aged male with a BMI of 31 kg/m2. Temperature 98.2 degrees Fahrenheit, blood pressure 142/76, pulse 77, respiratory rate 16, and O2 saturation 98 percent. Patient has no lymphadenopathy. Negative for carotid bruits. Lungs were clear to auscultation and percussion without wheezes. Heart was regular rate and rhythm without murmur, rubs, or gallops. Extremities are without significant clubbing, cyanosis, or edema. Pulses grossly intact.

Recent laboratory tests revealed mildly elevated total cholesterol at 237 mg/dL and LDL at 162 mg/dL.

Impression and plan: The diagnosis is left jaw pain with unknown etiology. In addition, the patient is obese and has a significant family history of cardiovascular disease with his father's death at age 52. I am scheduling the patient for an ECG and stress test to rule out cardiovascular origin based on patient history and presenting symptoms.

How This Level of E/M Service Was Assigned:

- **History:** Medically appropriate as deemed by the provider.
- **Physical Examination:** Medically appropriate as deemed by the provider.
- **Medical Decision Making:** Diagnosis made by the physician is lower left jaw pain, obesity, and significant family history of cardiovascular disease with his father's death at age 52. Using the redefined MDM table published by the AMA and adopted by CMS, the note indicates that one undiagnosed new problem with uncertain prognosis was addressed, which equates to moderate number and complexity of problems addressed. Two unique tests (ECG and stress test) are ordered/reviewed and the provider reviewed the patient's dental records for a combination of three items under Category 1, which equate to a moderate amount and/or complexity of data reviewed and analyzed. The level of MDM is based on two out of three elements; two elements in this case equate to Moderate MDM and code 99214.

99215

Documentation Requirements

Medical Decision Making: High

- High number and complexity of problems addressed
- Extensive amount and complexity of data reviewed and analyzed
- High risk of complications and/or morbidity

History: Medically appropriate

Examination: Medically appropriate

Key Point

The nature and extent of the patient history and physical examination are determined by the treating provider reporting the service.

Code Indicators (from the MDM table)

Number and Complexity of Problem(s)

- One or more chronic illnesses with severe exacerbation, progression, or side effects of treatment
- One acute or chronic illness or injury that poses a threat to life or bodily function

Amount and/or Complexity of Data

**Each unique test, order, or document contributes to the combination of two or combination of three in Category 1 below.*

- Extensive

(Must meet the requirements of at least two of the three categories.)

Category 1: Tests, documents, or independent historian(s)

- Any combination of three from the following:
  - review of prior external note(s) from each unique source*
  - review of the result(s) of each unique test*
  - ordering of each unique test*
  - assessment requiring an independent historian(s)

  or

Category 2: Independent interpretation of tests

- Independent interpretation of a test performed by another physician/other qualified health care professional (not separately reported)

  or

Category 3: Discussion of management or test interpretation

- Discussion of management or test interpretation with external physician/other qualified health care professional/appropriate source (not separately reported)

Risk of Complications/Morbidity or Mortality

High risk of morbidity from additional diagnostic testing or treatment.

Examples only:

- Drug therapy requiring intensive monitoring for toxicity
- Decision regarding elective major surgery with identified patient or procedure risk factors
- Decision regarding emergency major surgery
- Decision regarding hospitalization or escalation of hospital level care
- Decision not to resuscitate or to de-escalate care because of poor prognosis
- Parenteral controlled substances

Time Spent on Date of the Encounter

- 40 minutes

Sample Documentation—99215

Level V Established Patient Office Visit
Chief Complaint: A 61 y.o. white female with fever, weakness, weight loss and headaches x 3 weeks.

HPI: This patient reports fevers up to 102 degrees, no chills or sweats. Complains of bilateral headaches, worse in the morning. Denies having any of these symptoms prior to this illness. Has lost seven days of work in the past three weeks due to "just feeling bad." Notes anorexia, no dysphasia. Denies cough, rhinitis, ear pain or photophobia. Denies shortness of breath, sputum production, pleuritic or chest pain. Denies nausea, vomiting, diarrhea or abdominal pain. Denies flank pain, dysuria or urgency. Denies skin rashes.

Notes recent pain and stiffness in neck, shoulders and hips, not relieved by aspirin. Has had one episode of jaw pain while chewing. Admits to left-sided scalp tenderness.

Meds: Estrogen/Progesterone replacement, OTC multivitamins.
PMH: G4, P3, AB1, three children alive and well. Lives with her husband. No tobacco, uses alcohol socially, denies illicit drugs. Appendectomy age 15; fracture of right femur 20 years ago, no sequelae. No allergies. Prior to this illness, walked 5–7 miles a week and played tennis twice a week.

ROS: HEENT: Recent blurred vision such that she is afraid to drive. No dental problems.
Pulmonary See HPI.
Cardiovascular: No pressure, pain, palpitations, syncope. No orthopnea, paroxysmal nocturnal dyspnea or dyspnea on exertion. O/W neg.
G.I.: See HPI.
GU: Menopause 10 Years ago. See HPI.
Musculoskeletal: No history of arthritis or joint problems. Now stiff and painful neck, shoulders, hips. Neurologic: See HPI. No focal weakness, numbness, paresthesias. No seizure history. Difficulty walking due to painful joints and weakness.

Physical Exam: Height 5'4". Weight 118 lbs. (-6 lbs. in 6 months). BP: 110/70 T: 100.5 P: 65 R: l8. General Appearance: Well developed, obviously fatigued white female in no acute distress.

HEENT: PERRLA, EOMI, conjunctiva and sclerae clear. TM's intact, nasal passages clear. Teeth in good repair without signs of infection. Swelling and tenderness over both temporal arteries. Artery on left no pulse is palpable. Bilateral temporal bruits 1/4.
Neck: Muscular stiffness noted. No bony tenderness, bilateral carotid bruits. No masses.
Lungs: Normal respiratory excursion, clear to percussion and auscultation.
Heart: Normal PMI, regular rate and rhythm; no gallops, murmurs or rubs. No neck vein distention. Abdomen flat, healed appendectomy scar RLQ, soft, no masses, organomegaly or tenderness.
Spine/Back: Non-tender, flexes to 90 degrees with effort, no CVA tenderness.
GU: Deferred to her gynecologist. Last exam 3 months ago reported as normal.
Musculoskeletal: Diffuse rigidity of hips and shoulders bilaterally. No redness, heat, effusions or focal deformities. Neck and deltoid areas markedly tender. No edema.
Skin: Warm, dry, no rashes, normal turgor.
Neurological: Alert, oriented to person, place and time. No focal defects, DTR's + 2 upper, + 1 lower.

Rectal: Normal tone, no masses; stool heme negative.

Impression:
1. Temporal Arteritis with Polymyalgia Rheumatica.
2. R/O occult infection, specifically UTI, abscess.

Plan:
1. CBC with Diff, ESR, UA.
2. If ESR is elevated and CBC and UA do not show infection, start prednisone 60mg daily x 2 weeks and re-check. Clinical presentation precludes temporal biopsy at this time.

I personally spent a total of 45 minutes with this patient today, including examination and a significant discussion regarding temporal arteritis causes, treatments, and outcomes.

Sample Documentation—99215 (Continued)

Level V Established Patient Office Visit

S: This 62-year-old female presents with a chief complaint of progressive weight loss, loss of appetite, fatigue, constipation associated with vague abdominal pain, vaginal itching and white discharge, occasional headaches and blurry vision. The patient reports these symptoms have been ongoing and steadily increasing over the past 6–8 months.

The vaginal itching is severe at times and the constipation occurs at least once/week; she describes her stool as "rock hard." She occasionally notices blood on the toilet paper after defecating. The weight loss and decreased appetite are described as having been "noticed more by my family than me." The patient's diet consists of breakfast and lunch; no dinner is consumed. She snacks throughout the day consuming fruits, pastries and processed sweets. The patient states she has chronic hypertension and high cholesterol for which she takes medications. She has not modified her diet to accommodate the hypercholesterolemia because she says "the medicine makes up for it."

Past, Family and Social history reviewed and updated per chart entry September 18, 2019.

ROS: Blurry vision, especially noticeable while driving and watching TV. Headaches generally occur after these activities. Resp: no SOB. No cough. Cardio: no complaints except hypertension. GI: See HPI. GU: See HPI. Last Pap four years ago, normal. Pt. does report slight burning upon urination and reports this complaint for today at this time. Musculoskeletal: joints occasionally ache, more in the a.m. and subsiding as the day wears on. Neuro: no complaints. Endo: increased cholesterol, as noted. Denies diabetic history. General: fatigue, weight loss and decreased appetite as noted. Chronically cold. No fever, chills, diaphoresis. All other systems negative.

O: Weight: 155 lbs. Ht: 5'4". BP 140/110. Temp: 98.6. R: 16; P: 80. Slight gaunt appearance. Eyes: pupils round, reactive to light and accommodation. Sclerae/conjunctivae clear. Retinae: macular degeneration bilaterally. Fundi flat. Venous pulsations with arteriolar narrowing. Ears/EACs: WNL. Tympanic membranes WNL. Nose: nasal mucosa pink, healthy. No discharge. Throat: Tonsils absent. Posterior pharyngeal wall slightly erythematous. No exudate. Dentition poor; partially edentulous. Neck: no lymphadenopathy; thyroid nonpalpable. Heart: RRR; No murmur, gallop or rubs. Chest: normal breath sounds. No rales/rhonchi. Breasts: pedunculated; symmetrical; no mass/ tenderness; nipples without discharge. Abdomen: soft, nontender. No organomegaly. Bowel sounds diminished. Musculoskeletal: normal gait. No tender joints. No muscle atrophy but pt. is extremely slender. Trace ankle pitting. Neuro: no deficits. Reflexes 2+. GU: vulva slightly erythematous. No gross discharge noted. Vagina: some whitish exudate noted—culture obtained. Mucosa slightly dry; no lesions. Cervical cuff WNL. Pap taken. No inguinale lymphadenopathy. Rectal: one external nonthrombosed hemorrhoid noted. Rectal vault: full, hard feces palpable. Several medium sized hemorrhoids noted. No visible blood. Hemoccult taken—positive.

LABS: UA—dipstick/microscopic: glucose +4; proteins 3+; ketones neg; all other neg. Micro: no WBCs. No RBCs or casts. No bacteria; rare candida albicans noted. Urine culture sent to outside lab. Fingerstick glucose—320 mg/dL. Hemoccult and Pap taken as noted. Vaginal culture/wet mount sent to lab. Blood/chemistry panel ordered via outside lab including thyroid profile. HgA1c pending. Creatinine clearance; 24-hour urine.

Review of medical records reveals hypertension and hypercholesterolemia, treated as noted previously. No elevated glucose at that time.

A: (1) New onset hyperglycemia; R/O diabetes mellitus. (2) Diastolic hypertension, uncontrolled on Monopril. (3) Proteinuria. R/O nephrotic syndrome; (4) Vulvovaginitis. (5) Weight loss. (6) Constipation. (7) Possible diabetic retinopathy with macular degeneration. (8) Internal/external hemorrhoids, bleeding occult. (9) Hypercholesterolemia, by history.

P: This patient had multiple issues that left untreated could be very dangerous to her well-being. My plan of treatment is as follows: (1) Hyperglycemia: patient counseled regarding proper diet and provided an ADA daily diet plan. The properties and progressive nature of NIDDM were discussed at length. HgA1c pending. Return for repeat glucose level when urine collection is complete. (2) Hypertension: add HCTZ 12.5 mg q.o.d. (3) Vulvovaginitis: Monistat vag cream, apply b.i.d. for five days. Add yogurt to diet. (4) Constipation/hemorrhoids: Colace 100 mg q.d. for 5 days; ProctoFoam: as directed. (5) Referral to ophthalmology for diabetic retinopathy consultation. (6) Nephrotic range proteinuria—testing as above. Will order renal US and/or refer to Nephrology as needed. (7) Make appointment with GYN physician for complete exam. Pap smear/vaginal culture info will be provided to pt. (8) Follow up in three weeks. Will discuss labs at that time and will determine efficacy of Mevacor. Will discuss ophthalmology findings with pt. when results are received.

I personally spent 50 to 55 minutes on this patient's case today, including review of past history, physical examination, and a lengthy discussion regarding the importance of controlling her hypertension and the effects of uncontrolled blood glucose levels on other organ systems (i.e., eyes and kidneys).

Knowledge Assessment Chapter 6

See chapter 21 for answers and rationale.

1. History and physical examination elements are no longer used in selection of the level of office or other outpatient visits and therefore don't have to be documented in the medical record.
   a. True
   b. False
2. Total time on the date of the encounter includes non-face-to-face time. Which of the following activities personally performed by the treating provider may count toward the total time reported for purposes of code level selection? Select all that apply.
   a. Reviewing tests or other records
   b. Documenting clinical information in the medical record
   c. Ordering tests/procedures or medications
   d. Counseling and educating the patient or caregiver
3. Based on the time documented at the end of the sample documentation for 99205 that starts on page 53, code 99205 could be reported based on time alone.
   a. True
   b. False
4. A new patient presents to the office with two stable chronic illnesses. Limited data is reviewed, and changes are made to the patient's prescription drug regimen. Based on MDM elements, what level of service should be reported?
   a. 99203
   b. 99204
   c. 99214
   d. 99205

Chapter 7. Telemedicine Services (98000-98016)

Synchronous Audio-Video Evaluation and Management Services (98000-98007)

New Patient (98000-98003)

E/M Code	Medical Decision Making	History	Exam	Time Spent on Date of Encounter
98000	Straightforward	Medically appropriate	Medically appropriate	15 min.
98001	Low	Medically appropriate	Medically appropriate	30 min.
98002	Moderate	Medically appropriate	Medically appropriate	45 min.
98003	High	Medically appropriate	Medically appropriate	60 min.

General Guidelines

- Use these CPT® codes to report E/M services provided to a new patient via synchronous, real-time, audio-video interactive telecommunication.
- The provider and patient interact from different locations using real-time communication in which they can see and hear each other.
- These services may be provided in lieu of an in-person visit, when medically appropriate and when the patient and/or family/caregiver agree to receive care utilizing telecommunication services.
- These telehealth services may be initiated by the patient, family, caregiver, physician, or other qualified health care professional (OQHP), and do not require a specific time interval from the last in-person visit or telemedicine visit.
- Code selection is based on the extent of medical decision making (MDM) or total time, including face-to-face and non-face-to-face time spent on the date of the encounter.
- Simple tests, such as UA, CBC, and quick strep, which are results only tests and do not require separate interpretation, can be counted as ordered or reviewed as part of the Data element for MDM.
- History and physical examination elements are not required for code level selection. However, a medically appropriate history and/or physical examination should still be documented. The nature and degree of the history and/or physical examination is determined by the treating physician or other qualified health care professional reporting the service.
- Total time for these services includes total face-to-face and non-face-to-face time personally spent by the physician or OQHP on the day of the encounter.
- Physician or OQHP time may include the following activities:
  - preparing to see the patient (e.g., review of tests)
  - obtaining and/or reviewing separately obtained history
  - performing a medically appropriate examination and/or evaluation
  - counseling and educating the patient/family/caregiver
  - ordering medications, tests, or procedures
  - referring and communicating with other health care professionals (when not separately reported)
  - documenting clinical information in the electronic or other health record
  - independently interpreting results (not separately reported) and communicating results to the patient/family/caregiver
  - care coordination (not separately reported)
- These codes should not be reported solely to communicate laboratory results or other routine telecommunications related to a previous E/M service.
- Do not report these on the same day as an in-person E/M visit; add the elements and time of each visit together and report only one E/M service.
- Report prolonged service code 99417 with 98003 when the service runs 15 minutes beyond the time specified in the CPT code narrative. The time must be clearly documented in the medical record.

Key Point

If audio-video connections are lost during an encounter and only audio is restored, report the service that accounted for the majority of the time of the interactive portion of the service.

98000

Documentation Requirements

Medical Decision Making: Straightforward

- Minimal number and complexity of problems addressed
- No or minimal amount and complexity of data reviewed and analyzed
- Minimal risk of complications and/or morbidity or mortality

History: Medically appropriate

Examination: Medically appropriate

Key Point

The nature and extent of the patient history and physical examination are determined by the treating provider reporting the service.

Code Indicators (from the MDM table)

Number and Complexity of Problem(s)

- One self-limited or minor problem

Amount and/or Complexity of Data

- Minimal or none

Risk of Complications/Morbidity or Mortality

Minimal risk of morbidity from additional diagnostic tests or treatment

Time Spent on Date of the Encounter

- 15 minutes

Quick Tip

CMS documentation guidelines indicate that documentation should include the reason for the encounter and relevant history and physical examination findings.

98001

Documentation Requirements

Medical Decision Making: Low
- Low number and complexity of problems addressed
- Limited amount and complexity of data reviewed and analyzed
- Low risk of complications and/or morbidity or mortality

History: Medically appropriate

Examination: Medically appropriate

Key Point

The nature and extent of the patient history and physical examination are determined by the treating provider reporting the service.

Code Indicators (from the MDM table)

Number and Complexity of Problem(s)
- Two or more self-limited or minor problems
- One stable, chronic illness
- One acute, uncomplicated illness or injury
- One stable, acute illness
- One acute, uncomplicated illness or injury requiring hospital inpatient or observation level of care

Amount and/or Complexity of Data
**Each unique test, order, or document contributes to the combination of two or combination of three in Category 1 below.*
- Limited

(Must meet the requirements of at least one of the two categories.)

Category 1: Tests and documents
- Any combination of two from the following:
  - review of prior external note(s) from each unique source*
  - review of the result(s) of each unique test*
  - ordering of each unique test*

  or

Category 2: Assessment requiring an independent historian(s)
(For the categories of independent interpretation of tests and discussion of management or test interpretation, see moderate or high)

Risk of Complications/Morbidity or Mortality
Low risk of morbidity from additional diagnostic tests or treatment

Time Spent on Date of the Encounter
- 30 minutes

98002

Documentation Requirements

Medical Decision Making: Moderate

- Moderate number and complexity of problems addressed
- Moderate amount and complexity of data reviewed and analyzed
- Moderate risk of complications and/or morbidity or mortality

History: Medically appropriate

Examination: Medically appropriate

Key Point

The nature and extent of the patient history and physical examination are determined by the treating provider reporting the service.

Code Indicators (from the MDM table)

Number and Complexity of Problem(s)

- One or more chronic illnesses with exacerbation, progression, or side effects of treatment
- Two or more stable chronic illnesses
- One undiagnosed new problem with uncertain prognosis
- One acute illness with systemic symptoms
- One acute, complicated injury

Amount and/or Complexity of Data

**Each unique test, order, or document contributes to the combination of two or combination of three in Category 1 below.*

- Moderate

(Must meet the requirements of at least one of the three categories.)

Category 1: Tests, documents, or independent historian(s)

- Any combination of three from the following:
  - review of prior external note(s) from each unique source*
  - review of the result(s) of each unique test*
  - ordering of each unique test*
  - assessment requiring an independent historian(s)

  or

Category 2: Independent interpretation of tests

- Independent interpretation of a test performed by another physician/other qualified health care professional (not separately reported)

  or

Category 3: Discussion of management or test interpretation

- Discussion of management or test interpretation with external physician/other qualified health care professional/appropriate source (not separately reported)

Risk of Complications/Morbidity or Mortality

Moderate risk of morbidity from additional diagnostic testing or treatment

Examples only:

- Prescription drug management
- Decision regarding minor surgery with identified patient or procedure risk factors
- Decision regarding elective major surgery without identified patient or procedure risk factors
- Diagnosis or treatment significantly limited by social determinants of health

Time Spent on Date of the Encounter

- 45 minutes

98003

Documentation Requirements

Medical Decision Making: High

- High number and complexity of problems addressed
- Extensive amount and complexity of data reviewed and analyzed
- High risk of complications and/or morbidity or mortality

History: Medically appropriate

Examination: Medically appropriate

> **Key Point**
>
> **The nature and extent of the patient history and physical examination are determined by the treating provider reporting the service.**

Code Indicators (from the MDM table)

Number and Complexity of Problem(s)

- One or more chronic illnesses with severe exacerbation, progression, or side effects of treatment
- One acute or chronic illness or injury that poses a threat to life or bodily function

Amount and/or Complexity of Data

**Each unique test, order, or document contributes to the combination of two or combination of three in Category 1 below.*

- Extensive

(Must meet the requirements of at least two of the three categories.)

Category 1: Tests, documents, or independent historian(s)

- Any combination of three from the following:
  - review of prior external note(s) from each unique source*
  - review of the result(s) of each unique test*
  - ordering of each unique test*
  - assessment requiring an independent historian(s)

  or

Category 2: Independent interpretation of tests

- Independent interpretation of a test performed by another physician/other qualified health care professional (not separately reported)

  or

Category 3: Discussion of management or test interpretation

- Discussion of management or test interpretation with external physician/other qualified health care professional/appropriate source (not separately reported)

Risk of Complications/Morbidity or Mortality

High risk of morbidity from additional diagnostic testing or treatment

Examples only:

- Drug therapy requiring intensive monitoring for toxicity
- Decision regarding elective major surgery with identified patient or procedure risk factors
- Decision regarding emergency major surgery
- Decision regarding hospitalization or escalation of hospital-level care
- Decision not to resuscitate or to de-escalate care because of poor prognosis
- Parenteral controlled substances

Time Spent on Date of the Encounter

- 60 minutes

Established Patient (98004-98007)

E/M Code	Medical Decision Making	History	Exam	Time Spent on Date of Encounter
98004	Straightforward	Medically appropriate	Medically appropriate	10 min.
98005	Low	Medically appropriate	Medically appropriate	20 min.
98006	Moderate	Medically appropriate	Medically appropriate	30 min.
98007	High	Medically appropriate	Medically appropriate	40 min.

General Guidelines

- Use these CPT codes to report E/M services provided to an established patient via synchronous, real-time, audio-video interactive telecommunication.
- The provider and patient interact from different locations using real-time communication in which they can see and hear each other.
- These services may be provided in lieu of an in-person visit, when medically appropriate and when the patient and/or family/caregiver agree to receive care utilizing telecommunication services.
- These telehealth services may be initiated by the patient, family, caregiver, physician, or other qualified health care professional (OQHP), and do not require a specific time interval from the last in-person visit or telemedicine visit.
- Code selection is based on the extent of medical decision making (MDM) or total time spent by the provider on the date of the encounter.
- Simple tests, such as UA, CBC, and quick strep, which are results only tests and do not require separate interpretation, can be counted as ordered or reviewed as part of the Data element for MDM.
- History and physical examination elements are not required for code level selection. However, a medically appropriate history and/or physical examination should still be documented. The nature and degree of the history and/or physical examination is determined by the treating physician or other qualified health care professional reporting the service.
- Total time for these services includes time personally spent by the physician or OQHP on the day of the encounter.
- Physician or OQHP time may include the following activities:
  - preparing to see the patient (e.g., review of tests)
  - obtaining and/or reviewing separately obtained history
  - performing a medically appropriate examination and/or evaluation
  - counseling and educating the patient/family/caregiver
  - ordering medications, tests, or procedures
  - referring and communicating with other health care professionals (when not separately reported)
  - documenting clinical information in the electronic or other health record
  - independently interpreting results (not separately reported) and communicating results to the patient/family/caregiver
  - care coordination (not separately reported)
- These codes should not be reported solely to communicate laboratory results or other routine telecommunications related to a previous E/M service.
- These codes may be used to report regular follow-up in lieu of an in-person visit if the patient requires reassessment for a condition related to a treatment plan from a previous E/M visit.
- Do not report these on the same day as an in-person E/M visit; add the elements and time of each visit together and report only one E/M service.
- Report prolonged service code 99417 with 98007 when the service runs 15 minutes beyond the time specified in the CPT code narrative. The time must be clearly documented in the medical record.

Key Point

If audio-video connections are lost during an encounter and only audio is restored, report the service that accounted for the majority of the time of the interactive portion of the service.

98004

Documentation Requirements

Medical Decision Making: Straightforward
- Minimal number and complexity of problems addressed
- No or minimal amount and complexity of data reviewed and analyzed
- Minimal risk of complications and/or morbidity

History: Medically appropriate

Examination: Medically appropriate

Key Point

The nature and extent of the patient history and physical examination are determined by the treating provider reporting the service.

Code Indicators (from the MDM table)

Number and Complexity of Problem(s)
- One self-limited or minor problem

Amount and/or Complexity of Data
- Minimal or none

Risk of Complications/Morbidity or Mortality
Minimal risk of morbidity from additional diagnostic tests or treatment

Time Spent on Date of the Encounter
- 10 minutes

98005

Documentation Requirements

Medical Decision Making: Low

- Low number and complexity of problems addressed
- Limited amount and complexity of data reviewed and analyzed
- Low risk of complications and/or morbidity

History: Medically appropriate

Examination: Medically appropriate

> **Key Point**
>
> **The nature and extent of the patient history and physical examination are determined by the treating provider reporting the service.**

Code Indicators (from the MDM table)

Number and Complexity of Problem(s)

- Two or more self-limited or minor problems
- One stable, chronic illness
- One acute, uncomplicated illness or injury
- One stable, acute illness
- One acute, uncomplicated illness or injury requiring hospital inpatient or observation level of care

Amount and/or Complexity of Data

**Each unique test, order, or document contributes to the combination of two or combination of three in Category 1 below.*

- Limited

(Must meet the requirements of at least one of the two categories.)

Category 1: Tests and documents

- Any combination of two from the following:
  - review of prior external note(s) from each unique source*
  - review of the result(s) of each unique test*
  - ordering of each unique test*

  or

Category 2: Assessment requiring an independent historian(s)

(For the categories of independent interpretation of tests and discussion of management or test interpretation, see moderate or high)

Risk of Complications/Morbidity or Mortality

Low risk of morbidity from additional diagnostic testing or treatment

Time Spent on Date of the Encounter

- 20 minutes

98006

Documentation Requirements

Medical Decision Making: Moderate

- Moderate number and complexity of problems addressed
- Moderate amount and complexity of data reviewed and analyzed
- Moderate risk of complications and/or morbidity

History: Medically appropriate

Examination: Medically appropriate

> **Key Point**
>
> **The nature and extent of the patient history and physical examination are determined by the treating provider reporting the service.**

Code Indicators (from the MDM table)

Number and Complexity of Problem(s)

- One or more chronic illnesses with exacerbation, progression, or side effects of treatment
- Two or more stable, chronic illnesses
- One undiagnosed new problem with uncertain prognosis
- One acute illness with systemic symptoms
- One acute, complicated injury

Amount and/or Complexity of Data

**Each unique test, order, or document contributes to the combination of two or combination of three in Category 1 below.*

- Moderate

(Must meet the requirements of at least one of the three categories.)

Category 1: Tests, documents, or independent historian(s)

- Any combination of three from the following:
  - review of prior external note(s) from each unique source*
  - review of the result(s) of each unique test*
  - ordering of each unique test*
  - assessment requiring an independent historian(s)

  or

Category 2: Independent interpretation of tests

- Independent interpretation of a test performed by another physician/other qualified health care professional (not separately reported)

  or

Category 3: Discussion of management or test interpretation

- Discussion of management or test interpretation with external physician/other qualified health care professional/appropriate source (not separately reported)

Risk of Complications/Morbidity or Mortality

Moderate risk of morbidity from additional diagnostic testing or treatment.

Examples only:

- Prescription drug management
- Decision regarding minor surgery with identified patient or procedure risk factors
- Decision regarding elective major surgery without identified patient or procedure risk factors
- Diagnosis or treatment significantly limited by social determinants of health

Time Spent on Date of the Encounter

- 30 minutes

98007

Documentation Requirements

Medical Decision Making: High
- High number and complexity of problems addressed
- Extensive amount and complexity of data reviewed and analyzed
- High risk of complications and/or morbidity

History: Medically appropriate

Examination: Medically appropriate

Key Point

The nature and extent of the patient history and physical examination are determined by the treating provider reporting the service.

Code Indicators (from the MDM table)

Number and Complexity of Problem(s)
- One or more chronic illnesses with severe exacerbation, progression, or side effects of treatment
- One acute or chronic illness or injury that poses a threat to life or bodily function

Amount and/or Complexity of Data
**Each unique test, order, or document contributes to the combination of two or combination of three in Category 1 below.*

- Extensive

(Must meet the requirements of at least two of the three categories.)

Category 1: Tests, documents, or independent historian(s)
- Any combination of three from the following:
  - review of prior external note(s) from each unique source*
  - review of the result(s) of each unique test*
  - ordering of each unique test*
  - assessment requiring an independent historian(s)

  or

Category 2: Independent interpretation of tests
- Independent interpretation of a test performed by another physician/other qualified health care professional (not separately reported)

  or

Category 3: Discussion of management or test interpretation
- Discussion of management or test interpretation with external physician/other qualified health care professional/appropriate source (not separately reported)

Risk of Complications/Morbidity or Mortality
High risk of morbidity from additional diagnostic testing or treatment.

Examples only:

- Drug therapy requiring intensive monitoring for toxicity
- Decision regarding elective major surgery with identified patient or procedure risk factors
- Decision regarding emergency major surgery
- Decision regarding hospitalization or escalation of hospital level care
- Decision not to resuscitate or to de-escalate care because of poor prognosis
- Parenteral controlled substances

Time Spent on Date of the Encounter
- 40 minutes

Synchronous Audio-Only Evaluation and Management Services (98008-98015)

New Patient (98008-98011)

E/M Code	Medical Decision Making	History	Exam	Time Spent on Date of Encounter
98008	Straightforward	Medically appropriate	Medically appropriate	15 min.
98009	Low	Medically appropriate	Medically appropriate	30 min.
98010	Moderate	Medically appropriate	Medically appropriate	45 min.
98011	High	Medically appropriate	Medically appropriate	60 min.

General Guidelines

- Use these CPT codes to report E/M services provided to a new patient via synchronous, real-time, audio only interactive telecommunication.
- The provider and patient interact from different locations using real-time communication in which they can hear each other but do not utilize video communication.
- These services may be provided in lieu of an in-person visit, when medically appropriate and when the patient and/or family/caregiver agree to receive care utilizing telecommunication services.
- Synchronous audio-only E/M services require more than 10 minutes of medical discussion defined as synchronous (real-time) interactive verbal communication. It does not include online digital communications, except via a telecommunication technology device for the deaf.
- These telehealth services may be initiated by the patient, family, caregiver, physician, or other qualified health care professional (OQHP), and do not require a specific time interval from the last in-person visit or telemedicine visit.
- Code selection is based on the extent of medical decision making (MDM) or total time, including face-to-face and non-face-to-face time spent on the date of the encounter.
- Simple tests, such as UA, CBC, and quick strep, which are results only tests and do not require separate interpretation, can be counted as ordered or reviewed as part of the Data element for MDM.
- History and physical examination elements are not required for code level selection. However, a medically appropriate history and/or physical examination should still be documented. The nature and degree of the history and/or physical examination is determined by the treating physician or other qualified health care professional reporting the service.
- Total time for these services includes total face-to-face and non-face-to-face time personally spent by the physician or OQHP on the day of the encounter.
- Physician or OQHP time may include the following activities:
  - preparing to see the patient (e.g., review of tests)
  - obtaining and/or reviewing separately obtained history
  - performing a medically appropriate examination and/or evaluation
  - counseling and educating the patient/family/caregiver
  - ordering medications, tests, or procedures
  - referring and communicating with other health care professionals (when not separately reported)
  - documenting clinical information in the electronic or other health record
  - independently interpreting results (not separately reported) and communicating results to the patient/family/caregiver
  - care coordination (not separately reported)
- These codes should not be reported solely to communicate laboratory results or other routine telecommunications related to a previous E/M service.
- Do not report these on the same day as an in-person E/M visit; add the elements and time of each visit together and report only one E/M service.
- Report prolonged service code 99417 with 98011 when the service runs 15 minutes beyond the time specified in the CPT code narrative. The time must be clearly documented in the medical record.

98008

Documentation Requirements

Medical Decision Making: Straightforward

- Minimal number and complexity of problems addressed
- No or minimal amount and complexity of data reviewed and analyzed
- Minimal risk of complications and/or morbidity or mortality

History: Medically appropriate

Examination: Medically appropriate

Key Point

The nature and extent of the patient history and physical examination are determined by the treating provider reporting the service.

Code Indicators (from the MDM table)

Number and Complexity of Problem(s)

- One self-limited or minor problem

Amount and/or Complexity of Data

- Minimal or none

Risk of Complications/Morbidity or Mortality

Minimal risk of morbidity from additional diagnostic tests or treatment

Time Spent on Date of the Encounter

- 15 minutes

Quick Tip

CMS documentation guidelines indicate that documentation should include the reason for the encounter and relevant history and physical examination findings.

98009

Documentation Requirements

Medical Decision Making: Low

- Low number and complexity of problems addressed
- Limited amount and complexity of data reviewed and analyzed
- Low risk of complications and/or morbidity or mortality

History: Medically appropriate

Examination: Medically appropriate

Key Point

The nature and extent of the patient history and physical examination are determined by the treating provider reporting the service.

Code Indicators (from the MDM table)

Number and Complexity of Problem(s)

- Two or more self-limited or minor problems
- One stable, chronic illness
- One acute, uncomplicated illness or injury
- One stable, acute illness
- One acute, uncomplicated illness or injury requiring hospital inpatient or observation level of care

Amount and/or Complexity of Data

**Each unique test, order, or document contributes to the combination of two or combination of three in Category 1 below.*

- Limited

(Must meet the requirements of at least one of the two categories.)

Category 1: Tests and documents

- Any combination of two from the following:
  - review of prior external note(s) from each unique source*
  - review of the result(s) of each unique test*
  - ordering of each unique test*

  or

Category 2: Assessment requiring an independent historian(s)

(For the categories of independent interpretation of tests and discussion of management or test interpretation, see moderate or high)

Risk of Complications/Morbidity or Mortality

Low risk of morbidity from additional diagnostic tests or treatment

Time Spent on Date of the Encounter

- 30 minutes

98010

Documentation Requirements

Medical Decision Making: Moderate
- Moderate number and complexity of problems addressed
- Moderate amount and complexity of data reviewed and analyzed
- Moderate risk of complications and/or morbidity or mortality

History: Medically appropriate

Examination: Medically appropriate

Key Point

The nature and extent of the patient history and physical examination are determined by the treating provider reporting the service.

Code Indicators (from the MDM table)

Number and Complexity of Problem(s)
- One or more chronic illnesses with exacerbation, progression, or side effects of treatment
- Two or more stable chronic illnesses
- One undiagnosed new problem with uncertain prognosis
- One acute illness with systemic symptoms
- One acute, complicated injury

Amount and/or Complexity of Data
**Each unique test, order, or document contributes to the combination of two or combination of three in Category 1 below.*
- Moderate

(Must meet the requirements of at least one of the three categories.)

Category 1: Tests, documents, or independent historian(s)
- Any combination of three from the following:
  - review of prior external note(s) from each unique source*
  - review of the result(s) of each unique test*
  - ordering of each unique test*
  - assessment requiring an independent historian(s)

  or

Category 2: Independent interpretation of tests
- Independent interpretation of a test performed by another physician/other qualified health care professional (not separately reported)

  or

Category 3: Discussion of management or test interpretation
- Discussion of management or test interpretation with external physician/other qualified health care professional/appropriate source (not separately reported)

Risk of Complications/Morbidity or Mortality
Moderate risk of morbidity from additional diagnostic testing or treatment

Examples only:
- Prescription drug management
- Decision regarding minor surgery with identified patient or procedure risk factors
- Decision regarding elective major surgery without identified patient or procedure risk factors
- Diagnosis or treatment significantly limited by social determinants of health

Time Spent on Date of the Encounter
- 45 minutes

98011

Documentation Requirements

Medical Decision Making: High

- High number and complexity of problems addressed
- Extensive amount and complexity of data reviewed and analyzed
- High risk of complications and/or morbidity or mortality

History: Medically appropriate

Examination: Medically appropriate

> **Key Point**
>
> **The nature and extent of the patient history and physical examination are determined by the treating provider reporting the service.**

Code Indicators (from the MDM table)

Number and Complexity of Problem(s)

- One or more chronic illnesses with severe exacerbation, progression, or side effects of treatment
- One acute or chronic illness or injury that poses a threat to life or bodily function

Amount and/or Complexity of Data

**Each unique test, order, or document contributes to the combination of two or combination of three in Category 1 below.*

- Extensive

(Must meet the requirements of at least two of the three categories.)

Category 1: Tests, documents, or independent historian(s)

- Any combination of three from the following:
  - review of prior external note(s) from each unique source*
  - review of the result(s) of each unique test*
  - ordering of each unique test*
  - assessment requiring an independent historian(s)

  or

Category 2: Independent interpretation of tests

- Independent interpretation of a test performed by another physician/other qualified health care professional (not separately reported)

  or

Category 3: Discussion of management or test interpretation

- Discussion of management or test interpretation with external physician/other qualified health care professional/appropriate source (not separately reported)

Risk of Complications/Morbidity or Mortality

High risk of morbidity from additional diagnostic testing or treatment

Examples only:

- Drug therapy requiring intensive monitoring for toxicity
- Decision regarding elective major surgery with identified patient or procedure risk factors
- Decision regarding emergency major surgery
- Decision regarding hospitalization or escalation of hospital-level care
- Decision not to resuscitate or to de-escalate care because of poor prognosis
- Parenteral controlled substances

Time Spent on Date of the Encounter

- 60 minutes

Established Patient (98012-98015)

E/M Code	Medical Decision Making	History	Exam	Time Spent on Date of Encounter
98012	Straightforward	Medically appropriate	Medically appropriate	10 min.
98013	Low	Medically appropriate	Medically appropriate	20 min.
98014	Moderate	Medically appropriate	Medically appropriate	30 min.
98015	High	Medically appropriate	Medically appropriate	40 min.

General Guidelines

- Use these CPT codes to report E/M services provided to an established patient via synchronous, real-time, audio only interactive telecommunication.
- The provider and patient interact from different locations using real-time communication in which they can hear each other but do not utilize video communication.
- These services may be provided in lieu of an in-person visit, when medically appropriate and when the patient and/or family/caregiver agree to receive care utilizing telecommunication services.
- Synchronous audio-only E/M services require more than 10 minutes of medical discussion defined as synchronous (real-time) interactive verbal communication. It does not include online digital communications, except via a telecommunication technology device for the deaf.
- These telehealth services may be initiated by the patient, family, caregiver, physician, or other qualified health care professional (OQHP), and do not require a specific time interval from the last in-person visit or telemedicine visit.
- Code selection is based on the extent of medical decision making (MDM) or total time, including face-to-face and non-face-to-face time spent on the date of the encounter.
- Simple tests, such as UA, CBC, and quick strep, which are results only tests and do not require separate interpretation, can be counted as ordered or reviewed as part of the Data element for MDM.
- History and physical examination elements are not required for code level selection. However, a medically appropriate history and/or physical examination should still be documented. The nature and degree of the history and/or physical examination is determined by the treating physician or other qualified health care professional reporting the service.
- Total time for these services includes total face-to-face and non-face-to-face time personally spent by the physician or OQHP on the day of the encounter.
- Physician or OQHP time may include the following activities:
  - preparing to see the patient (e.g., review of tests)
  - obtaining and/or reviewing separately obtained history
  - performing a medically appropriate examination and/or evaluation
  - counseling and educating the patient/family/caregiver
  - ordering medications, tests, or procedures
  - referring and communicating with other health care professionals (when not separately reported)
  - documenting clinical information in the electronic or other health record
  - independently interpreting results (not separately reported) and communicating results to the patient/family/caregiver
  - care coordination (not separately reported)
- These codes should not be reported solely to communicate laboratory results or other routine telecommunications related to a previous E/M service.
- These codes may be used to report regular follow-up in lieu of an in-person visit if the patient requires reassessment for a condition related to a treatment plan from a previous E/M visit.
- Do not report these on the same day as an in-person E/M visit; add the elements and time of each visit together and report only one E/M service.
- Report prolonged service code 99417 with 98015 when the service runs 15 minutes beyond the time specified in the CPT code narrative. The time must be clearly documented in the medical record.
- When home and outpatient INR monitoring is evaluated during a synchronous telemedicine service, do not report these codes separately.
- If providing care plan oversight (CPO) during the same call(s), do not report these codes in addition to 99374-99380.
- These codes should not be reported during the same month as complex chronic care management services 99487 or 99489.
- These codes should not be reported if performed during the service time of transition care management services 99495 or 99496.

98012

Documentation Requirements

Medical Decision Making: Straightforward

- Minimal number and complexity of problems addressed
- No or minimal amount and complexity of data reviewed and analyzed
- Minimal risk of complications and/or morbidity

History: Medically appropriate

Examination: Medically appropriate

Key Point

The nature and extent of the patient history and physical examination are determined by the treating provider reporting the service.

Code Indicators (from the MDM table)

Number and Complexity of Problem(s)

- One self-limited or minor problem

Amount and/or Complexity of Data

- Minimal or none

Risk of Complications/Morbidity or Mortality

Minimal risk of morbidity from additional diagnostic tests or treatment

Time Spent on Date of the Encounter

- 10 minutes

98013

Documentation Requirements

Medical Decision Making: Low

- Low number and complexity of problems addressed
- Limited amount and complexity of data reviewed and analyzed
- Low risk of complications and/or morbidity

History: Medically appropriate

Examination: Medically appropriate

Key Point

The nature and extent of the patient history and physical examination are determined by the treating provider reporting the service.

Code Indicators (from the MDM table)

Number and Complexity of Problem(s)

- Two or more self-limited or minor problems
- One stable, chronic illness
- One acute, uncomplicated illness or injury
- One stable, acute illness
- One acute, uncomplicated illness or injury requiring hospital inpatient or observation level of care

Amount and/or Complexity of Data

**Each unique test, order, or document contributes to the combination of two or combination of three in Category 1 below.*

- Limited

(Must meet the requirements of at least one of the two categories.)

Category 1: Tests and documents

- Any combination of two from the following:
  - review of prior external note(s) from each unique source*
  - review of the result(s) of each unique test*
  - ordering of each unique test*

  or

Category 2: Assessment requiring an independent historian(s)

(For the categories of independent interpretation of tests and discussion of management or test interpretation, see moderate or high)

Risk of Complications/Morbidity or Mortality

Low risk of morbidity from additional diagnostic testing or treatment

Time Spent on Date of the Encounter

- 20 minutes

98014

Documentation Requirements

Medical Decision Making: Moderate
- Moderate number and complexity of problems addressed
- Moderate amount and complexity of data reviewed and analyzed
- Moderate risk of complications and/or morbidity

History: Medically appropriate

Examination: Medically appropriate

> **Key Point**
> **The nature and extent of the patient history and physical examination are determined by the treating provider reporting the service.**

Code Indicators (from the MDM table)

Number and Complexity of Problem(s)
- One or more chronic illnesses with exacerbation, progression, or side effects of treatment
- Two or more stable, chronic illnesses
- One undiagnosed new problem with uncertain prognosis
- One acute illness with systemic symptoms
- One acute, complicated injury

Amount and/or Complexity of Data
**Each unique test, order, or document contributes to the combination of two or combination of three in Category 1 below.*

- Moderate

(Must meet the requirements of at least one of the three categories.)

Category 1: Tests, documents, or independent historian(s)
- Any combination of three from the following:
  - review of prior external note(s) from each unique source*
  - review of the result(s) of each unique test*
  - ordering of each unique test*
  - assessment requiring an independent historian(s)

  or

Category 2: Independent interpretation of tests
- Independent interpretation of a test performed by another physician/other qualified health care professional (not separately reported)

  or

Category 3: Discussion of management or test interpretation
- Discussion of management or test interpretation with external physician/other qualified health care professional/appropriate source (not separately reported)

Risk of Complications/Morbidity or Mortality
Moderate risk of morbidity from additional diagnostic testing or treatment.

Examples only:

- Prescription drug management
- Decision regarding minor surgery with identified patient or procedure risk factors
- Decision regarding elective major surgery without identified patient or procedure risk factors
- Diagnosis or treatment significantly limited by social determinants of health

Time Spent on Date of the Encounter
- 30 minutes

98015

Documentation Requirements

Medical Decision Making: High

- High number and complexity of problems addressed
- Extensive amount and complexity of data reviewed and analyzed
- High risk of complications and/or morbidity

History: Medically appropriate

Examination: Medically appropriate

> **Key Point**
>
> **The nature and extent of the patient history and physical examination are determined by the treating provider reporting the service.**

Code Indicators (from the MDM table)

Number and Complexity of Problem(s)

- One or more chronic illnesses with severe exacerbation, progression, or side effects of treatment
- One acute or chronic illness or injury that poses a threat to life or bodily function

Amount and/or Complexity of Data

**Each unique test, order, or document contributes to the combination of two or combination of three in Category 1 below.*

- Extensive

(Must meet the requirements of at least two of the three categories.)

Category 1: Tests, documents, or independent historian(s)

- Any combination of three from the following:
  - review of prior external note(s) from each unique source*
  - review of the result(s) of each unique test*
  - ordering of each unique test*
  - assessment requiring an independent historian(s)

  or

Category 2: Independent interpretation of tests

- Independent interpretation of a test performed by another physician/other qualified health care professional (not separately reported)

  or

Category 3: Discussion of management or test interpretation

- Discussion of management or test interpretation with external physician/other qualified health care professional/appropriate source (not separately reported)

Risk of Complications/Morbidity or Mortality

High risk of morbidity from additional diagnostic testing or treatment.

Examples only:

- Drug therapy requiring intensive monitoring for toxicity
- Decision regarding elective major surgery with identified patient or procedure risk factors
- Decision regarding emergency major surgery
- Decision regarding hospitalization or escalation of hospital level care
- Decision not to resuscitate or to de-escalate care because of poor prognosis
- Parenteral controlled substances

Time Spent on Date of the Encounter

- 40 minutes

Brief Synchronous Communication Technology Service (eg, Virtual Check-In) (98016)

E/M Code	Patient Type	Audio	Video	Time Spent on Date of Encounter
98016	Established	Yes	Not required	5-10 min.

General Guidelines

- Use this CPT code to report an E/M service of five to 10 minutes of medical discussion provided to an established patient via synchronous, real-time, audio only interactive telecommunication.
- This service is based on time of the medical discussion only; MDM is not applicable.
- This telehealth service is patient initiated and used to determine if a more extensive E/M service may be required (i.e., 99212-99215).
- When this check-in telehealth service leads to another E/M service on the same date and time is used to select the level of E/M service, the time of each visit is added together, and one E/M is reported for the total time on the date of the encounter.
- Do not report this service if a related E/M service has been provided in the prior seven days.
- Do not report this service if the provider sees the patient within the next 24 hours or soonest available appointment.
- Less than five minutes of medical discussion should not be reported.
- Do not report 98016 in addition to 98000-98015.

Knowledge Assessment Chapter 7

See chapter 21 for answers and rationale.

1. An established patient is evaluated in real-time, using an interactive audio-video system. The patient is complaining of headache and ear pain. The provider documents that a total of 35 minutes was spent on the date of the encounter reviewing records, documenting the visit, ordering a prescription, and visiting with the patient. Using time to report the service, what telemedicine service should be reported?
   a. 98001
   b. 98006
   c. 98009
   d. 98014
2. Codes 98000-98015 require a specific time interval from the last in-person visit or telemedicine visit of at least seven days.
   a. True
   b. False
3. How many minutes of medical discussion are required to report new and established synchronous audio-only services (98008-98015)?
   a. Five to 10 minutes
   b. At least five minutes
   c. 10 minutes
   d. More than 10 minutes
4. Which of the following components are applicable to code 98016 *Brief communication technology-based service*? Select all that apply.
   a. Patient-initiated service
   b. Five to 10 minutes of medical discussion
   c. Requires video technology
   d. MDM does not apply

Chapter 8. Hospital Services (99221–99239)

Hospital Inpatient or Observation Care Services—Initial Care, New or Established Patient (99221–99223)

E/M Code	Medical Decision Making	History	Exam	Time Spent on Date of Encounter
99221	Straightforward or low	Medically appropriate	Medically appropriate	40 min.
99222	Moderate	Medically appropriate	Medically appropriate	55 min.
99223	High	Medically appropriate	Medically appropriate	75 min.

General Guidelines

- Code selection is based on MDM or total time, including face-to-face and non-face-to-face time spent on the date of the encounter.

Coding Axiom

Medicare does not accept consultation codes. Use initial hospital care codes to report the first inpatient encounter by a physician. The admitting physician should append modifier AI Principal physician of record, to the initial hospital care code.

- History and physical examination elements are not required for code level selection. However, a medically appropriate history and/or physical examination should still be documented. The nature and degree of the history and/or physical examination is determined by the treating physician or other qualified health care professional reporting the service.
- Total time for these services includes total face-to-face and non-face-to-face time personally spent by the physician or other qualified health care professional on the day of the encounter.
- Physician or other qualified health care professional time may include the following activities:
  - preparing to see the patient (e.g., review of tests)
  - obtaining and/or reviewing separately obtained history
  - performing a medically appropriate examination and/or evaluation
  - counseling and educating the patient/family/caregiver
  - ordering medications, tests, or procedures
  - referring and communicating with other health care professionals (when not separately reported)
  - documenting clinical information in the electronic or other health record
  - independently interpreting results (not separately reported) and communicating results to the patient/family/caregiver
  - care coordination (not separately reported)
- Comorbidities or other underlying conditions should not be considered when selecting the level of service unless they are addressed during the encounter and their presence increases the amount and/or complexity of data to be reviewed and analyzed or the risk of complications and/or morbidity or mortality.
- Use these codes if the patient has not been seen or had a professional service provided by this physician/qualified health care professional or any other physician/qualified health care professional from the same practice and exact same specialty and subspecialty during the stay.
- Transition from observation status to inpatient care does not constitute a new stay.

Key Point

When determining the amount and/or complexity of data reviewed and analyzed, each unique test ordered is counted once; the review of that test is included within the order.

- Consider using the appropriate critical care code instead of these codes if the physician/qualified health care professional provided constant care to a critically ill patient. Critical care codes are based on the patient's condition, not the site of service, and are selected according to time spent in attending the patient.
- Consider assigning the appropriate consultation code instead of these codes if the provider provided an opinion or advice about a specific problem at the request of another provider or other appropriate source.
- Report only the appropriate initial hospital or observation care, or comprehensive nursing facility assessment code if the patient was admitted to the hospital or nursing facility on the same day as another visit.
- Do not include the time spent by any other staff (e.g., nurse, nurse practitioner or physician assistant) toward the time thresholds. Face-to-face and non-face-to-face time is the time the treating provider spent on the date of the encounter.
- A service that spans two calendar dates is a single service and is reported on one calendar date. For Medicare, report the date the encounter starts and select a code that encompasses all the services provided, including admission and discharge.

- Use case management codes when coordination of care is provided on a date without a patient encounter.
  - Case management codes are "bundled" according to Medicare and cannot be billed to the carrier
  - Other third-party payers may reimburse for these services
- Report prolonged service code 99418 with 99223 when the service runs 15 minutes beyond the time specified in the CPT® code narrative. The time must be clearly documented in the medical record. For Medicare, report prolonged services code G0316 with 99223 when the service runs 15 or more minutes beyond the total time indicated in the E/M code description. See Chapter 19 for more information on G0316.
- CPT guidelines indicate these codes are used to report initial services provided to hospital inpatients and hospital outpatients'"observation status"; all other providers should report 99231–99233 or 99252–99255.
- Use codes 99234–99236 for E/M services provided to an inpatient *or* an observation patient that is admitted and discharged on the same day.
  - The patient must be seen twice—an initial evaluation and at least one subsequent encounter on the same date to report 99234–99236
  - If the patient is evaluated only once, report 99221–99223 as appropriate without a discharge code
- Per Medicare, report 99221-99223 for a patient admitted to inpatient hospital or observation care for less than eight hours on the same day. For patients admitted to inpatient hospital or observation care and discharged on a different date, report 99238 or 99239, unless the patient is in observation care for less than eight hours. If less than eight hours, report only the initial hospital services.
- For a patient admitted to inpatient hospital or observation care for at least eight hours but not more than 24 hours, and discharged on the same calendar date, report 99234, 99235, or 99326.
- Combine all E/M services performed on the same date by the same physician that are related to the admission, no matter where they were provided (e.g., emergency department, office, or nursing facility), and report the appropriate initial hospital care code.
- Assign modifier 24 to indicate that an E/M service performed during the postoperative period was not related to the prior procedure. The claim should show a different diagnosis from that for the surgery.
- Append modifier 25 to report that a separately identifiable E/M service was performed by the same provider on the same date as a minor procedure or other service. Only the content of the note documenting the separate E/M service should be used to determine the level of an additional E/M service.
- Append modifier 57 to report that the decision to perform surgery was made during this visit. For Medicare patients, modifier 57 is used to report the fact that the decision was made to perform major surgery (a procedure with a 90-day postoperative period).

Key Point

Modifiers 24, 25, and 57 are to be appended to the E/M code and not to the codes for other procedures or services that may be performed.

- Performance of diagnostic tests or studies during an encounter that require separate interpretation are not included when determining the level of E/M service when reported separately. A separate code(s) for the diagnostic tests or studies performed in addition to the E/M codes may be reported.
- Simple tests, such as UA, CBC, and quick strep, that are results only tests and do not require separate interpretation can be counted as ordered or reviewed as part of the Data element for MDM even if the test is reported by the provider performing the office E/M visit.
- A test/study that is independently interpreted by the provider that is not separately reported but is part of the E/M service is considered part of MDM.

Issues in This Code Range

- Codes for high-level E/M services have been targeted in the CERT program as being overutilized. Medical necessity and the level of medical decision making should be verified for all high-level E/M services.

99221

Documentation Requirements

Medical Decision Making: Straightforward or Low

- Minimal or low number and complexity of problems addressed and analyzed
- No, minimal or limited amount and complexity of data reviewed and analyzed
- Minimal or low risk of complications and/or morbidity or mortality

History: Medically appropriate

Examination: Medically appropriate

> **Key Point**
> **The nature and extent of the patient history and physical examination are determined by the treating provider reporting the service.**

Code Indicators (from the MDM table)

Number and Complexity of Problem(s)

- One self-limited or minor problem
- Two or more self-limited or minor problems
- One stable, chronic illness
- One acute, uncomplicated illness or injury
- One stable, acute illness
- One acute, uncomplicated illness or injury requiring hospital inpatient or observation level of care

Amount and/or Complexity of Data

**Each unique test, order, or document contributes to the combination of 2 or combination of 3 in Category 1 below.*

- Minimal or none
- Limited

(Must meet the requirements of at least 1 of the 2 categories.)

Category 1: Tests and documents

- Any combination of 2 from the following:
  - Review of prior external note(s) from each unique source*;
  - Review of the result(s) of each unique test*;
  - Ordering of each unique test*

  or

Category 2: Assessment requiring an independent historian(s)

(For the categories of independent interpretation of tests and discussion of management or test interpretation, see moderate or high)

Risk of Complications/ Morbidity or Mortality

Minimal or low risk of morbidity from additional diagnostic testing or treatment

Time Spent On Date of the Encounter

- 40 minutes

Sample Documentation—99221

Level I Initial Hospital Care

Three-year old female admitted from office after presenting with three day history of fever, cough and malaise. Fevers to 102, cough worse at night described as 'wet and loose sounding'. OTC meds for cough and sinus ineffectual. Some night sweats, no chills, N/V, or GU problems. No Hx of respiratory problems, no prior surgeries. NKDA. Child attends daycare.

Physical Exam: Vitals per written chart WNL T: 103. Well-developed, well-nourished female child resting quietly, alert and oriented but somewhat lethargic. Head normocephalic. PERRLA-Fundi disc edges sharp. Both TMs red and injected. ENT: nose slight erythema, OP w/o exudates, neck supple, no nodes. No meningeal signs. Chest: breathing unlabored. CV RRR. ABD soft non-tender, no CVAT, no HSM. Neuro WNL. Skin warm to touch. Post tibial pulses +1 bilaterally. Muscle strength +2, and DTR's +1.

X-ray reveals clear lungs.

Impression: Dehydration

Plan: 1. Admit for IV hydration, pulse oximetry monitoring.

Hospital Services

99222

Documentation Requirements

Medical Decision Making: Moderate

- Moderate number and complexity of problems addressed
- Moderate amount and complexity of data reviewed and analyzed
- Moderate risk of complications and/or morbidity or mortality

History: Medically appropriate

Examination: Medically appropriate

Code Indicators (from the MDM table)

Number and Complexity of Problem(s)

- One or more chronic illnesses with exacerbation, progression, or side effects of treatment
- Two or more stable, chronic illnesses
- One undiagnosed new problem with uncertain prognosis
- One acute illness with systemic symptoms
- One acute, complicated injury

Amount and/or Complexity of Data

**Each unique test, order, or document contributes to the combination of two or combination of three in Category 1 below.*

- Moderate

(Must meet the requirements of at least one of the three categories.)

Category 1: Tests, documents, or independent historian(s)

- Any combination of three from the following:
  - review of prior external note(s) from each unique source*
  - review of the result(s) of each unique test*
  - ordering of each unique test*
  - assessment requiring an independent historian(s)

  or

Category 2: Independent interpretation of tests

- Independent interpretation of a test performed by another physician/other qualified health care professional (not separately reported)

  or

Category 3: Discussion of management or test interpretation

- Discussion of management or test interpretation with external physician/other qualified health care professional/appropriate source (not separately reported)

Risk of Complications/Morbidity or Mortality

Moderate risk of morbidity from additional diagnostic testing or treatment

Examples only:

- Prescription drug management
- Decision regarding minor surgery with identified patient or procedure risk factors
- Decision regarding elective major surgery without identified patient or procedure risk factors
- Diagnosis or treatment significantly limited by social determinants of health

Time Spent on Date of the Encounter

- 55 minutes

Sample Documentation—99222

Level II Initial Hospital Care

History: This is the fifth hospital admission for this 18-year-old female with significant history of chronic asthma since age eight. All of her prior admissions were for asthma. The patient is compliant with medication which currently includes Slo-bid 300 mg TID, Intal inhaler QID and PRN Albuterol inhaler. She was seen in the office two days ago with a flare-up of her chronic asthma requiring increased use of Albuterol. Chest x-ray and CBC were within normal limits; theophylline level was 12.0. Exam at that time showed bilateral expiratory wheezing with good air movement and no acute distress. At that time she was started on oral corticosteroids in addition to her usual drugs. She returned to our office today with no improvement of symptoms, and in fact, increased respiratory distress and dyspnea. She is admitted to the hospital in status asthmaticus. Denies fever, increased sputum, URI, or other asthma triggers. She lives with her parents and two siblings, and is a

Sample Documentation—99222 (Continued)

high-school senior. No prior surgery. No significant family illnesses. No known drug allergies. No alcohol, tobacco or drug use. She denies sexual activity and contraceptive use. Menstrual periods are regular. Immunizations are up to date. Review of systems is otherwise within normal limits except as noted.

Exam: BP 110/60, pulse 60, respiration 28 and labored, afebrile. Well-developed, well-nourished, anxious female in mild respiratory distress with audible expiratory wheezing. HEENT: Normocephalic; PERRLA; EOM intact; nasal septum midline, passages clear; dentition WNL; oropharynx clear. Neck supple with no JVD, adenopathy, bruits or thyromegaly. Chest is symmetrical with minimal costal retractions; nontender to palpation and percussion, breath sounds revealed bilateral expiratory wheezing with diminished air movement without rales or rhonchi. Heart shows S1 and S2 within normal limits without gallop, murmur, click or irregularity. Abdomen soft, nontender, no organomegaly. No CVA tenderness. Extremities revealed distal pulses intact; no cyanosis, clubbing or edema; no muscle atrophy. Skin WNL.

Labs: Admission chest x-ray within normal limits but with some evidence of pulmonary hyperaeration. No infiltrates noted. CBC within normal limits. Theophylline level 13.4.

Impression: Status asthmaticus
Chronic asthma

Plan:
1. Admit for intravenous corticosteroids, intravenous aminophylline
2. Hydration and continue Intal Inhaler
3. Supplemental oxygen
4. See admitting orders

History: Medically appropriate as deemed by the provider

Physical Examination: Medically appropriate as deemed by the provider

Medical Decision Making: Diagnoses made by the physician are Status asthmaticus and Chronic asthma. There are blood tests ordered as well as a CXR. The patient is admitted to the hospital, and IV medications are started. The patient's problem is a chronic illness with severe exacerbation (high risk), with prescription drug management the overall medical decision making is of "moderate complexity."

Final E/M Level of Service: CPT code 99222 is assigned.

Level II Initial Hospital Care

History: A 72-year-old white male admitted after falling down the stairs at home earlier today. He was in obvious pain in ED and was given sedating analgesics. Some of the history was obtained from his wife. He noted immediate severe pain in his left hip area and pain in his left shoulder. Denies head trauma, no LOC, no visual disturbances, no bleeding, neck or back pain. Past history is generally otherwise noncontributory. Family history non-contributory. He had an MI seven years ago followed by two-vessel CABG; he had gallbladder surgery at age 38 and a fractured ankle at age 19. He reports occasional problems with arthritis in his knees and shoulders. No medications and no allergies. All systems reviewed and are otherwise within normal limits. No dizziness, palpitations, tremor or muscle weakness; no GI or GU complaints.

Physical Exam: BP l40/85, temperature 98.7, pulse 80, respirations 22. Well-developed, well-nourished male, resting quietly in bed, alert, oriented and appropriate but drowsy secondary to administered med. HEENT: Head atraumatic. Negative Battles Sign. PERRLA-Fundi flat. ENT: no hemotympanum. Lungs clear with unlabored breathing. Neck/spine nontender. There is bruising over the left shoulder but no obvious deformity. Range of motion and muscle strength normal as far as can be assessed. Right shoulder and right and left upper extremities otherwise normal There is obvious deformity of the left lower extremity in the upper femoral area with eversion and foreshortening of the limb with marked tenderness and bruising over the area; knee and lower leg are normal; right lower extremity is normal. Both feet are warm to touch. Post tibial pulses +1 bilaterally. Normal finger to nose. No nystagmus. Muscle strength +2, and DTR's +1, with stocking response to touch and pinprick.

X-ray of both shoulders and upper extremities shows no bony or soft tissue abnormality. There are mild degenerative changes in the shoulder and elbow and generalized demineralization. X-ray of the left hip shows a comminuted fracture with dislocation of the fragments and subluxation of the shaft of the femur. The right hip is normal. There are mild degenerative changes in the hip joints, with some bony demineralization.

Impression: Comminuted fracture, left femur, as described on x-ray
Contusion, left shoulder

Plan:
1. Admit for open reduction, internal fixation of the left femur fracture after cardiology evaluation for cardiac risk.
2. UA for blood.
3. See admitting orders.

Quick Tip

It would be appropriate to append modifier 57 to indicate that this encounter determined the need for major surgery during this admission.

Hospital Services

Hospital Services

99223

Documentation Requirements

Medical Decision Making: High

- High number and complexity of problems addressed
- Extensive amount and complexity of data reviewed and analyzed
- High risk of complications and/or morbidity or mortality

History: Medically appropriate

Examination: Medically appropriate

Code Indicators (from the MDM table)

Number and Complexity of Problem(s)

- One or more chronic illnesses with severe exacerbation, progression, or side effects of treatment
- One acute or chronic illness or injury that poses a threat to life or bodily function

Amount and/or Complexity of Data

**Each unique test, order, or document contributes to the combination of two or combination of three in Category 1 below.*

- Extensive

(Must meet the requirements of at least two of the three categories.)

Category 1: Tests, documents, or independent historian(s)

- Any combination of three from the following:
  - review of prior external note(s) from each unique source*
  - review of the result(s) of each unique test*
  - ordering of each unique test*
  - assessment requiring an independent historian(s)

  or

Category 2: Independent interpretation of tests

- Independent interpretation of a test performed by another physician/other qualified health care professional (not separately reported)

  or

Category 3: Discussion of management or test interpretation

- Discussion of management or test interpretation with external physician/other qualified health care professional/appropriate source (not separately reported)

Risk of Complications/Morbidity or Mortality

High risk of morbidity from additional diagnostic testing or treatment

Examples only:

- Drug therapy requiring intensive monitoring for toxicity
- Decision regarding elective major surgery with identified patient or procedure risk factors
- Decision regarding emergency major surgery
- Decision regarding hospitalization or escalation of hospital-level care
- Decision not to resuscitate or to de-escalate care because of poor prognosis
- Parenteral controlled substances

Time Spent on Date of the Encounter

- 75 minutes

Key Point

Tests that are results only and are analyzed as part of MDM do not count as an independent interpretation but may count as one item when determining the amount/complexity of data reviewed and analyzed (e.g., dipstick UA, CBC, quick strep test).

Sample Documentation—99223

Level III Initial Hospital Care

History: This is a 49-year-old male presented to the ER with a 15-year history of alcohol abuse with known liver decompensation and cirrhosis. He came to the emergency room because of hematemesis which began about six hours before admission when he vomited three times. The first time he brought up bright red blood, the second and third times he brought up coffee-ground emesis. In the ED he was noted to be confused as to time and place and was febrile.

Past history: Reveals that his general health has otherwise been good with no hypertension, heart disease, renal disease, diabetes or other significant medical problems. He has two prior hospitalizations, one for nonspecific gastroenteritis with diarrhea and dehydration, and another episode about three years ago for mild liver decompensation with jaundice, ascites and peripheral ankle edema which responded to bed rest, diet and salt restriction. Review of systems at this time is otherwise within normal limits.

Family history: Father died at age 57 with acute varicocele hemorrhage with advanced Laennec's cirrhosis. His mother is age 69, in good health. One brother died at age 11 from complications of acute glomerulonephritis. No family history of hypertension, diabetes, coronary artery disease, or other hereditary or familial disorders. History was obtained primarily from his mother who accompanied him to the emergency room.

Social history: He is single, lives alone, and has a ninth-grade education; he is a construction worker but has been unemployed for seven months. He smokes a pack and one-half of cigarettes daily and uses alcohol on a daily basis, usually vodka. No regular medications; he drinks five or six cups of coffee daily.

Physical Exam: Well-developed/well-nourished male appearing older than his stated age. Temperature 100.1, blood pressure 112/84, pulse 68 and regular, respiration 28. He is lying in bed with purposeless movements of extremities, responds to questions but answers inappropriately. Conjunctivae pale, scleral icterus, PERRLA, EOMI. TM's intact; oral mucosa pale, teeth in poor repair, oropharynx not injected. Neck veins flat, no thyromegaly. Trachea midline. Lungs clear to percussion and auscultation. Heart regular rate and rhythm; no murmurs or thrills. Abdomen protuberant with a fluid wave; liver edge is 3 fingers below the right costal margin; spleen tip felt on the left; no tenderness. No abnormal venous pattern on the abdominal wall. No submandibular, cervical or inguinal adenopathy. 2+ pitting edema of the lower extremities; pulses normal. Cranial nerves intact; deep tendon reflexes diminished; Babinski negative, + Asterixis.

Labs: Lab results in the ED showed H&H of 6 and 19, WBC 21,000, with a shift to the left; bilirubin 6.2, 4.2 direct and 2 indirect; alkaline phosphatase 165; SGOT 310, SGPT 140; serum ammonia 174 (11-55); BUN 46; creat. 1.2; albumin 2.4; K 3-6; PT/PTT-prolonged.

Impression:

- Hepatic encephalopathy
- Laennec's cirrhosis
- Hepatic decompensation
- Portal hypertension
- Esophageal varices with hematemesis
- Rule out peptic ulcer disease
- Rule out alcoholic gastritis
- Rule out esophageal varices
- Rule out spontaneous bacterial peritonitis

Plan: He will be admitted and subsequently scheduled for immediate upper GI endoscopy. He will have blood cultures, urine cultures, peritoneal fluid culture, and chest x-ray to rule out infectious process. He will be transfused with packed RBCs to a hematocrit of at least 30. Lactulose enemas. NPO, careful diuresis. Follow electrolytes.

Hospital Services

Sample Documentation—99223 (Continued)

Level III Initial Hospital Care

This 42-year-old diabetic female Hispanic patient is admitted today with four-day history of fever, chills, harsh cough productive of moderate amounts of greenish and foul-smelling sputum, shortness of breath at rest and general malaise. Onset of symptoms occurred rather suddenly, though the patient admits to a mild dry cough for several weeks, changing to a productive cough over the last four days. Denies rhinorrhea or nasal congestion. Pt. fainted today after walking up a flight of steps; says she "could not find my breath and then got dizzy." Feeling weak and just "really sick." Temperature taken at home last night 102 degrees. Had TB as a child in her native country in South America. Was apparently treated successfully at that time without sequelae. No history of asthma.

ROS: Head: no complaints except for recent dizziness. Ears: no complaints. Eyes: wears glasses. Last exam five years ago in her native country. Nose: denies rhinitis, as above. Throat: extremely sore secondary to deep cough. Resp: Cough, SOB as above. Breasts: has never had mammograms; denies history of nodule/mass. Cardio: pt. is hypertensive, controlled with Monopril 20 mg/day. Takes her Bp every other day at local drug store. GI: no NVD. Appetite diminished. GU: no complaints. Last Pap some years ago—normal. Musculoskeletal: admits to general arthralgias with onset of fever. No history of arthritis. Neuro: Without complaint. Endo: pt. is diabetic; controlled on daily Glucophage 1500 mg/day. Last glucose level taken at home a few days ago by home glucometer—pt. doesn't remember the result. Admits to being less than compliant in taking the med and monitoring the blood glucose.

PMH: Hypertension and diabetes for years. No major surgeries. Usual childhood illnesses. Immunizations: unknown. Allergy: severely allergic to penicillins: hives, no anaphylaxis.

FH: Noncontributory. Mother was nonhypertensive; nondiabetic. Never knew her father and therefore history is unavailable. Three siblings, alive and well.

SH: No smoke/no ETOH. Doesn't exercise. Married, two children.

O: General: febrile-appearing female, short with barrel-shaped chest, lying supine in bed. T: 101.6; P: 72; R: 30, shallow, guarded. BP: 132/82. Head: normocephalic. No lesions, signs of trauma or fall. Eyes: PERRLA. Sclerae sl. yellow. Ears: Canals clear. TM's WNL. Nose: mucosa pale. No exudates. Turbinates sl. congested. Septum deviated to left. Throat: posterior pharyngeal wall erythematous. Tonsils small, red without exudates. Tongue geographic, thick. Dentition poor. Gold fillings throughout. Neck: +3 anterior cervical lymphadenopathy. Thyroid not palpable. Chest auscultation reveals LUL clear; LLL with high-pitched rales. RUL nonaudible; RML and RLL some wheezing. Chest percussion reveals dull sounds over RML/RLL but "tinny" sounds over RUL. Breasts: WNL. No mass or tenderness. Areolae WNL. No discharge. Cardio: Normal S1, S2. No murmur or rub. Abdomen: no hepato- or splenomegaly. Some tenderness over epigastrium. BS active. GU: deferred. Rectal: deferred. Skin: Dry; no petechiae or purpura. Extremities: Warm. No pedal edema. Pulses +2 in upper/lower extremities. No digital clubbing. No CVA tenderness. Neuro: no focal deficits. DTRs +2 upper extremities; +1 lower extremities.

STAT portable chest x-ray ordered. Laboratory tests ordered: SMA-12 including CBC w/diff. STAT ABG. Blood glucose; Hg A1c; UA; sputum culture/sensitivity, and gram stain, AFB x 3. Oximetry reported 90 percent.

A:
1. Community acquired pneumonia of LUL. Probably bacterial
2. R/O pneumothorax
3. R/O atypical pneumonitis
4. NIDDM
5. HTN

P: (1) Patient admitted today to Medical Service ward. (2) Await chest x-ray/labs. (3) Obtain pulmonary consult. (4) Begin IV antibiotics—erythromycin 500 mg q. 6 h. (5) Begin Tylenol for fever. (6) 1500 cal/day ADA diet. (7) Fingersticks before meals. (8) Lispro insulin before meals. (9) Hold Glucophage for now. (10) Resp. isolation. (11) Nasal oxygen 2 liters by nasal cannula.

Addendum: Patient now reports she thinks she has visited the ED about eight months ago for lower respiratory infection, at which time she underwent chest x-ray. Old films to be pulled for comparative review.

Hospital Inpatient or Observation Care and Hospital Discharge Services—Subsequent Care[1] (99231–99239)

E/M Code	Medical Decision Making	History	Exam	Time Spent on Date of Encounter
99231	Straightforward or low complexity	Medically appropriate	Medically appropriate	25 min.
99232	Moderate complexity	Medically appropriate	Medically appropriate	35 min.
99233	High complexity	Medically appropriate	Medically appropriate	50 min.
99234	Straightforward or low complexity	Medically appropriate	Medically appropriate	45 min.
99235	Moderate complexity	Medically appropriate	Medically appropriate	70 min.
99236	High complexity	Medically appropriate	Medically appropriate	85 min.
99238[2]	Hospital inpatient or observation discharge day management			30 minutes or less [2]
99239[2]	Hospital inpatient or observation discharge day management			more than 30 minutes [2]

1 All subsequent levels of service include reviewing the medical record, diagnostic studies and changes in patient's status, such as history, physical condition and response to treatment since last assessment.

2 These codes are not based on the level of medical decision making. These codes are correctly assigned based on time, as the CPT code description indicates.

Hospital Services

General Guidelines

- Use codes 99231–99233 for any inpatient or observation evaluation and management (E/M) services provided after the first encounter, including reviewing diagnostic studies and noting changes in the patient's status. These codes also are used to report preoperative medical evaluation and/or postoperative care before discharge when these services were provided by a physician other than the surgeon.
- Code selection is based on MDM or total time, including face-to-face and non-face-to-face time spent on the date of the encounter.
- History and physical examination elements are not required for code level selection. However, a medically appropriate history and/or physical examination should still be documented. The nature and degree of the history and/or physical examination is determined by the treating physician or other qualified health care professional reporting the service.
- Total time for these services includes total face-to-face and non-face-to-face time personally spent by the physician or other qualified health care professional on the day of the encounter.
- Physician or other qualified health care professional time may include the following activities:
  - preparing to see the patient (e.g., review of tests)
  - obtaining and/or reviewing separately obtained history
  - performing a medically appropriate examination and/or evaluation
  - counseling and educating the patient/family/caregiver
  - ordering medications, tests, or procedures
  - referring and communicating with other health care professionals (when not separately reported)
  - documenting clinical information in the electronic or other health record
  - independently interpreting results (not separately reported) and communicating results to the patient/family/caregiver
  - care coordination (not separately reported)
- Comorbidities or other underlying conditions should not be considered when selecting the level of service unless they are addressed during the encounter and their presence increases the amount and/or complexity of data to be reviewed and analyzed or the risk of complications and/or morbidity or mortality.
- Consider assigning the appropriate consultation code instead of these codes if the provider provided an opinion or advice about a specific problem at the request of another provider or other appropriate source.
- Do not include the time spent by any other staff (e.g., nurse, nurse practitioner or physician assistant) toward the time thresholds. Face-to-face and non-face-to-face time is the time the treating provider spent on the date of the encounter.
- A service that spans two calendar dates is a single service and is reported on one calendar date.
- Use case management codes when coordination of care is provided on a date without a patient encounter. Case management codes are "bundled" according to Medicare and cannot be billed to the carrier. Other third-party payers may reimburse for these services.

Report prolonged service code 99418 with 99233 when the service runs 15 minutes beyond the time specified in the CPT® code narrative. The time must be clearly documented in the medical record. For Medicare, report prolonged services code G0316 with 99233 and 99236 when the service runs 15 or more minutes beyond the total time indicated in the E/M code description. See Chapter 19 for more information on G0316.

- CPT guidelines state that when a service in a separate site is reported and initial inpatient or observation care is a consultation, the consultant will report one of these codes for the second service performed on the same date.
- Use codes 99234–99236 for E/M services provided to an inpatient *or* an observation patient that is admitted and discharged on the same day.
- Assign modifier 24 to indicate that an E/M service performed during the postoperative period was not related to the prior procedure. The claim should show a different diagnosis from that for the surgery.
- Append modifier 25 to report that a separately identifiable E/M service was performed by the same provider on the same date as a minor procedure or other service. Only the content of the note documenting the separate E/M service should be used to determine the level of an additional E/M service.
- Append modifier 57 to report that the decision to perform surgery was made during this visit. For Medicare patients, modifier 57 is used to report the fact that the decision was made to perform major surgery (a procedure with a 90-day postoperative period).
- Performance of diagnostic tests or studies during an encounter that require separate interpretation are not included when determining the level of E/M service when reported separately. A separate code(s) for the diagnostic tests or studies performed in addition to the E/M codes may be reported.
- Simple tests, such as UA, CBC, and quick strep, that are results only tests and do not require separate interpretation can be counted as ordered or reviewed as part of the Data element for MDM even if the test is reported by the provider performing the office E/M visit.
- A test/study that is independently interpreted by the provider that is not separately reported but is part of the E/M service is considered part of MDM.
- Per Medicare, if a patient is admitted as an inpatient with a discharge less than eight hours later on the same calendar date, codes 99221–99223 must be used for the admission, and no discharge service is billed.
- Codes 99238 and 99239 for hospital discharge services are appropriately assigned by the length of time devoted to performing the service (e.g., 99238 requires 30 minutes or less and 99239 requires more than 30 minutes).

Medicare requirements for observation codes: For a provider to use codes 99234–99236, the patient must be an inpatient or an observation care patient for a minimum of eight hours on the same calendar date. If the patient is admitted for less than eight hours, the appropriate codes are 99221—99223 and no discharge code.

The physician must satisfy the documentation requirements for both the admission to and discharge from inpatient or observation care to bill CPT codes 99234, 99235, or 99236. The length of time for observation care or treatment status must also be documented.

Issues in This Code Range

- Many providers have established conventions of coding inpatients by location in the hospital, for example, all patients in the ICU are critical care or 99233, while all patients on a general floor might be coded as 99231. Relative to coding, these types of conventions are a bad idea. The nature of the presenting problem for these codes is especially useful as they are typically one-line descriptors of the status of the patient, for example, "improving, inadequate response, serious complication," etc.
- In this section we find one of only a few E/M codes where the level of medical decision making is expressed as a range. Normally these levels are clearly indicated though the nature of presenting problem may state "low-moderate severity." In this case we see the level of decision making expressed as straightforward or low for codes 99231 and 99234.

99231

Documentation Requirements

Medical Decision Making: Straightforward or Low

- Minimal or low number and complexity of problems addressed
- No, minimal or limited amount and complexity of data reviewed and analyzed
- Minimal or low risk of complications and/or morbidity or mortality

History: Medically appropriate

Examination: Medically appropriate

Code Indicators (from the MDM table)

Number and Complexity of Problem(s)

- One self-limited or minor problem
- Two or more self-limited or minor problems
- One stable, chronic illness
- One acute, uncomplicated illness or injury
- One stable, acute illness
- One acute, uncomplicated illness or injury requiring hospital inpatient or observation level of care

Amount and/or Complexity of Data

**Each unique test, order, or document contributes to the combination of 2 or combination of 3 in Category 1 below.*

- Minimal or none
- Limited

(Must meet the requirements of at least 1 of the 2 categories.)

Category 1: Tests and documents

- Any combination of 2 from the following:
  - Review of prior external note(s) from each unique source*;
  - Review of the result(s) of each unique test*;
  - Ordering of each unique test*

  or

Category 2: Assessment requiring an independent historian(s)

(For the categories of independent interpretation of tests and discussion of management or test interpretation, see moderate or high)

Risk of Complications/ Morbidity or Mortality

Minimal or low risk of morbidity from additional diagnostic testing or treatment

Time Spent On Date of the Encounter

- 25 minutes

Sample Documentation—99231

Level I Subsequent Hospital Visit

Gastric ulcer, now stable. Since admission, she has received three units of packed RBCs; hematocrit 29.9, hemoglobin 9.2. Tolerating clear liquids well. No GI complaints at this time. NG tube was removed. Stools remain somewhat melanotic and heme +.

Blood pressure, pulse, respirations are stable; temperature normal. Abdominal exam is basically unchanged from yesterday.

Endoscopy yesterday showed a large gastric ulcer at the lesser curvature of the angulus covered with a large clot; ulcer was benign in appearance, pathology report pending.

She is now hungry and can be fed. I think that her acute bleed has stabilized, and she will be discharged in the next two to three days; there are no apparent cardiovascular or pulmonary complications.

99232

Documentation Requirements

Medical Decision Making: Moderate

- Moderate number and complexity of problems addressed
- Moderate amount and complexity of data reviewed and analyzed
- Moderate risk of complications and/or morbidity or mortality

History: Medically appropriate

Examination: Medically appropriate

Key Point

The nature and extent of the patient history and physical examination are determined by the treating provider reporting the service.

Code Indicators (from the MDM table)

Number and Complexity of Problem(s)

- One or more chronic illnesses with exacerbation, progression, or side effects of treatment
- Two or more stable, chronic illnesses
- One undiagnosed new problem with uncertain prognosis
- One acute illness with systemic symptoms
- One acute, complicated injury

Amount and/or Complexity of Data

**Each unique test, order, or document contributes to the combination of two or combination of three in Category 1 below.*

- Moderate

(Must meet the requirements of at least one of the three categories.)

Category 1: Tests, documents, or independent historian(s)

- Any combination of three from the following:
  - review of prior external note(s) from each unique source*
  - review of the result(s) of each unique test*
  - ordering of each unique test*
  - assessment requiring an independent historian(s)

Key Point

When determining the amount and/or complexity of data reviewed and analyzed, each unique test ordered is counted once; the review of that test is included within the order.

or

Category 2: Independent interpretation of tests

- Independent interpretation of a test performed by another physician/other qualified health care professional (not separately reported)

Key Point

Tests that are results only and are analyzed as part of MDM do not count as an independent interpretation but may count as one item when determining the amount/complexity of data reviewed and analyzed (e.g., dipstick UA, CBC, quick strep test).

or

Category 3: Discussion of management or test interpretation

- Discussion of management or test interpretation with external physician/other qualified health care professional/appropriate source (not separately reported)

Risk of Complications/Morbidity or Mortality
Moderate risk of morbidity from additional diagnostic testing or treatment

Examples only:

- Prescription drug management
- Decision regarding minor surgery with identified patient or procedure risk factors
- Decision regarding elective major surgery without identified patient or procedure risk factors
- Diagnosis or treatment significantly limited by social determinants of health

Time Spent on Date of the Encounter

- 35 minutes

Sample Documentation—99232

Level II Subsequent Hospital Visit

S: Both the patient and the nursing staff note increasing redness around venous stasis ulcers. The patient is complaining of more pain in the area of the pretibial ulcer on the right lower extremity.

O: The patient is resting quietly in bed, but he is increasingly anxious about his condition. Blood pressure, respiration and pulse stable; temperature now elevated to 100.6. Lungs clear, CV RRR, + S4, No S3, no murmur. Large stasis ulcer in the pretibial area of the right lower extremity measuring 1 x 2.5 cm, unchanged from the last exam 24 hours ago. There is obvious erythema covering the ulcerated area about 3 cm. with a definite red streak extending proximally to just below the level of the knee. Skin is warm to touch, exquisitely tender adjacent to the ulcer and moderately tender over the red streak. The left leg shows two 2-cm ulcers, unchanged from the last exam with no surrounding erythema. The ulcer craters are filled with dry, intact eschar and there is 1+ edema of the left lower extremity.

A: Hospital-acquired secondary infection of the stasis ulcer with surrounding cellulitis and early ascending lymphangitis. Edema due to local stasis.

P:
1. Debride eschar.
2. Swab ulcer crater for C&S of the purulent drainage, and stat gram stain.
3. Unasyn IV Q 6 hrs, pending results of gram stain and culture.
4. Elevate lower extremities on pillows to four inches above the level of the right atrium.
5. Start wet-to-dry dressings for large ulcer on the right lower extremity.

99233

Documentation Requirements

Medical Decision Making: High

- High number and complexity of problems addressed
- Extensive amount and complexity of data reviewed and analyzed
- High risk of complications and/or morbidity or mortality

History: Medically appropriate

Examination: Medically appropriate

Code Indicators (from the MDM table)

Number and Complexity of Problem(s)

- One or more chronic illnesses with severe exacerbation, progression, or side effects of treatment
- One acute or chronic illness or injury that poses a threat to life or bodily function

Amount and/or Complexity of Data

**Each unique test, order, or document contributes to the combination of two or combination of three in Category 1 below.*

- Extensive

(Must meet the requirements of at least two of the three categories.)

Category 1: Tests, documents, or independent historian(s)

- Any combination of three from the following:
  - review of prior external note(s) from each unique source*
  - review of the result(s) of each unique test*
  - ordering of each unique test*
  - assessment requiring an independent historian(s)

  or

Category 2: Independent interpretation of tests

- Independent interpretation of a test performed by another physician/other qualified health care professional (not separately reported)

  or

Category 3: Discussion of management or test interpretation

- Discussion of management or test interpretation with external physician/other qualified health care professional/appropriate source (not separately reported)

Risk of Complications/Morbidity or Mortality

High risk of morbidity from additional diagnostic testing or treatment

Examples only:

- Drug therapy requiring intensive monitoring for toxicity
- Decision regarding elective major surgery with identified patient or procedure risk factors
- Decision regarding emergency major surgery
- Decision regarding hospitalization or escalation of hospital-level care
- Decision not to resuscitate or to de-escalate care because of poor prognosis
- Parenteral controlled substances

Time Spent on Date of the Encounter

- 50 minutes

Sample Documentation—99233

Level III Subsequent Hospital Visit

History: The patient reports 20 minutes of squeezing, substernal chest pain associated with shortness of breath, diaphoresis, and nausea. Pain was not relieved by two sublingual nitroglycerin, does not change with position. There has been no sharp chest pain. The pain began when she went to the bathroom. This was her first BM since admission and she had to "strain" a fair amount. Otherwise, system review is negative and unchanged since admission.

Exam: She appears to be in moderate discomfort. Temperature 98.6, pulse 80, respirations 22 and blood pressure 122/84. HEENT: EOMI, PERRLA, TM's normal, oropharynx clear. Neck: no jugular venous distention or abdominal jugular reflux. Chest: clear to auscultation and percussion; Heart: PMI midline. Regular rate and rhythm, no gallop or murmur or rubs. Pulses are full and equal in all extremities. Abdomen flat and soft, bowel sounds normoactive; no hepatosplenomegaly. Extremities: no edema, full range of motion without cyanosis, clubbing or edema. Skin is cool and clammy.

EKG inverted T-waves laterally with acute I mm ST elevation and new reciprocal changes inferiorly.

Assessment: Four days status post subendocardial myocardial infarction with new onset of chest pain and EKG changes. Unstable angina, possibly extension of MI. Discussion with the patient and her family included discussion of diagnostic results, management options, potential medication side effects, and the need for consultation to evaluate patient for cardiovascular intervention.

Plan:
1. Nitroglycerin IV per protocol
2. Morphine IV per protocol
3. Stat cardiovascular surgery consultation
4. Begin heparin drip
5. Beta blocker, follow heart rate
6. Hold ace inhibitor

Note: This encounter could well require prolonged services or critical care by the time this day is over.

99234

Documentation Requirements

Medical Decision Making: Straightforward or Low

- Minimal or low number and complexity of problems addressed
- No, minimal or limited amount and complexity of data reviewed and analyzed
- Minimal or low risk of complications and/or morbidity or mortality

History: Medically appropriate

Examination: Medically appropriate

> **Key Point**
>
> **This code is used to report the admission and discharge of a patient to observation or inpatient status that is at least eight hours in duration but occurring on the same date.**

Code Indicators (from the MDM table)

Number and Complexity of Problem(s)

- One self-limited or minor problem
- Two or more self-limited or minor problems
- One stable, chronic illness
- One acute, uncomplicated illness or injury
- One stable, acute illness
- One acute, uncomplicated illness or injury requiring hospital inpatient or observation level of care

Amount and/or Complexity of Data

**Each unique test, order, or document contributes to the combination of 2 or combination of 3 in Category 1 below.*

- Minimal or none
- Limited

(Must meet the requirements of at least 1 of the 2 categories.)

Category 1: Tests and documents

- Any combination of 2 from the following:
  - Review of prior external note(s) from each unique source*;
  - Review of the result(s) of each unique test*;
  - Ordering of each unique test*

  or

Category 2: Assessment requiring an independent historian(s)

(For the categories of independent interpretation of tests and discussion of management or test interpretation, see moderate or high)

Risk of Complications/ Morbidity or Mortality

Minimal or low risk of morbidity from additional diagnostic testing or treatment

Time Spent On Date of the Encounter

- 45 minutes

99235

Documentation Requirements

Medical Decision Making: Moderate

- Moderate number and complexity of problems addressed
- Moderate amount and complexity of data reviewed and analyzed
- Moderate risk of complications and/or morbidity or mortality

History: Medically appropriate

Examination: Medically appropriate

> **Quick Tip**
>
> **Patients who are admitted and discharged on the same date should be seen by the provider at least twice, once for the decision to admit to observation or inpatient status, and once to determine that the patient is adequately improved for discharge.**

Code Indicators (from the MDM table)

Number and Complexity of Problem(s)

- One or more chronic illnesses with exacerbation, progression, or side effects of treatment
- Two or more stable, chronic illnesses
- One undiagnosed new problem with uncertain prognosis
- One acute illness with systemic symptoms
- One acute, complicated injury

> **Key Point**
>
> **When determining the amount and/or complexity of data reviewed and analyzed, each unique test ordered is counted once; the review of that test is included within the order.**

Amount and/or Complexity of Data

**Each unique test, order, or document contributes to the combination of two or combination of three in Category 1 below.*

- Moderate

(Must meet the requirements of at least one of the three categories.)

Category 1: Tests, documents, or independent historian(s)

- Any combination of three from the following:
  - review of prior external note(s) from each unique source*
  - review of the result(s) of each unique test*
  - ordering of each unique test*
  - assessment requiring an independent historia(s)

> **Key Point**
>
> **Tests that are results only and are analyzed as part of MDM do not count as an independent interpretation but may count as one item when determining the amount/complexity of data reviewed and analyzed (e.g., dipstick UA, CBC, quick strep test).**

or

Category 2: Independent interpretation of tests

- Independent interpretation of a test performed by another physician/other qualified health care professional (not separately reported)

or

Category 3: Discussion of management or test interpretation

- Discussion of management or test interpretation with external physician/other qualified health care professional/appropriate source (not separately reported)

Risk of Complications/Morbidity or Mortality
Moderate risk of morbidity from additional diagnostic testing or treatment

Examples only:

- Prescription drug management
- Decision regarding minor surgery with identified patient or procedure risk factors
- Decision regarding elective major surgery without identified patient or procedure risk factors
- Diagnosis or treatment significantly limited by social determinants of health

Time Spent on Date of the Encounter
- 70 minutes

99236

Documentation Requirements

Medical Decision Making: High

- High number and complexity of problems addressed
- Extensive amount and complexity of data reviewed and analyzed
- High risk of complications and/or morbidity or mortality

History: Medically appropriate

Examination: Medically appropriate

Code Indicators (from the MDM table)

Number and Complexity of Problem(s)

- One or more chronic illnesses with severe exacerbation, progression, or side effects of treatment
- One acute or chronic illness or injury that poses a threat to life or bodily function

Amount and/or Complexity of Data

**Each unique test, order, or document contributes to the combination of two or combination of three in Category 1 below.*

- Extensive

(Must meet the requirements of at least two of the three categories.)

Category 1: Tests, documents, or independent historian(s)

- Any combination of three from the following:
  - review of prior external note(s) from each unique source*
  - review of the result(s) of each unique test*
  - ordering of each unique test*
  - assessment requiring an independent historian(s)

  or

Category 2: Independent interpretation of tests

- Independent interpretation of a test performed by another physician/other qualified health care professional (not separately reported)

  or

Category 3: Discussion of management or test interpretation

- Discussion of management or test interpretation with external physician/other qualified health care professional/appropriate source (not separately reported)

Risk of Complications/Morbidity or Mortality

High risk of morbidity from additional diagnostic testing or treatment

Examples only:

- Drug therapy requiring intensive monitoring for toxicity
- Decision regarding elective major surgery with identified patient or procedure risk factors
- Decision regarding emergency major surgery
- Decision regarding hospitalization or escalation of hospital-level care
- Decision not to resuscitate or to de-escalate care because of poor prognosis
- Parenteral controlled substances

Time Spent on Date of the Encounter

- 85 minutes

Quick Tip

This code may be used to report the care of a patient who is admitted to the hospital and then, after a minimum of eight hours of treatment, is discharged from the current facility and may be transferred to the care of another provider at a different facility. For example, a patient might be admitted by an internist to a rural hospital, but his condition worsens and the patient is subsequently transferred to a regional or urban care center for care by a specialist.

99238

Documentation Requirements

Duration of Time

- 30 minutes or less
- Constitutes the total duration of time spent performing the discharge service, even if the time spent on that date was not continuous

Parameters

- Includes final physical examination
- Includes discussion regarding hospital stay and post-discharge patient care guidelines
- Includes preparation of discharge records, prescriptions, and referral forms, among other documentation

Coding Exclusions

- Excludes services performed for patients admitted and discharged on the same date from an observation unit, observation care, or inpatient hospitalization (see codes 99234–99236 for further information)
- Excludes "discharge" of a patient from a specialist's care when the specialist is not the attending physician. These providers must report the subsequent hospital care codes to appropriately report these services (see codes 99231–99233 for more information).
- Excludes nursing facility discharge (see codes 99315–99316 for further instruction)
- Excludes discharge services for newborns that are admitted and discharged on the same date (see code 99463 for more information)

Sample Documentation—99238

Hospital Discharge Day Management

S: This is the fourth hospital day for this 68-year-old white female admitted with congestive heart failure. She is totally symptom-free at this time. She has neither positional nor exertional dyspnea. She denies chest pain, she denies nausea. Her appetite has improved and is essentially back to normal.

O: This pleasant lady appears comfortable, she is neither dyspneic nor cyanotic. Inspection of the neck reveals no jugular venous distention. Auscultation of the heart is normal, sinus rhythm at 80 per minute without intermittencies or murmurs. Auscultation of the lungs: completely clear, no wheezes, rales or rhonchi. Examination of the lower extremities reveals no edema.

A: Congestive heart failure secondary to mild coronary artery disease, now compensated and stable.

P: Patient will be discharged home with the following discharge instructions:

1. RX furosemide 20 mg p.o. q. a.m.
2. RX Lanoxin 0.125 mg each a.m.
3. RX isosorbide 10 mg p.o. TID
4. Potassium chloride 6 mEq p.o. TID
5. Arrangements for Meals on Wheels with no-salt-added diet
6. Instruction sheet for no-salt-added diet given
7. Arrange for visiting nurse home evaluation within 24 hours of discharge
8. Arrange a follow-up visit at the office in one week, serum Lanoxin and potassium levels to be drawn at that time
9. Family conference completed. Family members agreed to arrange for assistance for the patient with laundry services and housecleaning.

(Final hospital discharge, 30 minutes or less)

Quick Tip

If the provider fails to indicate the time spent preparing the patient for discharge in the documentation, the time is presumed to be 30 minutes or less.

99239

Documentation Requirements

Duration of Time

- Thirty-one minutes or more
- Constitutes the total duration of time spent performing the discharge service, even if the time spent on that date was not continuous

Parameters

- Includes final physical examination
- Includes discussion(s) regarding hospital stay and post-discharge patient care guidelines
- Includes preparation of discharge records, prescriptions, and referral forms, among other documentation.

Coding Exclusions

- Excludes services performed for patients admitted and discharged on the same date from an observation unit, observation care, or inpatient hospitalization (see codes 99234–99236 for further information)
- Excludes "discharge" of a patient from a specialist's care when the specialist is not the attending physician. These providers must report the subsequent hospital care codes to appropriately report these services (see codes 99231–99233 for more information).
- Excludes nursing facility discharge (see codes 99315–99316 for further instruction).
- Excludes discharge services for newborns that are admitted and discharged on the same date. See code 99463 for more information.

Key Point

The provider must document that the time spent was more than 30 minutes to report this code.

Knowledge Assessment Chapter 8

See chapter 21 for answers and rationale.

1. Codes 99234–99236 are used to report E/M services provided to an observation patient or inpatient admitted and discharged on the same day.
   a. True
   b. False
2. What code is used to report a patient admitted to observation with a history, exam, and moderate MDM documented?
   a. 99221
   b. 99222
   c. 99231
   d. 99232
3. What codes are used to report a patient who is admitted and discharged the same date, and the provider had two encounters documented with the patient?
   a. 99221-99223
   b. 99231-99233
   c. 99234-99236
   d. 99238-99239

Hospital Services

Chapter 9. Consultations (99242–99255)

Office or Other Outpatient Consultations (99242–99245)

E/M Code	Medical Decision Making	History	Exam	Time Spent on Date of Encounter
99242	Straightforward	Medically appropriate	Medically appropriate	20 min.
99243	Low complexity	Medically appropriate	Medically appropriate	30 min.
99244	Moderate complexity	Medically appropriate	Medically appropriate	40 min.
99245	High complexity	Medically appropriate	Medically appropriate	55 min.

General Guidelines

Use these CPT® codes if the physician/qualified health care professional provided an opinion or gave advice regarding evaluation or management of a specific problem at the request of another physician/qualified health care professional or appropriate source. A consultation may also be necessary to determine whether the consultant is willing to accept transfer and ongoing management of the patient's entire care or for management of a specific problem. The consultant may initiate diagnostic or therapeutic services.

- Consultation codes are appropriate in many settings such as the physician's office, or outpatient site including patient's home or residence or emergency department.
- A written report must be sent to the requesting provider or source to be placed in the patient's permanent medical record. Required documentation includes the request for consultation, the need or reason for the consultation, consultant's opinion and any services that were ordered or performed.
- When a common chart is used, a separate report to the requesting provider does not need to be sent. Examples of a common chart include large multispecialty clinics with electronic medical records.
- Use the appropriate office consultation code if the consultant was asked again for an opinion or advice regarding the same problem or a new problem.
- Code selection is based on MDM or total time, including face-to-face and non-face-to-face time spent on the date of the encounter.
- History and physical examination elements are not required for code level selection for office and other outpatient consultation services. However, a medically appropriate history and/or physical examination should still be documented. The nature and degree of the history and/or physical examination is determined by the treating physician or other qualified health care professional reporting the service.
- Clinical staff may collect information pertaining to the history and exam and the patient and/or caregiver may provide information directly (e.g., by electronic health record [EHR] portal or questionnaire) that is reviewed by the reporting provider.
- Total time for these services includes total face-to-face and non-face-to-face time personally spent by the physician or other qualified health care professional on the day of the encounter.
- Physician or other qualified health care professional time may include the following activities:
  - preparing to see the patient (e.g., review of tests)
  - obtaining and/or reviewing separately obtained history
  - performing a medically appropriate examination and/or evaluation
  - counseling and educating the patient/family/caregiver
  - ordering medications, tests, or procedures
  - referring and communicating with other health care professionals (when not separately reported)
  - documenting clinical information in the electronic or other health record
  - independently interpreting results (not separately reported) and communicating results to the patient/family/caregiver
  - care coordination (not separately reported)
- Assign the appropriate critical care code instead of these codes if the physician provided constant attention to a critically ill patient.
- Assign the appropriate office visit code if the patient or family member and not another physician (or appropriate source) requested the consultation.
- Do not consider the time spent by other staff (e.g., nurse) as part of the total time.
- Append modifier 25 to report that a separately identifiable E/M service was performed by the same physician/qualified health care professional on the same day as a procedure or service. Only the work involved in the separate E/M service should be considered when determining the correct level of service.

Quick Tip

Modifiers 25, 32, and 57 are to be appended to the E/M code and not to the codes for the other procedures or services that may be performed.

- Use modifier 32 when the services were mandated, such as by a third-party payer, or as a result of a governmental, legislative or regulatory requirement.
- Append modifier 57 to indicate that the decision to perform major surgery has been made.
- Append modifier 95 to indicate that the E/M service was rendered to a patient at a distant site via a real-time interactive audio and video telecommunications system. The communication between the physician or other qualified health care professional and the patient should be commensurate with the same key components or requirements of those that would be required if the service had been rendered in a face-to-face setting.
- Report separately the codes for the diagnostic tests or studies performed.
- Codes for high-level E/M services have been targeted in the CERT program as being overutilized. Medical necessity and the level of medical decision making should be verified for all high-level E/M services.
- Follow-up visits initiated by the physician consultant or patient are reported with the appropriate site-of-service codes (e.g., office visits) for established patients. However, if an additional request is documented in the record for an additional opinion or advice for the same or separate problem, the consultation codes may be reported again.
- Transfer-of-care services (for either specific condition or the patient's entire care) are reported with the appropriate new or established patient codes for office or other outpatient visits or home or residence services.
- Report prolonged services code 99417 with 99245 when the service runs 15 minutes beyond the time specified in the CPT® code narrative. The time must be clearly documented in the medical record.
- Medicare eliminated the use of all consultation codes with the exception of telehealth inpatient consultation G codes. See chapter 19 for more information on G codes. Report outpatient consultations with the appropriate E/M service code for the site of service and new or established patient.

Consultations

99242

Documentation Requirements

Medical Decision Making: Straightforward

- Minimal number and complexity of problems addressed
- No or minimal amount and complexity of data reviewed and analyzed
- Minimal risk of complications and/or morbidity or mortality

History: Medically appropriate

Examination: Medically appropriate

Key Point

The nature and extent of the patient history and physical examination are determined by the treating provider reporting the service.

Code Indicators (from the MDM table)

Number and Complexity of Problem(s)

- One self-limited or minor problem

Amount and/or Complexity of Data

- Minimal or none

Risk of Complications/Morbidity or Mortality

Minimal risk of morbidity from additional diagnostic tests or treatment

Time Spent on Date of the Encounter

- 20 minutes

(See "General Guidelines" for additional documentation considerations.)

Key Point

Tests that are results only and are analyzed as part of MDM do not count as an independent interpretation but may count as one item when determining the amount/complexity of data reviewed and analyzed (e.g., dipstick UA, CBC, quick strep test).

Sample Documentation—99242

Level II Office/Outpatient Consultation

TO: Dr. Attending Psychiatrist

FROM: Dr. Consultant

RE: Admitting evaluation

Chief complaint: "They brought me for a checkup."

History: This 24-year-old white male is seen for the first time for medical evaluation at the request of Dr. Attending Psychiatrist at the County Mental Health Facility where he was sent from County Correctional Facility after being charged with assault. He was admitted to CMHF for treatment. He is seen today for an admitting H&P.

Past history: He states that he has had no serious medical problems. His only past illness was chickenpox and occasional upper respiratory infections. He smokes about a pack of cigarettes a day and drinks "some," but would not elaborate further.

Allergies: He states that he was given Haldol while in a reformatory eight years ago which caused him to choke and stutter. No other allergies.

Illicit drug use: He reports using cocaine and smoking marijuana in the past but "none in the past few months." Admitting drug screens at CCF were normal.

Family history: Father is 43, mother 41, both living and well.

Review of systems: No specific complaints on general review but admits to feeling anxious and depressed. Cardiorespiratory: No chest pain, shortness of breath, palpitations or hemoptysis. GI: No nausea, vomiting, diarrhea, constipation. GU: No dysuria, urgency, frequency. Neuromuscular: no myalgia, arthralgia.

Physical exam: This is a well-developed, well nourished, moderately obese white male in no acute distress. Height 5'6", weight 185, temperature 98.3, pulse 72, respirations 20, blood pressure l35/88.

HEENT: Some male pattern alopecia starting; he has a large sebaceous cyst on the scalp, midline, measuring about 2 cm in diameter. He states that this is getting larger and would like it removed because it is sometimes tender. Eyes: EOM intact. PERRLA, Snellen Chart tests reveal vision 20/ 25 on right and 20/20 on the left, uncorrected. Ears: TM's intact; hearing is grossly normal. Nose, mouth and throat: nose patent, tongue midline; pharynx not injected.

Neck: Supple; no bruits; no lymphadenopathy; thyroid normal.

Chest: Symmetrical expansion; lungs clear to auscultation and percussion.

Heart: regular sinus rhythm; no murmurs or gallops. S1, S2 normal.

Abdomen: Moderately obese; no organomegaly, masses, tenderness or hernia. Bowel sounds normal and active in all quadrants.

Rectal/genital: Circumcised, no lesions of penis; both testes descended; no inguinal hernia; rectal negative to inspection; sphincter tone normal; prostate normal; stool guaiac negative.

Neurological: Sensation to touch and pain normal. Cranial nerves II-XII intact; No pathological reflexes. Babinski negative. Deep tendon reflexes +2 and symmetrical.

Extremities: No varicosities or edema. Full range of motion in all extremities. Muscle strength normal.

Skin: Normal except for sebaceous cyst of scalp.

Impression:
1. Sebaceous cyst of scalp
2. Probable non-allergic intolerance to Haldol
3. R/O situational depression

Medical Management Recommendations:
1. Avoid Haldol.
2. Consider excision of scalp cyst in near future.
3. No other medical problems at this time.
4. Psychiatric consultation to follow.

Thank you for allowing me to see your patient.

(General multisystem)

Consultations

99243

Documentation Requirements

Medical Decision Making: Low
- Low number and complexity of problems addressed
- Limited amount and complexity of data reviewed and analyzed
- Low risk of complications and/or morbidity or mortality

History: Medically appropriate

Examination: Medically appropriate

Code Indicators (from the MDM table)

Number and Complexity of Problem(s)
- Two or more self-limited or minor problems
- One stable, chronic illness
- One acute, uncomplicated illness or injury
- One stable, acute illness
- One acute, uncomplicated illness or injury requiring hospital inpatient or observation level of care

Amount and/or Complexity of Data
**Each unique test, order, or document contributes to the combination of two or combination of three in Category 1 below.*
- Limited

(Must meet the requirements of at least one of the two categories.)

Category 1: Tests and documents
- Any combination of two from the following:
  - review of prior external note(s) from each unique source*
  - review of the result(s) of each unique test*
  - ordering of each unique test*

  or

Category 2: Assessment requiring an independent historian(s)
(For the categories of independent interpretation of tests and discussion of management or test interpretation, see moderate or high)

Risk of Complications/Morbidity or Mortality
Low risk of morbidity from additional diagnostic tests or treatment

Time Spent on Date of the Encounter
- 30 minutes

Consultations

Sample Documentation—99243

Level III Office/Outpatient Consultation

TO: Dr. Attending Physician

FROM: Dr. Consultant

RE: Evaluation of retinopathy

This is a 32-year-old insulin-dependent diabetic being seen at the request of her family physician for evaluation of diabetic retinopathy. Her diabetes was diagnosed at age 12, and she has been controlled with insulin since that time. Her diabetes is basically stable and controlled by diet and medication. She is periodically evaluated for retinopathy. With the last examination about one year ago, reportedly she had very minimal nonproliferative retinopathy. The patient is not hypertensive. She has had no visual changes or problems, no blurring of vision, vision loss, scotoma, floaters, pain or photophobia. No dizziness, unsteadiness, lightheadedness or impairment of night vision. Review of systems otherwise within normal limits; she has no other health problems. She checks her blood sugar daily and adheres to her diabetic regimen. She takes no medications except her sliding scale insulin.

Exam: Visual acuity good with current corrective lenses; conjunctivae are clear. No icterus. Gross visual fields intact. Extraocular movements intact; no nystagmus. Pupils equal, round react normally to light and accommodation. Pupils were dilated. Slit lamp examination showed no corneal abnormalities. Anterior chambers normal. Lenses clear. Intraocular pressures normal. Minimal nonproliferative retinopathy with a few very small areas of pinpoint exudate. Optic discs are flat and normal; posterior segments otherwise normal.

Assessment: Minimal nonproliferative retinopathy
Insulin dependent diabetes mellitus

Discussion & Recommendations: In comparing her current findings to my charts and mapping from her examination a year ago, I believe there has been no progression of her retinopathy in the past year. No intervention needs to be undertaken at this time. The patient should be cautioned to be particularly watchful for any change in visual symptomatology, to report any changes promptly, and to continue her efforts to follow her diabetic treatment plan faithfully. She should, of course, continue to receive yearly ophthalmologic evaluations.

Thank you for allowing me to participate in the care of your patient. I will be happy to see her again if any problems should arise.

Quick Tip

Note that specialists perform most consultations, as is the case with this ophthalmology consultation.

99244

Documentation Requirements

Medical Decision Making: Moderate
- Moderate number and complexity of problems addressed
- Moderate amount and complexity of data reviewed and analyzed
- Moderate risk of complications and/or morbidity or mortality

History: Medically appropriate

Examination: Medically appropriate

Code Indicators (from the MDM table)

Number and Complexity of Problem(s)
- One or more chronic illnesses with exacerbation, progression, or side effects of treatment
- Two or more stable chronic illnesses
- One undiagnosed new problem with uncertain prognosis
- One acute illness with systemic symptoms
- One acute, complicated injury

Amount and/or Complexity of Data
**Each unique test, order, or document contributes to the combination of two or combination of three in Category 1 below.*
- Moderate

(Must meet the requirements of at least one of the three categories.)

Category 1: Tests, documents, or independent historian(s)
- Any combination of three from the following:
  - review of prior external note(s) from each unique source*
  - review of the result(s) of each unique test*
  - ordering of each unique test*
  - assessment requiring an independent historian(s)

Key Point

When determining the amount and/or complexity of data reviewed and analyzed, each unique test ordered is counted once; the review of that test is included within the order.

or

Category 2: Independent interpretation of tests
- Independent interpretation of a test performed by another physician/other qualified health care professional (not separately reported)

Key Point

Tests that are results only and are analyzed as part of MDM do not count as an independent interpretation but may count as one item when determining the amount/complexity of data reviewed and analyzed (e.g., dipstick UA, CBC, quick strep test).

or

Category 3: Discussion of management or test interpretation
- Discussion of management or test interpretation with external physician/other qualified health care professional/appropriate source (not separately reported)

Risk of Complications/Morbidity or Mortality
Moderate risk of morbidity from additional diagnostic testing or treatment

Examples only:
- Prescription drug management
- Decision regarding minor surgery with identified patient or procedure risk factors
- Decision regarding elective major surgery without identified patient or procedure risk factors
- Diagnosis or treatment significantly limited by social determinants of health

Time Spent on Date of the Encounter
- 40 minutes

Sample Documentation—99244

Level IV Office/Outpatient Consultation
Dr. Internal Medicare Consult
1234 Anyway Place
Scottsville, Ohio 45111

January 6, 20XX

Dear Dr. Orthopaedic Surgeon:

Thank you for your request for an Internal Medicine consultation on this 49-year-old male, who presents for pre-operative physical examination and clearance, scheduled for a right hip replacement in two weeks. The patient is hypertensive, has multifocal osteoarthritis with femoral head and acetabular degeneration of the right hip, and status-post polypectomy of the large intestine one year ago. The patient presents today with no new complaints though does need refills on antihypertensive med. Currently takes Ziac 5mg/6.25 mg daily. Takes Motrin PRN, Voltaren 100 mg/day for arthritic exacerbation and pain. The OA of the right hip has grossly interfered with the patient's ADLs, and subjects him to constant pain and impaired gait.

PMH: Usual childhood diseases. T&A age 14; fracture right wrist at age eight. Degenerative arthritis for "years." Fell and injured the right hip some years ago, without apparent sequelae until recently.

ROS: HEENT: no complaints. Throat: T&A as noted. Ears: hears well without tinnitus. Cardio: HTN as noted, controlled on combination beta blocker/diuretic medication with good results. Denies other problems (angina, SOB). Resp/chest: no complaints. Musculoskeletal: Old fx as noted. OA as described, followed by orthopaedic surgeon. Takes meds as noted with some relief.

O: Ht. 5'11"; Wt. 195 lbs. T: 98.6; P: 68; BP: 136/88. General: well-developed, well-nourished adult male in no acute distress, who walks with guarded gait with slight limp, favoring to the left. Alert, oriented X 3. Head: WNL. No suspicious lesions. Ears, nose, throat: All WNL. Nasal mucosa pale; no exudates. Pharynx WNL. Ear canals hairy with minimal cerumen present. TM's clear. Eyes: PERRLA. EOMI. Sclerae and conjunctivae clear. Fundi: discs flat with narrowed arterioles. Neck: no cervical lymphadenopathy. No tenderness. FROM. No JVD or bruits. CV: normal heart sounds; S1, S2. Has S4 gallop. No murmur or rub noted. Resp: good breath sounds, clear to P&A. Abd: no mass, tenderness, organomegaly (spleen/liver). BS sl. hyperactive. Genitals: WNL. Testicles nontender and without mass. Some varicosities noted. Penis uncircumcised; several small papillomas in fold of prepuce noted but otherwise WNL. Rectal: no masses or hemorrhoids. Prostate nontender, +2 firm, not boggy. Skin: normal in color, turgor and without lesion.

Extremities/Joints: FROM though with obvious discomfort when performing SLR on the right. Hip ROM limited by pain. No arthritic changes noted over hands. There is minimal muscle atrophy noted at the right thigh, though not marked. Neuro: alert and oriented x 3. DTRs +2 in upper extremities and lower extremities.
The patient is accompanied by x-rays of the right and left hips, with a full report by Radiology. On re-view of the films, there is severe degenerative joint disease of the right hip with mild changes on the left. Report states "severe osteoarthritis of the right hip involving the femoral head and acetabular rim."

EKG: NSR at 70; PR 0.12; QRS 0.08. Normal axis; no ischemic changes. UA: neg for glucosuria; WBCs neg; RBCs neg; ketones neg; protein neg; neg for bacteria; color: light yellow, clear; specific gravity: 1.018; pH 7.5.

A: Cleared for surgery pending labs. Bilateral OA, worse in right hip vs. left. Mild HTN, med-controlled. S/P polypectomy.

P: OK for surgery. Follow HTN. Refill Ziac. Anesthesia will manage HTN perioperatively. Handicapped parking sticker application completed and provided to patient.

This comprises the consultation note for this patient. I have suggested to the patient, who recently moved to this area and does not have a preferred Internist, that I can follow him for the above IM findings. The patient's blood was drawn and sent to the health plan's lab for CBC w/diff, platelets, SMA-20, clotting studies. A pre-op CXR has been ordered. Results of these tests will be provided to the pre-op center upon their arrival. Thank you for your kind request of this most pleasant patient. If I can be of further service to you, please let me know.

Internal Medicine Physician

Consultations

99245

Documentation Requirements

Medical Decision Making: High

- High number and complexity of problems addressed
- Extensive amount and complexity of data reviewed and analyzed
- High risk of complications and/or morbidity or mortality

History: Medically appropriate

Examination: Medically appropriate

> **Key Point**
>
> **The nature and extent of the patient history and physical examination are determined by the treating provider reporting the service.**

Code Indicators (from the MDM table)

Number and Complexity of Problem(s)

- One or more chronic illnesses with severe exacerbation, progression, or side effects of treatment
- One acute or chronic illness or injury that poses a threat to life or bodily function

Amount and/or Complexity of Data

**Each unique test, order, or document contributes to the combination of two or combination of three in Category 1 below.*

- Extensive

(Must meet the requirements of at least two of the three categories.)

Category 1: Tests, documents, or independent historian(s)

- Any combination of three from the following:
  - review of prior external note(s) from each unique source*
  - review of the result(s) of each unique test*
  - ordering of each unique test*
  - assessment requiring an independent historian(s)

  or

Category 2: Independent interpretation of tests

- Independent interpretation of a test performed by another physician/other qualified health care professional (not separately reported)

  or

Category 3: Discussion of management or test interpretation

- Discussion of management or test interpretation with external physician/other qualified health care professional/appropriate source (not separately reported)

Risk of Complications/Morbidity or Mortality

High risk of morbidity from additional diagnostic testing or treatment

Examples only:

- Drug therapy requiring intensive monitoring for toxicity
- Decision regarding elective major surgery with identified patient or procedure risk factors
- Decision regarding emergency major surgery
- Decision regarding hospitalization or escalation of hospital-level care
- Decision not to resuscitate or to de-escalate care because of poor prognosis
- Parenteral controlled substance

Time Spent on Date of the Encounter

- 55 minutes

> **Quick Tip**
>
> **For services of 70 minutes or more, see prolonged services code 99417.**

Sample Documentation—99245

Level V Office/Outpatient Consultation

TO: Dr. Attending Physician

FROM: Dr. Consultant

RE: Evaluation of chest pain

History: This 63-year-old female is seen at the request of Dr. Attending Physician for evaluation of exertional chest pain. The patient reports upper chest pain radiating to the throat for the last 10 days with one episode a day; each episode lasts 10 to 15 minutes occurring with normal physical activity such as housework. Another episode occurred at rest in the early AM hours, awakening the patient from sleep, associated with shortness of breath and fatigue. Also complains of an episode of syncope lasting about three minutes, 48 hours ago while standing at the sink. Her husband says the patient suddenly fell to the floor, bruising herself, but she exhibits no seizure-like activity.

Past history: No allergies. She smokes a pack a day of cigarettes, and has borderline hypertension. No diabetes, hyperlipidemia or obesity. No other surgery or significant illnesses. She drinks three to four cups of coffee a day; ETOH socially.

Review of systems: She says a murmur was noted once on an insurance physical. She has aching in her legs below the calf, left more than right, on exertion such as walking up steps gradually increasing over the past three years, but the aching goes away with rest. No palpitations, shortness of breath, tremors, edema, dizziness, rheumatic fever, current GI or GU complaints, although she was treated for an ulcer in the past.

Physical Exam:

General: BP 140/90, no orthostatic changes, pulse 72, respirations 14, afebrile. Well developed, slender white female in no acute distress, well oriented, communicative, and verbalizing some apprehension about her health.

Neck: Jugular venous pressure normal. Carotid pulses full with bruit or transmitted murmur.

Lungs: Clear to percussion and auscultation. No intercostal retractions.

Cardiovascular: PMI normal, S1 and S2 and S4, present; no S3 or gallop or rub. Grade III/VI systolic murmur, radiates to carotids and a grade 1/6 diastolic blowing murmur radiating to the carotids. No abdominal bruits. No carotid bruits.

Abdomen shows no masses, tenderness, organomegaly.

Extremities: Bilateral soft femoral bruits. Pulses are diminished in DP/PT arteries bilaterally. No pedal edema or varicosities.

Skin: Normal in color, without lesions

EKG: Sinus rhythm at 72. PR 0.16, Axis +30, no old MI or ischemic changes. QRS 0.08.

Impression:

1. Crescendo Angina
   A. R/O CAD
   B. R/O Aortic Stenosis
2. Syncope
   A. due to cardiac arrhythmia secondary to ischemia
   B. R/O aortic stenosis
3. Aortic stenosis
   A. no history of rheumatic fever
   B. consider congenital bicuspid aortic valve type
4. Claudication
   A. consistent with peripheral atherosclerosis
   B. level below knee L>R

Recommendations:

1. Stat admission to CCU
2. R/O MI protocol
3. Check lipids, thyroid function, CBC
4. Stat echocardiogram
5. Possible cardiac catheterization
6. Smoking cessation emphasized

I discussed the above recommendations and risks with the patient and her husband, who both understand and agree with the need for emergency admission. As you recall, I telephoned your office and as per our discussion arranged for the emergency admission.

We also discussed various medications that may be used for angina with aortic stenosis and claudication before it is begun.

Thank you for allowing me to participate in the care of your patient.

Quick Tip

At the request of the consultant, the primary care physician arranged for admission and was the admitting physician; therefore, the consultation was a separate service.

Consultations

Inpatient or Observation Consultations (99252–99255)

E/M Code[1]	Medical Decision Making	History	Exam	Time Spent on Date of Encounter
99252	Straightforward	Medically appropriate	Medically appropriate	35 min.
99253	Low complexity	Medically appropriate	Medically appropriate	45 min.
99254	Moderate complexity	Medically appropriate	Medically appropriate	60 min.
99255	High complexity	Medically appropriate	Medically appropriate	80 min.

1 These codes are used for hospital inpatients, observation-level services, residents of nursing facilities or patients in a partial hospital setting.

General Guidelines

- Use these codes if the physician/qualified health care professional provided an opinion or gave advice regarding evaluation and/or management of a specific problem at the request of another physician/qualified health care professional or appropriate source. A consultation may also be necessary to determine whether the consultant is willing to accept transfer and ongoing management of the patient's entire care or for management of a specific problem.
- Consultation codes are appropriate only if the service was provided in the hospital, nursing facility or partial hospital setting. A written report must be sent to the requesting provider or source to be placed in the permanent medical record for that patient. Required documentation includes the request for consultation, need for the consultation, consultant's opinion and any services that were ordered or performed.

Coding Axiom

Medicare does not accept consultation codes. Use initial hospital care codes to report the first inpatient encounter by a physician.

- When a common chart is used, a separate report to the requesting provider does not need to be sent.
- Code selection is based on MDM or total time, including face-to-face and non-face-to-face time spent on the date of the encounter.
- History and physical examination elements are not required for code level selection. However, a medically appropriate history and/or physical examination should still be documented. The nature and degree of the history and/or physical examination is determined by the treating physician or other qualified health care professional reporting the service.
- Total time for these services includes total face-to-face and non-face-to-face time personally spent by the physician or other qualified health care professional on the day of the encounter.
- Physician or other qualified health care professional time may include the following activities:
  - preparing to see the patient (e.g., review of tests)
  - obtaining and/or reviewing separately obtained history
  - performing a medically appropriate examination and/or evaluation
  - counseling and educating the patient/family/caregiver
  - ordering medications, tests, or procedures
  - referring and communicating with other health care professionals (when not separately reported)
  - documenting clinical information in the electronic or other health record
  - independently interpreting results (not separately reported) and communicating results to the patient/family/caregiver
  - care coordination (not separately reported)
- Comorbidities or other underlying conditions should not be considered when selecting the level of service unless they are addressed during the encounter and their presence increases the amount and/or complexity of data to be reviewed and analyzed or the risk of complications and/or morbidity or mortality.
- Consider assigning the appropriate critical care code instead of these codes if the physician provided constant attention to a critically ill patient.
- Do not consider the time spent by other staff (e.g., nurse) as part of total time.
- A service that spans two calendar dates is a single service and is reported on one calendar date.
- Use case management codes when coordination of care is provided on a date without a patient encounter. Case management codes are "bundled" according to Medicare and cannot be billed to the carrier. Other third-party payers may reimburse for these services.

Key Point

These codes may be reported when the patient has not been seen or had a professional service provided by this physician/qualified health care professional or any other physician/qualified health care professional from the same practice and exact same specialty and subspecialty during the stay.

- Report prolonged service code 99418 with 99255 when the service runs 15 minutes beyond the time specified in the CPT® code narrative. The time must be clearly documented in the medical record.

Consultations

- CPT guidelines state that when a service in a separate site is reported and initial inpatient or observation care is a consultation, the consultant will report one of these codes for the second service performed on the same date.
- Use codes 99234–99236 for E/M services provided to an inpatient *or* an observation patient that is admitted and discharged on the same day.
- Transfer-of-care services (for either specific condition or the patient's entire care) are reported with the appropriate new or established patient codes for the site of service.
- Medicare eliminated the use of all consultation codes with the exception of telehealth inpatient consultation G codes. See chapter 19 for more information on G codes.
- Use modifier 32 when the services were mandated, such as by a third-party payer, or as a result of a governmental, legislative, or regulatory requirement.

Quick Tip

Modifiers 25, 32, and 57 are to be appended to the E/M code and not to the codes for the other procedures or services that may be performed.

- Append modifier 25 to report that a separately identifiable E/M service was performed by the same provider on the same date as a minor procedure or other service. Only the content of the note documenting the separate E/M service should be used to determine the level of an additional E/M service.
- Append modifier 57 to report that the decision to perform surgery was made during this visit. For Medicare patients, modifier 57 is used to report the fact that the decision was made to perform major surgery (a procedure with a 90-day postoperative period).
- Performance of diagnostic tests or studies during an encounter that require separate interpretation are not included when determining the level of E/M service when reported separately. A separate code(s) for the diagnostic tests or studies performed in addition to the E/M codes may be reported.
- Simple tests, such as UA, CBC, and quick strep, that are results only tests and do not require separate interpretation can be counted as ordered or reviewed as part of the Data element for MDM even if the test is reported by the provider performing the office E/M visit.
- A test/study that is independently interpreted by the provider that is not separately reported but is part of the E/M service is considered part of MDM.

Special Instructions for Consultations Performed in the Hospital or Nursing Facility

Medicare requires that the initial hospital care code (99221–99223) be reported for each physician's first visit with a patient during a specific hospitalization. As only one physician can be the admitting physician, CMS created HCPCS Level II modifier AI that is to be appended to the initial hospital care code by the attending physician. All other physicians and consultants report the initial hospital care code without appending a modifier. Subsequent inpatient encounters by any physician are reported using codes 99231–99233.

- For Medicare beneficiaries, append modifier AI to the initial hospital care code (99221–99223) or initial nursing facility care code (99304–99306) reported by the attending physician
- Only the admitting physician of record who oversees the patient's care reports modifier AI
- It is inappropriate for consulting physicians to report modifier AI with their initial hospital care code

Do not append modifier AI to subsequent hospital care codes (99231–99233) or inpatient consultation codes (99252–99255).

Admitting Provider vs. Consultant

Medicare allows only one physician to be the admitting physician of record for hospital inpatient and nursing facility admissions. To identify the admitting physician of record who oversees the patient's care, CMS requires the use of HCPCS Level II modifier AI Principal physician of record, be reported by the admitting physician on the initial hospital care or initial nursing facility care code. Note that private payers may choose whether to follow the CMS policy regarding modifier AI; therefore, providers should verify consultation code policies with individual payers before using AI.

99252

Documentation Requirements

Medical Decision Making: Straightforward

- Minimal number and complexity of problems addressed
- No or minimal amount and complexity of data reviewed and analyzed
- Minimal risk of complications and/or morbidity or mortality

History: Medically appropriate

Examination: Medically appropriate

Key Point

The nature and extent of the patient history and physical examination are determined by the treating provider reporting the service.

Code Indicators (from the MDM table)

Number and Complexity of Problem(s)

- One self-limited or minor problem

Amount and/or Complexity of Data

- Minimal or none

Risk of Complications/Morbidity or Mortality

Minimal risk of morbidity from additional diagnostic tests or treatment

Time Spent on Date of the Encounter

- 35 minutes

Sample Documentation—99252

Level II Inpatient Consultation

TO: Dr. Attending Physician

FROM: Dr. Consultant

RE: Evaluation of hearing loss

I was called in consultation to evaluate this 45-year-old male for progressive hearing loss. The patient was admitted four days ago for bleeding ulcers, and upon history and physical examination was noted to have decreased hearing. The patient denies any history of chronic middle ear disease as a child. He does report minimal tinnitus when he is sitting in a quiet room, but denies any dizziness. His wife has complained that she has to repeat things and wondered if he needed a hearing aid. He has a past history of noise exposure while hunting and while working in a manufacturing plant in his early 20s. He has worn ear protection while using firearms or around machinery for the past I2 years.

Physical exam: External auditory canals are clear; TM's are intact with no scarring or bulging. normal mobility. Rinne and Weber tests are normal. Exam of the nose and sinuses shows no obstructions, discharge, tenderness or other abnormalities. Oral cavity is clear; teeth are in good repair. Oropharynx and posterior pharynx all within normal limits.

Audiometry shows bilateral sloping, moderate high frequency sensorineural hearing loss from 2 kHz without an air-bone gap. Impedance studies were normal.

Impression:

Bilateral moderate high frequency sensorineural hearing loss

Recommendations:

Hearing aid evaluation and fitting
Hearing conservation program to reduce and protect him from noise trauma

Thank you for allowing me to see your patient.

Quick Tip

Append modifier 25 to the consultation code if reporting the audiology testing performed by the provider and not by the facility or facility staff.

99253

Documentation Requirements

Medical Decision Making: Low

- Low number and complexity of problems addressed
- Limited amount and complexity of data reviewed and analyzed
- Low risk of complications and/or morbidity or mortality

History: Medically appropriate

Examination: Medically appropriate

Code Indicators (from the MDM table)

Number and Complexity of Problem(s)

- Two or more self-limited or minor problems
- One stable, chronic illness
- One acute, uncomplicated illness or injury
- One stable, acute illness
- One acute, uncomplicated illness or injury requiring hospital inpatient or observation level of care

Amount and/or Complexity of Data

**Each unique test, order, or document contributes to the combination of two or combination of three in Category 1 below.*

- Limited

(Must meet the requirements of at least one of the two categories.)

Category 1: Tests and documents

- Any combination of two from the following:
  - review of prior external note(s) from each unique source*
  - review of the result(s) of each unique test*
  - ordering of each unique test*

  or

Category 2: Assessment requiring an independent historian(s)

(For the categories of independent interpretation of tests and discussion of management or test interpretation, see moderate or high)

Risk of Complications/Morbidity or Mortality

Low risk of morbidity from additional diagnostic tests or treatment

Time Spent on Date of the Encounter

- 45 minutes

Sample Documentation—99253

Level III Inpatient Consultation

TO: Dr. Attending Physician

FROM: Dr. Consultant

RE: Evaluation of cataracts

History: This 79-year-old white female with multiple problems was transferred from her nursing home two days ago for chest pain, nausea and vomiting which are being treated by her attending physician. He has requested that I evaluate the patient for possible cataract surgery. The patient is somewhat difficult to communicate with, and history is taken from the hospital record and from her daughter. The daughter states that her mother was diagnosed with cataracts some time ago and had declined surgery although she was warned about the possibility of losing her sight if the cataracts progressed. The daughter states that her mother's vision has gradually gotten worse over the past few years, and her mother has recently indicated that she can no longer read, see the television, or distinguish among utensils at the table. The patient has stated that she would be willing to have the procedure done.

No known allergies; no other significant history or complaints.

Physical examination: Elderly, thin, well-developed white female, oriented to time and place, BP 148/86. The patient is pleasant but clearly prefers that her daughter speak for her. She responds appropriately to direct questions. The patient hears well.

Examination of the eyes shows limited visual acuity due to mature cataracts in both eyes. Extraocular movements intact. Conjunctivae pink. Pupils' equal, reactive to light and accommodation. Slit lamp exam shows normal anterior chambers, mature posterior subcapsular cataracts. Discs and posterior segments normal as far as can be determined at this time but examination is obscured by the cataract. Intraocular pressures normal.

Impression: Bilateral mature posterior subcapsular cataracts

Recommendations: The patient will clearly benefit from removal of the cataracts and replacement with intraocular lens. After discussion with the patient and her daughter, we decided to schedule the first cataract procedure as soon as possible, with the second to follow at a suitable interval. Intraocular lens will be placed at the time of surgery with anticipated visual correction to 20/25. The daughter asked whether or not the first procedure could be done before her mother was discharged. I advised her that surgery would not be done until her GI symptoms are completely resolved, and therefore she would be discharged prior to the procedure.

Thank you for allowing me to see this patient.

99254

Documentation Requirements

Medical Decision Making: Moderate

- Moderate number and complexity of problems addressed
- Moderate amount and complexity of data reviewed and analyzed
- Moderate risk of complications and/or morbidity or mortality

History: Medically appropriate

Examination: Medically appropriate

Code Indicators (from the MDM table)

Number and Complexity of Problem(s)

- One or more chronic illnesses with exacerbation, progression, or side effects of treatment
- Two or more stable chronic illnesses
- One undiagnosed new problem with uncertain prognosis
- One acute illness with systemic symptoms
- One acute, complicated injury

Amount and/or Complexity of Data

**Each unique test, order, or document contributes to the combination of two or combination of three in Category 1 below.*

- Moderate

(Must meet the requirements of at least one of the three categories.)

Category 1: Tests, documents, or independent historian(s)

- Any combination of three from the following:
  - review of prior external note(s) from each unique source*
  - review of the result(s) of each unique test*
  - ordering of each unique test*
  - assessment requiring an independent historian(s)

  or

Category 2: Independent interpretation of tests

- Independent interpretation of a test performed by another physician/other qualified health care professional (not separately reported)

  or

Category 3: Discussion of management or test interpretation

- Discussion of management or test interpretation with external physician/other qualified health care professional/appropriate source (not separately reported)

Risk of Complications/Morbidity or Mortality

Moderate risk of morbidity from additional diagnostic testing or treatment

Examples only:

- Prescription drug management
- Decision regarding minor surgery with identified patient or procedure risk factors
- Decision regarding elective major surgery without identified patient or procedure risk factors
- Diagnosis or treatment significantly limited by social determinants of health

Time Spent on Date of the Encounter

- 60 minutes

Consultations

Sample Documentation—99254

Level IV Inpatient Consultation
TO: Dr. Attending Physician
FROM: Dr. Consultant:
RE: New onset—seizure activity

History: This 7-year-old male was admitted because he experienced three episodes of seizure activity in the week prior to admission. All three episodes occurred early in the morning, shortly after awakening, and all were observed by family members. The episodes reportedly lasted from two to three minutes on each occasion and involved generalized tonic-clonic movements and loss of consciousness; with loss of bladder control. The patient experienced a definite postictal state, sleeping for three hours and complaining of muscle aches and pains upon awakening with no memory of the seizure activity. The family states that they believe that each episode seems progressively longer. The patient has had no seizures observed in the hospital. The only aura-type prodrome that may be present is tingling in the left leg the night before each event. No fevers in association with the seizures.

Past History: Product of a normal pregnancy, labor and delivery. Normal developmental milestones. Detailed history from both parents elicited no etiology for seizure onset. The patient's immunizations are up to date. He has no past history of chronic conditions including infections, asthma or any other conditions. He sprained an ankle last fall. He is active, participating in sports activities, has a normal diet, and has no past or recent history of other trauma, especially head trauma. He has had no illnesses within the past several weeks, no colds, fevers, flu, GI or GU disturbances and no neurological symptoms. He lives with his family, is a second grader and does well in school, and has no learning difficulties. No one in the family has been ill with the past several weeks. No alcohol, tobacco or drug use. Past, family, social history and review of systems is otherwise within normal limits. No known exposure to toxic substances.

Physical examination: Vitals including blood pressure, pulse, temperature, respirations, height and weight all within normal limits for age. Well developed, well-nourished child. Alert and oriented, lying quietly in bed, somewhat mischievous, but cooperative and relaxed.

HEENT: Eyes show flat discs, EOMI, PERRLA, no abnormalities. ENT clear. Neck supple, no masses or tenderness. Lungs clear. Heart regular rhythm, no murmur.

Neurological: Gait and station are normal. Muscle strength and tone equal and age-appropriate in all extremities. Recent and distant memory appropriate. Attention span excellent for his age. Language and fund of knowledge appropriate for his age group. Cranial nerves II through XII all completely normal. Sensation normal to touch and pinprick. Deep tendon reflexes +2 in all four extremities. Cerebellar finger to nose, upper and lower rapid alternating movements, heel to shin all normal for age. Fine motor coordination appropriate for his age.

Lab: EEG done as an outpatient prior to last seizure showed spike discharges from left temporal lobe.

Impression: Tonic-clonic seizure. Possibly following a partial seizure with secondary generalization.

Discussion: Workup will include fasting glucose, calcium, magnesium and electrolyte. Further investigation with neuro-imaging in a child with a normal history and neuro exam is not indicated at this time. Will begin phenobarbital 4mgm/KG/Day.

I have discussed these recommendations with his parents, and they agree to proceed with the workup and treatment plan if you agree. Thank you for allowing me to participate in the care of your patient.

99255

Documentation Requirements

Medical Decision Making: High

- High number and complexity of problems addressed
- Extensive amount and complexity of data reviewed and analyzed
- High risk of complications and/or morbidity or mortality

History: Medically appropriate

Examination: Medically appropriate

Key Point

The nature and extent of the patient history and physical examination are determined by the treating provider reporting the service.

Code Indicators (from the MDM table)

Number and Complexity of Problem(s)

- One or more chronic illnesses with severe exacerbation, progression, or side effects of treatment
- One acute or chronic illness or injury that poses a threat to life or bodily function

Amount and/or Complexity of Data

**Each unique test, order, or document contributes to the combination of two or combination of three in Category 1 below.*

- Extensive

(Must meet the requirements of at least two of the three categories.)

Category 1: Tests, documents, or independent historian(s)

- Any combination of three from the following:
  - review of prior external note(s) from each unique source*
  - review of the result(s) of each unique test*
  - ordering of each unique test*
  - assessment requiring an independent historian(s)

  or

Category 2: Independent interpretation of tests

- Independent interpretation of a test performed by another physician/other qualified health care professional (not separately reported)

  or

Category 3: Discussion of management or test interpretation

- Discussion of management or test interpretation with external physician/other qualified health care professional/appropriate source (not separately reported)

Risk of Complications/Morbidity or Mortality

High risk of morbidity from additional diagnostic testing or treatment

Examples only:

- Drug therapy requiring intensive monitoring for toxicity
- Decision regarding elective major surgery with identified patient or procedure risk factors
- Decision regarding emergency major surgery
- Decision regarding hospitalization or escalation of hospital-level care
- Decision not to resuscitate or to de-escalate care because of poor prognosis
- Parenteral controlled substances

Time Spent on Date of the Encounter

- 80 minute

Quick Tip

For services of 95 minutes or more, see prolonged services code 99418.

Consultations

Sample Documentation—99255

Level V Inpatient Consultation
TO: Dr. Attending Physician
FROM: Dr. Consulting Gastroenterologist
RE: Evaluation for GI bleed

History: This is the first Community Hospital admission for this 76-year-old female who noted the onset of black, tarry stools and lightheadedness some three days prior to admission. She has a known history of recurrent peptic ulcer disease over the past 10 years for which she has been treated with the usual dietary restrictions, H2 blockers and antacids. She also is a long-standing hypertensive, without complications, for which she is presently on Vasotec 10 mg a day and HCTZ 25 mg a day. There is no past history of renal involvement or cardiac involvement. The day prior to admission, her lightheadedness increased with dizziness on mild exertion. Her black stools became more frequent. She had the onset of the sensation of substernal chest pressure, which on the morning of admission progressed to anterior chest pain with some radiation into the neck and toward the left shoulder.

On admission to the hospital in the ER, she was noted to have hematocrit and hemoglobin of 22 and 7. Her EKG revealed ST depression and T-wave inversion in the lateral precordial leads, consistent with subendocardial ischemia. Her blood pressure was 98/64. She responded to the use of sublingual nitrates and the addition of parenteral calcium channel blocker to her regimen. She also received three units of packed RBC's with her hematocrit now 30 and hemoglobin of 10, with resolution of her angina.

Past History: Previous hospitalization was for hysterectomy at age 42, for menometrorrhagia. No other surgery. Only other hospitalization was for childbirth, gravida 2, para 1, AB 1. No other significant medical problems or chronic illness. All systems reviewed and are otherwise within normal limits.

Family History: Father died at age 81, acute myocardial infarction; he was hypertensive with NIDDM controlled by diet. Mother died at age 59 of ovarian cancer. Three brothers, all deceased, one of complications of alcohol abuse, one of coronary heart disease and one of complications of diabetes. Her sister, age 69, is living with mild hypertension, controlled with medications. No other relevant family history. She is married; her husband is 77 and in good health except for diffuse degenerative joint disease. She has one living daughter, age 50, mild hypertensive. She is a high-school graduate, retired clerk. Uses alcohol sparingly; uses caffeine moderately. Regular medications include H2 blockers, Vasotec and HCTZ as noted above. She occasionally uses enteric-coated aspirin to relieve aches and pains.

Physical Exam: Respirations 22 and somewhat labored, temperature 99.3, pulse 96, BP 112/78. The patient is pale and somewhat dyspneic, otherwise in no acute distress.

HEENT: Eyes: PERRLA; EOMI; Ears, nose, mouth and throat all clear with no signs of infection. Neck supple, trachea midline; no thyromegaly; no cervical or submandibular nodes. Neck vein distension to 14cm. Normal carotids. Breasts are negative with no masses, no nipple discharge. Lungs reveal occasional fine rales at both bases, otherwise clear to auscultation and percussion; no use of accessory muscles of respiration. Heart: PMI, normal sinus rhythm, soft third heart sound, no murmurs. Abdomen soft, nontender, without palpable masses or organomegaly. Bowel sounds are normal. Extremities are negative with good pulses, no edema. cyanosis or clubbing. Neurological exam is grossly normal; cranial nerves intact. DTR's equal. Pelvic exam deferred. Rectal exam revealed soft, mushy black stool strongly heme positive.

Impression:
1. Massive upper GI hemorrhage, probable secondary to reactivation of known peptic ulcer disease
2. Hypotension, resolved with transfusions
3. Angina pectoris, secondary to acute anemia and hypotension
4. Mild CHF secondary to blood transfusion fluid overload

Recommendations:
1. Admit to ICU R/O MI protocol
2. Transfuse with RBC's to maintain hematocrit of 30 or above
3. Once the patient is stabilized, therapeutic endoscopy for management of GI bleed
4. Hold antihypertensives until needed
5. Bumetanide for fluid overload/CHF
6. Biopsy for H. Pylori during endoscopy

Thank you for asking me to see your patient.

(General multisystem)

Key Point

The documentation supports a consultation noting who requested the consult and the purpose of the consult; this report is part of the patient's permanent hospital record. The consultant has made recommendations and will initiate treatment when the patient is stable.

Knowledge Assessment Chapter 9

See chapter 21 for answers and rationale.

1. Which of the following are appropriate places of service for use of office or other outpatient consultation codes (99241–99245)?
   a. Physician office
   b. Patient's home
   c. Hospital inpatient
   d. Emergency department
2. Codes 99241–99255 may be used to report consults initiated by a physician or the patient themselves.
   a. True
   b. False
3. Medicare no longer recognizes consultation codes but they are still used and reimbursable by some carriers.
   a. True
   b. False
4. Based on the documentation for code 99243, what is the level for number and complexity of problems addressed?
   a. Straightforward
   b. Low
   c. Moderate
   d. High

Chapter 10. Other Hospital-Based Services (99281–99292)

Emergency Department Services, New or Established Patient (99281–99288)

E/M Code	Medical Decision Making	History	Exam	Time Spent Face to Face (avg.)[1]
99281	May not require the presence of a physician	Medically appropriate	Medically appropriate	N/A
99282	Straightforward complexity	Medically appropriate	Medically appropriate	N/A
99283	Low complexity	Medically appropriate	Medically appropriate	N/A
99284	Moderate complexity	Medically appropriate	Medically appropriate	N/A
99285	High complexity			N/A
99288[2]	Physician direction of EMS			N/A

1 Time is not a component for selecting emergency department levels.
2 Code 99288 is used to report two-way communication with emergency medical services personnel in the field.

General Guidelines

- Use these CPT® codes when an unscheduled, episodic evaluation and management (E/M) service was rendered to a patient who needed immediate medical attention. The services must have been provided in a hospital-based facility open 24 hours a day. These codes apply to new and established patients.
- Consider assigning the appropriate consultation code instead of these codes when an opinion or advice was provided about a patient for a specific problem at the request of another physician or other appropriate source.
- Report only the appropriate initial hospital inpatient or observation care (99221–99223), or comprehensive nursing facility assessment code if the patient was admitted to the hospital or a nursing facility on the same day as the emergency department visit.
- Consider assigning the appropriate critical care codes (99291, 99292) instead of these codes if the physician provided constant attention to a critically ill patient.
- Append modifier 25 to report that a separately identifiable E/M service was performed by the same physician/qualified health care professional on the same day as a procedure or service. Only the content of the work associated with the separate E/M service should be considered when assigning the correct E/M level.
- Append modifier 57 to indicate that the decision to perform surgery was made at the visit. For Medicare, the decision must be to perform major surgery.

Issues in This Code Range

- Greater use of the critical care codes would be expected as these providers routinely deal with unstable patients. When the level of patient care supports the use of critical care services it is imperative that the documentation supports the service and that time spent providing critical care services is documented in the record. When using these codes, coders must be cognizant of all the codes that are bundled in to these services to avoid unbundling. Critical care codes have a greater RVU value and are reported in lieu of emergency department codes. For detailed information on critical care codes and services included with these services, refer to the critical care services section later in this chapter.
- Codes for high-level E/M services have been targeted in the CERT program as being overutilized. Medical necessity and the level of medical decision making should be verified for all high-level E/M services.

Quick Tip

Services by nonemergency department providers are usually reported with other category E/M services. Some payers restrict the use of codes 99281–99285 to ED-based physicians only.

99281

Documentation Requirements

Problem Severity

- Problem not requiring the presence of the physician, but service provided under physician's supervision.

Special Coding and Documentation Considerations

- The concept of the level of MDM does not apply and time is not used in reporting this service.
- Report separately the codes for the diagnostic test or studies performed.
- Documentation of these nonphysician visits should be individualized to the patient, relevant to the problem present and include evidence of the evaluation and management of the patient and the presenting problem.
- The management documentation should clearly state the treatment or care plan related to the identified problem. It should also state who was involved in the development and initiation of the care plan and follow standard documentation guidelines, including date, patient name, and provider's signature with credentials. This documentation is to be part of the patient's permanent medical record.
- This code has been erroneously used to report nonphysician services that do not have an evaluation and/or a management component. Examples include:
  - taking of any or all of the routine vital signs (e.g., blood pressure check)
  - administering previously prescribed medication only
  - filling out forms
  - collecting blood or other specimens
  - dispensing educational material without further evaluation or management of the patient
- Do not bill this code with any other E/M service provided on the same day.

Sample Documentation—99281

Level I Emergency Department Visit

A 7-year-old black male presents to the emergency department with his mother for a burn recheck. He was seen in this department two days ago after picking up an expended sparkler and sustaining a minor burn to the right palm which was cleaned and dressed.

He is a well-developed, well-nourished black child in no acute distress. He has had no fever and examination of the palmate surface shows a healing 5 centimeter linear area of burn. Neurovascularly intact, good range of motion all digits.

Apply clean dressing. Burn care sheet provided. Follow up as needed or if signs of infection appear. (**Note:** Patient seen by clinical staff only.)

99282

Documentation Requirements

Medical Decision Making: Straightforward

- Minimal number and complexity of problems addressed
- No or minimal amount and complexity of data reviewed and analyzed
- Minimal risk of complications and/or morbidity or mortality

History: Medically appropriate

Examination: Medically appropriate

Code Indicators (from the MDM table)

Number and Complexity of Problem(s)

- One self-limited or minor problem

Amount and/or Complexity of Data

- Minimal or none

Risk of Complications/Morbidity or Mortality
Minimal risk of morbidity from additional diagnostic tests or treatment

Sample Documentation—99282

Level II Emergency Department Visit
This 33-year-old male presents today in the ED for evaluation and treatment of NVD, fever, and chills of over four-hour duration. Patient noticed symptoms began about six hours after ingesting a buffet "all you can eat" meal at a local restaurant. Had various dishes at that time including chicken, chicken casseroles, spaghetti and meatballs, and fresh salad. Tried an OTC antiemetic to no avail.

ROS: Negative for other GI or CV indications. Past Medical Hx: no history gastritis; appendicitis.

O: T: 99.4; R: 24; P: 60; BP: 124/76. General: adult male in obvious distress; worried. Mouth: pharynx WNL. Heart: RSR, no murmurs. Chest: clear. Abd: muscular with sl. epigastric tenderness. BS hyperactive.

Laboratory Findings: Blood profile: normal chemistries. WBCs 7,500 with no shift.

A: Probable staphylococci gastroenteritis.

P: Compazine 25 mg IM. Encourage p.o. fluids. Prescription for Lomotil sig: 2 tabs q.i.d. #32. Follow up with Primary Care Physician if no improvement. If worsening occurs return to ED.

99283

Documentation Requirements

Medical Decision Making: Low

- Low number and complexity of problems addressed
- Limited amount and complexity of data reviewed and analyzed
- Low risk of complications and/or morbidity or mortality

History: Medically appropriate

Examination: Medically appropriate

Code Indicators (from the MDM table)

Number and Complexity of Problem(s)

- Two or more self-limited or minor problems
- One stable, chronic illness
- One acute, uncomplicated illness or injury
- One stable, acute illness
- One acute, uncomplicated illness or injury requiring hospital inpatient or observation level of care

Amount and/or Complexity of Data

**Each unique test, order, or document contributes to the combination of two or combination of three in Category 1 below.*

- Limited

(Must meet the requirements of at least one of the two categories.)

Category 1: Tests and documents

- Any combination of two from the following:
  - review of prior external note(s) from each unique source*
  - review of the result(s) of each unique test*
  - ordering of each unique test*

  or

Category 2: Assessment requiring an independent historian(s)

(For the categories of independent interpretation of tests and discussion of management or test interpretation, see moderate or high)

Risk of Complications/Morbidity or Mortality

Low risk of morbidity from additional diagnostic tests or treatment

Sample Documentation—99283

Level III Emergency Department Visit

S: A 52-year-old female present today in the ED after the sudden onset of left-sided renal colic this a.m. She is a known hypercalcemic stone former, from primary hyperparathyroidism, and has passed eight calculi in the past six years. She underwent a resection of her parathyroid adenoma four mos. ago, without complications. At that time, two nonobstructing calculi were seen in the left renal pelvis by x-ray. She has mild parathyroid bone disease without bone pain. Her pain is intermittent, severe and radiates to the vulva. She has vomited four times and is unable to keep down any liquids or oral pain meds. The pain is not relieved by any position, and she finds it difficult to lie still. Today's presentation is "exactly like my other episodes" of renal colic.

She has urinated several times today, small amounts, without dysuria or hematuria noted. No fever, sweats, chills, shakes. No diarrhea/constipation. No history of pyelonephritis. Pulmonary: no cough. Heart: no pain, palpitations, or SOB. Current medications include Os-Cal and Rocaltrol, on taper.

FH: Renal calculi in father; mother died of MI at age 70. NKA.

O: T: 97.4; R: 24; P: 104; BP: 138/84. General: well-developed, well-nourished slightly heavyset female in acute distress. Skin is dry without rashes; normal turgor. HEENT: unremarkable. Neck: parathyroidectomy scar midline below thyroid, healing well. No masses. Lungs: clear to percussion and auscultation. Heart: regular rate and rhythm. No gallops, murmurs, or rubs. Spine: nontender. Mild left flank tenderness. Abdomen: rounded, healed appendectomy scar RLQ, without tenderness; no hepatosplenomegaly. No mass. Rare bowel sounds. GU: deferred due to pain. Rectal: normal tone, nontender. Stool heme negative. Extremities: no clubbing, cyanosis, edema, tenderness. Pulses normal. Neuro: alert; oriented x 3. No gross focal deficits.

Labs: UA: pH 6; color clear yellow; Spec gravity 1.022; trace blood; 0-4 WBC/HPF; no bacteria; no casts. Stat KUB: radiopaque calculus, 0.6 diameter, at the utero-vesicular junction. CBC w/ diff and chemistries pending.

A:
1. Recurrent renal colic; no signs infection.
2. S/P partial parathyroidectomy for adenoma.

P:
1. Patient is unable to maintain hydration or take oral pain medications secondary to vomiting.
2. IV hydration, parenteral analgesia.
3. Strain urine for stone passage. No need to send the calculus for analysis as we already know the composition of previous stones, the etiology, and she has received definitive treatment (partial parathyroidectomy).
4. Urine C&S.
5. Urology consultation requested.

Other Hospital-based Services

99284

Documentation Requirements

Medical Decision Making: Moderate

- Moderate number and complexity of problems addressed
- Moderate amount and complexity of data reviewed and analyzed
- Moderate risk of complications and/or morbidity or mortality

History: Medically appropriate

Examination: Medically appropriate

Code Indicators (from the MDM table)

Number and Complexity of Problem(s)

- One or more chronic illnesses with exacerbation, progression, or side effects of treatment
- Two or more stable chronic illnesses
- One undiagnosed new problem with uncertain prognosis
- One acute illness with systemic symptoms
- One acute, complicated injury

Amount and/or Complexity of Data

**Each unique test, order, or document contributes to the combination of two or combination of three in Category 1 below.*

- Moderate

(Must meet the requirements of at least one of the three categories.)

Category 1: Tests, documents, or independent historian(s)

- Any combination of three from the following:
  - review of prior external note(s) from each unique source*
  - review of the result(s) of each unique test*
  - ordering of each unique test*
  - assessment requiring an independent historian(s)

  or

Category 2: Independent interpretation of tests

- Independent interpretation of a test performed by another physician/other qualified health care professional (not separately reported)

  or

Category 3: Discussion of management or test interpretation

- Discussion of management or test interpretation with external physician/other qualified health care professional/appropriate source (not separately reported)

Risk of Complications/Morbidity or Mortality

Moderate risk of morbidity from additional diagnostic testing or treatment

Examples only:

- Prescription drug management
- Decision regarding minor surgery with identified patient or procedure risk factors
- Decision regarding elective major surgery without identified patient or procedure risk factors
- Diagnosis or treatment significantly limited by social determinants of health

Sample Documentation—99284

Level IV Emergency Department Visit

This is a 23-year-old female, on active duty in the military but home at this time on military leave, with a three-day history of lower right back pain secondary to muscle strain she thinks. Several hours prior to her presentation here, she developed rapid onset of fever, severe shaking chills and nausea and vomiting. No diarrhea. She also c/o headaches at this time. Denies dysuria, polyuria, and change in urine color or stool color/consistency. Denies any real injury to her back, just thought she might have strained something carrying her suitcase. Positive history of frequent UTIs. Has not self-treated. No increase in fluid intake.

ROS: Feels well in general except for this episode. CV: history of heart murmur present since a child. She has been told by her military doctors that this murmur presents no problems for her. No resp. problems. Neg. GI or GU symptomatology, but frequent UTIs as noted. Psych: likes the military, relatively happy as she is stationed close to home.

PMH: gravida 1, para 1 vaginal delivery three years ago.

SH: Taking BCPs now. Smokes 1/2 pack cigarettes/day. Drinks occasionally. Unmarried. Child lives with the patient's mother.

O: Vitals: T; 104.4; BP: 124/82; R: 22. General: well-developed, well-nourished female appearing her stated age. HEENT: unremarkable. Nasopharynx normal. Eyes WNL. Ears WNL. Throat WNL. Chest: clear to P&A. Heart auscultation reveals grade II/VI holosystolic murmur along the left sternal border; otherwise WNL. GI: Sl. tenderness over epigastrium referred to the right flank region. No guarding or rebound. Negative psoas sign. No organomegaly. No mass. Right CVA tenderness. Unable to touch her chin to her chest. Negative Kernig's sign. Musculoskeletal exam: entirely WNL. No muscle spasm.

Labs: CBC, UA with culture and sensitivity, and blood chemistries ordered. KUB ordered. (all STAT labs)

A: Right acute pyelonephritis.

P: Patient is well hydrated and tolerating oral agents well; therefore, begin Cipro 500 mg q.12h. for two weeks. Re-check in three to four days. PRN sooner. Tylenol for temperature elevations. Encourage fluids.

99285

Documentation Requirements

Medical Decision Making: High

- High number and complexity of problems addressed
- Extensive amount and complexity of data reviewed and analyzed
- High risk of complications and/or morbidity or mortality

History: Medically appropriate

Examination: Medically appropriate

> **Key Point**
>
> **The nature and extent of the patient history and physical examination are determined by the treating provider reporting the service.**

Code Indicators (from the MDM table)

Number and Complexity of Problem(s)

- One or more chronic illnesses with severe exacerbation, progression, or side effects of treatment
- One acute or chronic illness or injury that poses a threat to life or bodily function

> **Key Point**
>
> **When determining the amount and/or complexity of data reviewed and analyzed, each unique test ordered is counted once; the review of that test is included within the order.**

Amount and/or Complexity of Data

**Each unique test, order, or document contributes to the combination of two or combination of three in Category 1 below.*

- Extensive

(Must meet the requirements of at least two of the three categories.)

Category 1: Tests, documents, or independent historian(s)

- Any combination of three from the following:
  - review of prior external note(s) from each unique source*
  - review of the result(s) of each unique test*
  - ordering of each unique test*
  - assessment requiring an independent historian(s)

  or

Category 2: Independent interpretation of tests

- Independent interpretation of a test performed by another physician/other qualified health care professional (not separately reported)

  or

Category 3: Discussion of management or test interpretation

- Discussion of management or test interpretation with external physician/other qualified health care professional/appropriate source (not separately reported)

Risk of Complications/Morbidity or Mortality

High risk of morbidity from additional diagnostic testing or treatment

Examples only:

- Drug therapy requiring intensive monitoring for toxicity
- Decision regarding elective major surgery with identified patient or procedure risk factors
- Decision regarding emergency major surgery
- Decision regarding hospitalization or escalation of hospital-level care
- Decision not to resuscitate or to de-escalate care because of poor prognosis
- Parenteral controlled substances

Sample Documentation—99285

Level V Emergency Department Visit

A 73-year-old male presents this morning in the Emergency Department for evaluation and treatment of fever, chills and headache of one week duration. Patient had a home temperature of 103 degrees last evening. Also c/o productive cough, general malaise and muscle/joint aching. Occasional sputum, which is yellow-green in color, without blood and thick in consistency. The patient has had nocturnal diaphoresis and a several pound weight loss over the previous week. No history of previous pneumonitis or TB. The patient also c/o of concomitant symptoms of sore throat, mild earaches and decreased appetite. Other than this episode, he feels he has been in general good health and has a good sense of well-being.

ROS: Resp: does admit to SOB when coughing and with physical exertion over the last few days. Blames sore throat on cough. Heart: c/o some chest pain with deep inspiration over the last several days. Denies paroxysmal nocturnal dyspnea, orthopnea or dyspnea on exertion. No history MI or angina. GI: No NVD. No dark or clay-colored stools. GU: decreased urination this past week. Reports his urine seems darker during past week. No neuro complaints. Musculoskeletal: only "old age" complaints. O/w neg.

PE: General: well-developed male who appears ill and extremely fatigued. Answers all questions promptly; no signs disorientation. Alert. T: 103. Pulse 100. Resp: 20. Blood pressure 138/72. Skin is hot to touch without lesions or petechiae. Head normocephalic. Pupils are equal, round and reactive to light and accommodation. EOMs intact. Fundi: disc edges sharp. Ears: right TM red and injected; left TM WNL. Nose: mucosa slightly erythemic. Pharynx: erythematous without exudates. Neck supple without mass. Nontender, small cervical lymph nodes. No meningeal signs. Lungs: rhonchi audible bilaterally, lower lobes. Heart: regular rate and rhythm. There is a grade I/VI ejection murmur noted at the 5th left intercostal space without radiation. Abd: scaphoid, soft. Tenderness to percussion in RUQ. No mass. No rebound. Rectal within normal limits. Stool guaiac negative. Neuro: cranial nerves intact. Motor/sensory intact.

Laboratory tests ordered are blood chemistries, H&H and STAT CXR. UA also ordered as well as sputum culture and sensitivity, gram stain. ABGs: pH 7.0; PO2 65; PCO2 36.

STAT CXR reveals patchy infiltrate in the right and left lower lobes; remainder of lung fields is otherwise clear.

Admission Impression: 73-y/o male with probable community acquired pneumonia. Diff. dxs' include mycoplasma, Legionella, pneumococcus and gram negative infections.

P: (1) Admit due to age, temperature greater 101 degrees, and multi-lobe involvement. (2) Begin Erythromycin 500 mg q.i.d. (3) Patient unable to produce sputum—induce sputum for gram stain, C&S. (4) IV hydration. (5) Oxygen two liters by nasal cannula. Monitor with oximetry.

Quick Tip

Although the patient will be admitted, the emergency department physician is not the admitting physician and it is appropriate to report code 99285.

99288

Documentation Requirements

Physician direction of emergency medical systems (EMS) emergency care, advanced life support

Parameters:

- Two-way voice communication by a physician or other qualified health care professional in a hospital emergency or critical care department with ambulance or rescue personnel outside the hospital
- Physician directs performance of necessary medical procedures taking place in the field
- Includes telemetry, cardiopulmonary resuscitation, intubation, administration of intravenous fluids and/or administration of intramuscular, intratracheal, or subcutaneous drugs, and/or defibrillation/electrical conversion of arrhythmia

Documentation:

- Typically, these communications are recorded, as well as entered into a written log.

Coding Issues:

- Medicare, as well as most other third-party payers, considers this service bundled into the evaluation and management (E/M) code billed by the emergency department physician at the time the patient arrives at the facility. Therefore, it would not typically be coded separately.

Special Instructions for E/M Coding of Trauma Care

The American College of Surgeons (ACS) published a bulletin titled "Effectively Using E/M Codes for Trauma Care." The bulletin provides coding guidance for surgeons on how to appropriately report E/M codes related to care rendered to injured or critically ill patients in the emergency department or inpatient setting including critical care services.

Highlights from the article are bulleted below:

- The ACS recommends the creation of a standardized evaluation form for the history and physical for both admissions and consultations. The Advanced Trauma Life Support (ATLS) initial assessment and management tool may be incorporated into the creation of the surgeon's initial assessment and management document to ensure capture of all necessary elements to code at the highest levels of E/M codes.
- Trauma admission forms usually cover a multisystem exam as the majority of trauma patients would receive a comprehensive evaluation.
- Complete, accurate, and detailed documentation is essential and should include times for time-based codes such as critical care services as well as the history, exam, and medical decision making for non-time-based codes.
- Because trauma care typically involves an evaluation in the ED and/or admission to the hospital, or transfer to another facility of observation, it is vitally important to ensure proper reporting of the patient's status and the corresponding E/M code as well as the appropriate place of service code.
- In some circumstances, critical care services may be provided and reported in conjunction with other E/M codes for the same patient on the same date of service; for example, a patient may be admitted to the hospital (99223) and later in the day the patient's condition deteriorates to a degree where the physician must provide critical care to stabilize the patient. The total duration of time spent providing the critical care may also be reported.

Critical Care Services (99291–99292)

E/M Code	Patient Status	Physician Attendance	Time
99291[1]	Critically ill or critically injured	Constant	First 30–74 min.
99292[2]	Critically ill or critically injured	Constant	Each additional 30 minutes beyond the first 74 minutes

1 Under outpatient prospective payment rules, only 99291 is submitted for critical care services in a hospital setting.
2 Under outpatient prospective payment rules, 99292 is not an appropriate code for hospital outpatient use.

Note: For critical care services provided in a facility to patients less than 71 months of age, see codes 99471–99476.

Note: Inpatient critical care for 29 days to 24 months is reported with codes 99471 and 99472.

General Guidelines

- A minimum of 30 minutes must be rendered and appropriately documented in order to report the first hour of critical care. If total time documented is less than 30 minutes, report the appropriate level of E/M code. Critical care of less than 15 minutes duration is not reported separately.
- Record in the patient's record the time spent with the patient and the service provided.
- Append modifier 24 to code 99291 or 99292 to report postoperative critical care services that were unrelated to the surgery performed.
- Assign modifier 25 to code 99291 or 99292 to report preoperative critical care services that were unrelated to surgery but provided by the same physician on the same day as the surgery.
- A critical illness or injury acutely impairs one or more vital organ systems such that there is a high probability of imminent or life threatening deterioration in the patient's condition.
- Critical care involves high-complexity decision making to assess, manipulate, and support vital system functions to treat single or multiple vital organ system failure and/or to prevent further life threatening deterioration of the patient's condition.
- Examples of vital organ system failure include but are not limited to central nervous system failure, circulatory failure, shock, and renal, hepatic, metabolic, and/or respiratory failure. Although critical care typically requires interpretation of multiple physiologic parameters and/or application of advanced technologies, critical care may be provided in life threatening situations when these elements are not present.
- Providing medical care to a critically ill, injured, or postoperative patient qualifies as a critical care service only if both the illness and injury and the treatment being provided meet the above requirements.
- Critical care is usually, but not always, given in a critical care area, such as the coronary care unit, intensive care unit, pediatric intensive care unit, respiratory care unit, or the emergency care facility.
- Outpatient critical services for pediatric patients through 71 months old are reported with codes 99291 and 99292. See codes 99468–99476 for inpatient neonatal and pediatric critical services.
- Codes 99291 and 99292 should be used for physician attendance during a transport of a critically ill patient older than 24 months.
- Critical care and other E/M services may be provided to the same patient on the same date by the same physician based on CPT guidelines. However, there are NCCI edits in place bundling emergency room services and critical care services together. With appropriate modifiers and supporting documentation, they can be reported together on the same day, assuming they were provided at separate times and are separately identifiable services.
- Critical care services codes are time-based codes; thus, they are used to report the total amount of time spent by the physician providing critical care services to the patient.
- Critical care time does not have to be continuous and may encompass several critical care encounters per day.
- Per Medicare, for providers in the same specialty and group providing care concurrently to a patient on the same date, combine the total time spent by each provider to meet the time thresholds for 99291 and 99292.
- Time spent, per day, is added together for a total amount that aids in appropriate code selection. Note that a physician does not need to be in constant attendance at the patient's bedside, but does have to be directly involved in work related to the patient's care.The first hour of critical care can only be reported once per day. Assign the correct code for critical care provided to a hospital inpatient according to the following guidelines:
  - less than 30 minutes—Appropriate E/M code
  - 30–74 minutes—99291 x 1
  - 75–104 minutes—99291 x 1 and 99292 x 1
  - 105–134 minutes—99291 x 1 and 99292 x 2
  - 135–164 minutes—99291 x 1 and 99292 x 3
  - 165–194 minutes—99291 x 1 and 99292 x 4

Key Point

For Medicare patients, the provider must spend 104 minutes providing critical care services to report add-on code 99292. This differs from CPT Guidelines. See the CMS Evaluation and Management Services Guide for more information: https://www.cms.gov/outreach-and-education/medicare-learning-network-mln/mlnproducts/downloads/eval-mgmt-serv-guide-icn006764.pdf.

Other Hospital-based Services

Special Instructions for Reporting Critical Care Services

There are no absolute limits on the amount of critical care time that can be billed per day or hospital stay as long as the medical records can support the need for all critical care services provided. However, time spent performing procedures or services that can be reported separately should not be included in the time reported as critical care time.

- If, outside of the critical care period, the physician performs and adequately documents a complete E/M service, assignment of an additional E/M code reflecting this service is appropriate. Append modifier 25 to the additional E/M code to indicate that this was a medically necessary separately identifiable service.
- Time spent providing services that do not directly relate and contribute to the care and treatment of the critical patient is not reported as critical care. This may include time spent outside of the unit, phone calls with other providers or patients, and remote supervision of a patient.
- For Medicare, however, only one physician may bill for a given hour of critical care even if more than one physician provided care to a critically ill or injured patient.
- According to *CPT 2025*, the following CPT codes are included in critical care codes and may not be billed on dates when critical care is billed:

36000	Introduction of needle or intracath, vein
36410	Venipuncture, over age 3, requiring physician's skill
36415	Venipuncture
36591	Collection of blood specimen from a completely implantable venous access device
36600	Arterial puncture
43752	Naso- or oro-gastric tube placement, necessitating physician's skill
43753	Therapeutic gastric intubation and aspiration(s), necessitating physician's skill
71045	Radiologic examination, chest; single view
71046	Radiologic examination, chest; 2 views
92953	Temporary transcutaneous pacing
93598	Cardiac output measurement(s), thermodilution or other indicator dilution method, performed during cardiac catheterization for the evaluation of congenital heart defects
94002	Ventilation assist and management, initiation of pressure or volume preset ventilators for assisted or controlled breathing; hospital inpatient/observation, initial day
94003	Ventilation assist and management, initiation of pressure or volume preset ventilators for assisted or controlled breathing; hospital inpatient/observation, each subsequent day
94004	Ventilation assist and management, initiation of pressure or volume preset ventilators for assisted or controlled breathing; nursing facility, per day
94660	Continuous positive airway pressure ventilation (CPAP) initiation and management
94662	Continuous negative pressure ventilation initiation and management
94760	Noninvasive ear or pulse oximetry for oxygen saturation; single determination
94761	Noninvasive ear or pulse oximetry for oxygen saturation; multiple determinations (e.g., during exercise)
94762	Noninvasive ear or pulse oximetry for oxygen saturation; by continuous overnight monitoring (separate procedure)

- When additional procedures are reported on the same date as critical care services, the time involved in the procedures may not be included in total critical care time. For Medicare beneficiaries, the list of inclusive CPT codes when critical care is rendered may vary slightly from that published in *CPT 2025*. Check with your Medicare carrier for a correct listing of inclusive services when critical care is provided.
- CMS and other commercial carriers have been quite explicit in stating that physicians must be clear and thorough in notating the amount of time actually spent providing critical care services to a patient. Failure to accurately and appropriately document critical care times can result in a carrier downcoding the service or outright denying the claim. Remember, the physician must devote his/her complete and full attention to the patient during the time specified as providing critical care.
- There are a number of templates and forms that can be used to capture all of the relevant information necessary to properly and correctly report critical care services. These forms and templates can be customized to the specific needs of a practice. A sample template is shown below.

Sample Documentation of Critical Care Time

Patient's Name:____________________________.

Patient's Medical Record Number:________________________.

The services I provided to this patient were provided to treat________________________

____

(State the condition the patient was treated for)

The services I provided required the highest level of my skills with direct and personal management of the patient's treatment. These services included:

- Medical record documentation
- Vital sign assessments
- Medication orders and management
- Reviewing all notes and previous visits
- Collaborating with other physicians on treatment options
- Care, transfer of care, and discharge plans
- Interpreting/reviewing all tests and studies
- Discussions with family or surrogate decision makers
- Other
- ____

The total critical care time was__________hours ________minutes. The total time does not include treating other patients, performing separately reportable procedures, or activities that were not directly related to the care of the patient.

Physician's signature:____________________________Date:________________.

99291

Documentation Requirements

Patient Status:
- Lack of stability
- Conditions pose significant threat to life or risk of prolonged impairment

Physician Attendance
- Constant/intermittent
- Full attention devoted to the unstable critically ill or unstable critically injured patient

Time Spent Face to Face (average)
- First 30–74 minutes

Special Coding and Documentation Considerations
- Use this code to report critical care services rendered for a total of 30–74 minutes on a given day, even if the time spent by the physician is not continuous.
- Critical care performed on neonatal or pediatric patients less than 71 months of age may be reported with codes 99291 and 99292 when performed in an outpatient setting.
- Only report 99291 once per date even if the time spent on that date is not continuous.

Key Point

Time spent rendering critical care must be documented in the medical record. Documentation should support the need for constant attendance by the provider.

99292

Documentation Requirements

Patient Status

- Lack of stability
- Conditions pose significant threat to life or risk of prolonged impairment

Physician Attendance

- Constant/intermittent
- Full attention devoted to the unstable critically ill or unstable critically injured patient

Time Spent Face to Face (average)

- Each additional 30 minutes beyond the first 74 minutes

Special Coding and Documentation Considerations

- Never assign 99292 alone—it should be reported only with 99291
- Critical care performed on neonatal or pediatric patients less than 71 months of age may be reported with codes 99291 and 99292 when performed in an outpatient setting.

Knowledge Assessment Chapter 10

See chapter 21 for answers and rationale.

1. To qualify as an emergency department service, the encounter must be performed in a hospital-based facility that is open 24 hours a day.
   a. True
   b. False
2. What code would be reported when a physician or other qualified health professional at the hospital is in two-way communication with rescue workers on site at a major traffic accident?
   a. This is not a billable service
   b. 99288
   c. 99285
   d. 99291
3. The physician documented that 75 minutes was spent monitoring a critical patient who was given fluids and pressors after becoming hypoxic and hypotensive. What critical-care code(s) would be reported?
   a. 99291 and 99292
   b. 99291
   c. 99292
   d. 99291, 99292 x 2
4. When additional procedures are performed by the same physician on the same date as critical care services, the time spent performing the additional procedures is counted toward the total critical-care time.
   a. True
   b. False
5. What code is assigned for 25 minutes of total critical-care time?
   a. 99291
   b. 99292
   c. Not reportable
   d. Another appropriate level of E/M but not a critical-care code

Other Hospital-based Services

Chapter 11. Nursing Facility Services (99304–99316)

Initial Nursing Facility Care—Comprehensive Nursing Facility Assessments (99304–99306)

E/M Code	Medical Decision Making	History	Exam	Time Spent on Date of Encounter
99304	Straightforward or low covmplexity	Medically appropriate	Medically appropriate	25 min.
99305	Moderate complexity	Medically appropriate	Medically appropriate	35 min.
99306	High complexity	Medically appropriate	Medically appropriate	50 min.

General Guidelines

- Nursing facility and skilled nursing facility care are reported using these codes.
- Use these codes to report initial E/M services provided in a psychiatric residential treatment center and intermediate care facility for individuals with intellectual disabilities.
- Code selection is based on MDM or total time, including face-to-face and non-face-to-face time spent on the date of the encounter.
- History and physical examination elements are not required for code level selection. However, a medically appropriate history and/or physical examination should still be documented. The nature and degree of the history and/or physical examination is determined by the treating physician or other qualified health care professional reporting the service.
- Total time for these services includes total face-to-face and non-face-to-face time personally spent by the physician or other qualified health care professional on the day of the encounter.
- Physician or other qualified health care professional time may include the following activities:
  - preparing to see the patient (e.g., review of tests)
  - obtaining and/or reviewing separately obtained history
  - performing a medically appropriate examination and/or evaluation
  - counseling and educating the patient/family/caregiver
  - ordering medications, tests, or procedures
  - referring and communicating with other health care professionals (when not separately reported)
  - documenting clinical information in the electronic or other health record
  - independently interpreting results (not separately reported) and communicating results to the patient/family/caregiver
  - care coordination (not separately reported)
- Comorbidities or other underlying conditions should not be considered when selecting the level of service unless they are addressed during the encounter and their presence increases the amount and/or complexity of data to be reviewed and analyzed or the risk of complications and/or morbidity or mortality.
- Consider assigning the appropriate consultation code instead of these codes if the provider provided an opinion or advice about a specific problem at the request of another provider or other appropriate source.
- Do not include the time spent by any other staff (e.g., nurse, nurse practitioner or physician assistant) toward the time thresholds. Face-to-face and non-face-to-face time is the time the treating provider spent on the date of the encounter.
- A service that spans two calendar dates is a single service and is reported on one calendar date.
- Report prolonged service code 99418 with 99306 when the service runs 15 minutes beyond the time specified in the CPT® code narrative. The time must be clearly documented in the medical record. For Medicare, report prolonged services code G0317 with 99306 when the service runs 15 or more minutes beyond the total time. See Chapter 19 for more information on G0317.
- Per CPT guidelines, initial nursing facility assessment must be performed by the principal (or admitting) physician or other qualified health care professional (OQHP) overseeing the patients' care in the facility. Some payers may require the use of modifiers to identify the role of the principal or admitting physician.
- Hospital inpatient or observation discharge services performed on the same date as initial nursing facility admission may be reported separately.
- Physician(s) or OQHP should only report 99304–99306 once per admission.
- Initial nursing facility services provided by consulting provider(s) may be reported using 99304–99306 or 99252–99255.

- Append modifier 95 to indicate that the E/M service was rendered to a patient at a distant site via a real-time interactive audio and video telecommunications system. The communication between the physician or other qualified health care professional and the patient should be commensurate with the same key components or requirements of those that would be required if the service had been rendered in a face-to-face setting.
- Performance of diagnostic tests or studies during an encounter that require separate interpretation are not included when determining the level of E/M service when reported separately. A separate code(s) for the diagnostic tests or studies performed in addition to the E/M codes may be reported.
- Simple tests, such as UA, CBC, and quick strep, that are results only tests and do not require separate interpretation can be counted as ordered or reviewed as part of the Data element for MDM even if the test is reported by the provider performing the office E/M visit.
- A test/study that is independently interpreted by the provider that is not separately reported but is part of the E/M service is considered part of MDM.
- When using MDM to determine the level of service for nursing facility E/M visits, effective January 1, 2023, a new category specific to initial nursing facility care has been added to the "Number and Complexity of Problems Addressed" section: *Multiple morbidities requiring intensive management:* for patients with diagnoses likely to require frequent medication or treatment changes and/or re-evaluations, and patients at risk of worsening medical status or risk of hospital admission. This category is only used for code selection in the nursing facility services section.
- These codes include the services formerly known as residential care, skilled nursing facility (SNF), intermediate care facility (ICF) or long-term care facility (LTCF) services.

99304

Documentation Requirements

Medical Decision Making: Straightforward or Low

- Minimal or low number and complexity of problems addressed
- No, minimal or limited amount and complexity of data reviewed and analyzed
- Minimal or low risk of complications and/or morbidity or mortality

History: Medically appropriate

Examination: Medically appropriate

Code Indicators (from the MDM table)

Number and Complexity of Problem(s)

- One self-limited or minor problem
- Two or more self-limited or minor problems
- One stable, chronic illness
- One acute, uncomplicated illness or injury
- One stable, acute illness
- One acute, uncomplicated illness or injury requiring hospital inpatient or observation level of care

Amount and/or Complexity of Data

**Each unique test, order, or document contributes to the combination of 2 or combination of 3 in Category 1 below.*

- Minimal or none
- Limited

(Must meet the requirements of at least 1 of the 2 categories.)

Category 1: Tests and documents

- Any combination of 2 from the following:
  - Review of prior external note(s) from each unique source*;
  - Review of the result(s) of each unique test*;
  - Ordering of each unique test*

  or

Category 2: Assessment requiring an independent historian(s)

(For the categories of independent interpretation of tests and discussion of management or test interpretation, see moderate or high)

Risk of Complications/Morbidity or Mortality

Minimal or low risk of morbidity from additional diagnostic testing or treatment

Time Spent On Date of the Encounter

- 25 minutes

Quick Tip

The purpose of this encounter should be the assessment or reassessment of a nursing facility patient. The same codes are used for new or established patients.

Sample Documentation—99304

Level I Initial Nursing Facility

S: The patient is a 78-year-old female who has been cared for at home by an extended family member. The patient fell out of her chair today and injured her left arm. The patient has been uncooperative of late, not taking her medications for hypothyroid, arthritis, constipation, and hypertension. The family is concerned and determined it was appropriate to arrange for admission to the nursing facility as her needs have progressed.

The patient is calm and responds appropriately to questions. She states that she has been taking her medications although the care taker has found them throughout the house. The family is unsure how long she has been noncompliant with her medications. She states her arm is feeling better after taking Tylenol. Patient states she is sluggish throughout the day and has general joint aches and is otherwise doing okay.

ROS: General: no other complaints, HEENT: without com plaints. CV: no complaints, GI: c/o constipation, MS: as above, Psych: is slightly depressed and upset that some family members have not been to visit.

PMH/SH/FH: As above, widowed for 5 years, quit smoking 20+ years ago.

O: General: alert; feels well, except as above. T: 97.4. P: 78; R: 18; BP: 144/88. HEENT: head normocephalic. Atraumatic. Eyes: PERRLA. EOMI. Conjunctivae clear. Bilateral cataracts. Fundi flat. Ears: WNL. Nose/Throat/Mouth: Oral cavity is dry. Throat WNL. No exudates. Resp: lung fields clear to P&A. Heart: normal S1, S2. NSR. No murmurs. S4 gallop present. GI: Soft, nontender. No organomegaly. BS hypoactive. GU: deferred. Rectal: vault full of hard feces. No hemorrhoids or blood. Musculoskeletal: left upper extremity ecchymotic just above the elbow, outer aspect. Some tenderness with palpation. No gross deformity. FROM. Remainder WNL except for global general discomfort with decreased ROM in all joints. Skin: pale, cool and dry. Neuro: alert and oriented x 2. DTRs +1 lower extremities and upper extremities. Delayed relaxation. Babinski equivocal. Motor/ sensory diffuse weakness 1/4.

A: (1) Noncompliant patient with contusion LUE. (2) hypothyroidism; (3) dementia; (4) bowel impaction, poss. secondary to hypothyroidism; (5) HTN

P: (1) Orders for T4, TSH; (2) ice to arm; acetaminophen for pain; (3) manual disimpaction followed by tap water enemas; (4) when patient is euthyroid, reevaluate for dementia work up; (5) admit to NF

99305

Documentation Requirements

Medical Decision Making: Moderate
- Moderate number and complexity of problems addressed
- Moderate amount and complexity of data reviewed and analyzed
- Moderate risk of complications and/or morbidity or mortality

History: Medically appropriate

Examination: Medically appropriate

Code Indicators (from the MDM table)

Number and Complexity of Problem(s)
- One or more chronic illnesses with exacerbation, progression, or side effects of treatment
- Two or more stable, chronic illnesses
- One undiagnosed new problem with uncertain prognosis
- One acute illness with systemic symptoms
- One acute, complicated injury

Amount and/or Complexity of Data
**Each unique test, order, or document contributes to the combination of two or combination of three in Category 1 below.*

- Moderate

(Must meet the requirements of at least one of the three categories.)

Category 1: Tests, documents, or independent historian(s)
- Any combination of three from the following:
  - review of prior external note(s) from each unique source*
  - review of the result(s) of each unique test*
  - ordering of each unique test*
  - assessment requiring an independent historian(s)

  or

Category 2: Independent interpretation of tests
- Independent interpretation of a test performed by another physician/other qualified health care professional (not separately reported)

  or

Category 3: Discussion of management or test interpretation
- Discussion of management or test interpretation with external physician/other qualified health care professional/appropriate source (not separately reported)

Risk of Complications/Morbidity or Mortality
Moderate risk of morbidity from additional diagnostic testing or treatment

Examples only:

- Prescription drug management
- Decision regarding minor surgery with identified patient or procedure risk factors
- Decision regarding elective major surgery without identified patient or procedure risk factors
- Diagnosis or treatment significantly limited by social determinants of health

Time Spent on Date of the Encounter
- 35 minutes

Nursing Facility Services

Sample Documentation—99305

Level II Initial Nursing Facility

This is a 73-year-old female. She has severe hypertension, mixed arthritis secondary to rheumatoid and degenerative changes, and psoriasis. The staff telephoned my office this morning to report the patient has had nausea, vomiting and diarrhea during the night. Cannot correlate these symptoms with food ingestion. Patient began feeling nauseated an hour before bedtime, felt feverish and then awakened with the urge to vomit. Brown diarrhea culminated with fresh blood on the toilet paper. A few hours ago the patient reports cramping across the lower quadrants of the abdomen, relieved only with defecation and occurring every 45 minutes to an hour. Has vomited several times throughout the night without hematemesis; last episode of emesis about three hours ago. Now also c/o dizziness and slight disorientation. Has been unable to take anything p.o., including meds and liquids. Missed one dose HCTZ last evening.

ROS: General: On Cognex for dementia but seems unhappy with its effects; c/o "losing my memory." HEENT: without complaint with the exception of psoriatic lesions over forehead, with pruritus and some flaking of skin. Using Elocon cream with good response. Occasional dry mouth. Neck: no complaints except for stiffness. Chest/Resp: no cough. No real complaints. Heart: HTN, as above. On HCTZ 25 mg q.i.d. and Cardizem 240 mg q.d. without consistent control. Abdomen: as above. Reports early satiety at times. GU: without complaint. Skin: psoriasis, as stated. Psoriatic lesions also over elbows; these sometimes get tender as she leans on her elbows while doing some ADLs. Musculoskeletal: arthritis as described. Has been on various NSAIDS; now has good relief of symptoms by Daypro. Neuro: occasional peripheral paresthesias but no complaints at this time.

PMH: Partial salpingo-oophorectomy, right, 30 years ago. T&A in childhood. Last year was hospitalized secondary to malignant hypertension with CHF, peripheral edema and SOB.

SH: Married for over 50 years; husband deceased. Four children, none in immediate area.

FH: Mother had a history of hypertension and diabetes. Father killed in accident.

O: T: 100.8. BP: 148/98. R: 24. P: 96. General: feverish-appearing female in slight distress, not vomiting at this time. Head: no signs of active psoriasis. Normocephalic. A few benign-appearing senile keratotic lesions over forehead at margins of eyebrows, bilaterally. Eyes: clear. Fundi WNL. Some crusting over lower palpebral border, OD. Conjunctiva sl. erythematous, OD. Patient does admit to itching and watery eye. OS within normal limits. Nasal mucosa dry. No exudates. Pharynx: sl. irritation apparent at posterior pharyngeal wall with adherent mucus, probably due to vomiting. Yellowed dentition. Lips: sl. dry, especially at corners. No lesions. Neck: no lymphadenopathy. Thyroid without nodule. Chest: clear to A&P. No signs aspirate. Abdomen: flat, without rebound. Some discomfort RLQ/LLQ. Minimal distention. No signs obstruction/ peritonitis. BS normal tones. No organomegaly. Skin: warm, dry. Flaking at elbows where active psoriasis is apparent. Musculoskeletal: Guarded ROM at elbows, knees. Muscle atrophy in quadriceps. Extremities: no peripheral edema. Circ: good. Neuro: DTRs diminished +1. Motor/sensory intact. Rectal: no signs hemorrhage. No hemorrhoids. By digital exam—vault clean. No internal hemorrhoids palpated. Stool guaiac negative. Anoscopy not performed. Psych: good spirits other than for immediate complaints. Memory testing not administered at this time.

Labs: UA WNL. CBC w/diff ordered; chem profile; stool for WBC, O&P, C&S.

Discussed patient's care and health care status with daughter who has power of attorney. As patient has exceeded the care available at assisted living facility, it was determined that it would be appropriate to admit the patient to the nursing facility for care of ongoing and acute health issues.

A: (1) R/O gastroenteritis. (2) Probable dizziness secondary dehydration by vomiting/diarrhea and n.p.o. status. (3) On Cognex—reassess efficacy; schedule testing after GI symptoms resolution. (4) Severe HTN. (5) OD blepharitis/conjunctivitis. (6) Psoriasis, active at elbows, bilat. (7) Arthritis, as described. Care plan includes plan below and is placed in chart.

P: (1) Tetracycline 250 mg t.i.d. for gastroenteritis; (2) Imodium capsules 4 mg and then 2 mg t.i.d. until stool forms; (3) Tigan 200 mg IM. If no improvement, another 200 mg in four hours; (4) Neosporin ophthalmic ung—apply t.i.d. to OD, affected area; (5) continue HCTZ/Cardizem; (6) continue Elocon; (7) continue Cognex; (8) hold Daypro until GI distress subsides. Labs pending—fax results to my office. (9) When nausea subsides, begin clear liquid diet, progress to light meals as directed in orders on chart.

99306

Documentation Requirements

Medical Decision Making: High

- High number and complexity of problems addressed
- Extensive amount and complexity of data reviewed and analyzed
- High risk of complications and/or morbidity or mortality

History: Medically appropriate

Examination: Medically appropriate

> **Key Point**
> **The nature and extent of the patient history and physical examination are determined by the treating provider reporting the service.**

Code Indicators (from the MDM table)

Number and Complexity of Problem(s)

- One or more chronic illnesses with severe exacerbation, progression, or side effects of treatment
- One acute or chronic illness or injury that poses a threat to life or bodily function

Amount and/or Complexity of Data

**Each unique test, order, or document contributes to the combination of two or combination of three in Category 1 below.*

- Extensive

(Must meet the requirements of at least two of the three categories.)

Category 1: Tests, documents, or independent historian(s)

- Any combination of three from the following:
  - review of prior external note(s) from each unique source*
  - review of the result(s) of each unique test*
  - ordering of each unique test*
  - assessment requiring an independent historian(s)

  or

Category 2: Independent interpretation of tests

- Independent interpretation of a test performed by another physician/other qualified health care professional (not separately reported)

  or

Category 3: Discussion of management or test interpretation

- Discussion of management or test interpretation with external physician/other qualified health care professional/appropriate source (not separately reported)

Risk of Complications/Morbidity or Mortality

High risk of morbidity from additional diagnostic testing or treatment

Examples only:

- Drug therapy requiring intensive monitoring for toxicity
- Decision regarding elective major surgery with identified patient or procedure risk factors
- Decision regarding emergency major surgery
- Decision regarding hospitalization or escalation of hospital-level care
- Decision not to resuscitate or to de-escalate care because of poor prognosis
- Parenteral controlled substances

Time Spent on Date of the Encounter

- 50 minutes

Sample Documentation—99306

Level III Initial Nursing Facility

This is a patient who is well-known to me. She is 84-years-of-age, and lived alone with minimal ADL/medical assistance. On the day of admission to the hospital, she slipped and fell in her home and fractured her right femur, lying on the floor until her part-time medical aide found her several hours later. She was admitted to the hospital via the ER with an uneventful hospital course, undergoing right femoral pinning by Dr. Orthopaedic Surgeon. Please see note detailing pt.'s hospital course and hospital discharge on this date for additional information.

She is admitted to the NH at this time for continued care of her femoral fracture as well as for her other medical ailments including HTN, hypothyroidism, polyarthritis and refractory left otitis externa. Upon admission to the nursing facility, the patient states she is feeling physically well but is "depressed and not looking forward to being in a nursing home." She is in a right long-leg cast and is not ambulatory. She says her leg periodically throbs during the night, especially over the incision. She is on p.o. 100 mg Ultram PRN pain, which she takes continually, with good relief of pain but with some sedation.

ROS: General: feels fatigued at times. Eats three meals/day, all prepared by her without assistance. HEENT: Wears dentures. No complaints with the exception of the otitis externa, AS, with intense pruritus as the primary symptoms. Some otorrhea on pillow in a.m.'s—whitish in color; not on meds at this time. Chest/Resp: no complaints. CV: No SOB. Some lightheadedness. HTN as stated, controlled with Norvasc 5 mg p.o. q.d. GI: No complaints. GU: no incontinence. Musculoskeletal: mild degenerative arthritis in major joints including hips, knees, shoulders. Worse in a.m.'s. Takes an occasional Motrin with some relief prior to fall but otherwise prefers not to take meds for this. Right femoral fracture as described. Skin: no complaints except for incisional discomfort over right upper thigh. Says ankles and feet constantly feel cold. Endo: On Synthroid 88 mcg daily. Admits to not being very compliant with her thyroid medicine as she doesn't "see the need any-more."

PMH: Chronic conditions as listed. Noncontributory otherwise. NKDA.

SH: Widowed; lives alone with assistance coordinated through Social Services three days per week, for approximately four hours each day. Has three children, 10 grandchildren. Her family visits her every week and takes her to church each Sunday.

FH: Thyroid disease and hypertension.

O: General: well-developed, well-nourished female in no acute distress, lying passively in bed. BP: 138/86; P: 60; R: 20 and regular. T: 99.2. Height and weight will be recorded later today. Affect: Patient feels "very down" about being shifted to a nursing facility from the hospital, and wants to go home ASAP. Head: normocephalic. Patchy alopecia areata. No scalp lesions. Ears: AS canal erythemic with traces of frothy otorrhea. No signs of excoriations. TM thickened without perforation. AD: some cerumen. TM appears WNL. Pharynx: pale mucosa. Uvula appears long and brushes posterior pharynx and tongue (apparently this does not elicit the cough reflex). Dentition: patient is edentulous. Gingivae appear healthy. Neck: no lymphadenopathy. Thyroid palpable and without nodule or mass. Chest is clear to A/P. Heart: regular rate, rhythm. S4 gallop but no murmurs, rubs. Abdomen: no mass or tenderness. Spleen, liver without tenderness or organomegaly. Normal BS. Genitalia: normal female. Skin: clear, cool. Buttocks: no signs of decubitus ulcer. Musculoskeletal: right femoral fracture, in long-leg cast. No muscle atrophy noted. Pedal pulse good on right. Joints with full passive ROM with some guarded resistance. Motor/sensory intact. Left extremity WNL with intact neuro. DTRs delayed at left knee +1.

A: (1) S/P open reduction internal fixation, right femoral fracture. (2) Hypertension, controlled. Fall possibly due to orthostasis on Norvasc. (3) Hypothyroid, on Synthroid. (4) Otitis externa, chronic, refractory, left. (5) Osteoarthritis. (6) Mild reactive depression.

P: Patient's convalescence should take about six weeks, at which point she may be transitioned to another setting. Will coordinate with her family and SS to determine the best course. She will begin to ambulate in a few weeks. Will coordinate physical therapy at that time. Follow hypertension, continue on Norvasc 5 mg q.d. and check for orthostatic hypotension; follow hypothyroid, continue on Synthroid 88 mcg q.d. and follow on T4/TSH levels. Rx—begin (1) Domeboro otic solution two drops t.i.d.; (2) decrease Ultram to 50 mg p.o. q.6h. PRN pain. Add acetaminophen for pain, q.4 h. Monitor BMs—will switch to Duract two capsules q.6h. if constipation develops; (3) check Beck's depression scale when patient is on Ultram and euthyroid; consider antidepressant if no change. The patient's family will be coming by today. Have full disclosure consent and will apprise them of the details. Detailed new care plan to be placed in chart, Ortho will be by to see the patient in 10 days. A total of 55 minutes was spent in reviewing this case and assessing the patient.

Subsequent Nursing Facility Care, Discharge, and Annual Nursing Assessment (99307–99316)

E/M Code	Medical Decision Making	History	Exam	Time Spent on Date of Encounter
99307	Straightforward	Medically appropriate	Medically appropriate	10 min.
99308	Low complexity	Medically appropriate	Medically appropriate	20 min.
99309	Moderate complexity	Medically appropriate	Medically appropriate	30 min.
99310	High complexity	Medically appropriate	Medically appropriate	45 min.
99315	Nursing facility discharge day management			30 minutes or less
99316	Nursing facility discharge day management			More than 30 minutes

General Guidelines

- Use these codes to report initial E/M services provided in a psychiatric residential treatment center and intermediate care facility for individuals with intellectual disabilities.
- Code selection is based on MDM or total time, including face-to-face and non-face-to-face time spent on the date of the encounter.

Quick Tip

Report these services for subsequent nursing facility services. Note that some payers may evaluate frequency of services for coverage.

- History and physical examination elements are not required for code level selection. However, a medically appropriate history and/or physical examination should still be documented. The nature and degree of the history and/or physical examination is determined by the treating physician or other qualified health care professional reporting the service.
- Total time for these services includes total face-to-face and non-face-to-face time personally spent by the physician or other qualified health care professional on the day of the encounter.
- Physician or other qualified health care professional time may include the following activities:
  - preparing to see the patient (e.g., review of tests)
  - obtaining and/or reviewing separately obtained history
  - performing a medically appropriate examination and/or evaluation
  - counseling and educating the patient/family/caregiver
  - ordering medications, tests, or procedures
  - referring and communicating with other health care professionals (when not separately reported)
  - documenting clinical information in the electronic or other health record
  - independently interpreting results (not separately reported) and communicating results to the patient/family/caregiver
  - care coordination (not separately reported)
- Comorbidities or other underlying conditions should not be considered when selecting the level of service unless they are addressed during the encounter and their presence increases the amount and/or complexity of data to be reviewed and analyzed or the risk of complications and/or morbidity or mortality.
- Consider assigning the appropriate consultation code instead of these codes if the provider provided an opinion or advice about a specific problem at the request of another provider or other appropriate source.
- Do not include the time spent by any other staff (e.g., nurse, nurse practitioner or physician assistant) toward the time thresholds. Face-to-face and non-face-to-face time is the time the treating provider spent on the date of the encounter.
- Performance of diagnostic tests or studies during an encounter that require separate interpretation are not included when determining the level of E/M service when reported separately. A separate code(s) for the diagnostic tests or studies performed in addition to the E/M codes may be reported.
- Simple tests, such as UA, CBC, and quick strep, that are results only tests and do not require separate interpretation can be counted as ordered or reviewed as part of the Data element for MDM even if the test is reported by the provider performing the office E/M visit.
- A test/study that is independently interpreted by the provider that is not separately reported but is part of the E/M service is considered part of MDM.

- When using MDM to determine the level of service for nursing facility E/M visits, effective January 1, 2023, a new category specific to initial nursing facility care has been added to the "Number and Complexity of Problems Addressed" section: *Multiple morbidities requiring intensive management:* for patients with diagnoses likely to require frequent medication or treatment changes and/or re-evaluations, and patients at risk of worsening medical status or risk of hospital admission. This category is only used for code selection in the nursing facility services section.
- A service that spans two calendar dates is a single service and is reported on one calendar date.
- Report prolonged services code 99418 with 99310, when the service runs 15 minutes beyond the time specified in the CPT® code narrative. The time must be clearly documented in the medical record. For Medicare, report prolonged services code G0317 with 99310 when the service runs 15 or more minutes beyond the total time. See Chapter 19 for more information on G0317.
- CPT guidelines state that when a service in a separate site is reported and initial nursing facility care is a consultation, the consultant will report one of these codes for the second service performed on the same date.
- Nursing facility and skilled nursing facility care are reported using these codes.
- Physician(s) or OQHP should only report 99304–99306 once per admission.
- Initial nursing facility services provided by consulting provider(s) may be reported using 99304–99306 or 99252–99255.
- For codes 99307–99310: Append modifier 95 to indicate that the E/M service was rendered to a patient at a distant site via a real-time interactive audio and video telecommunications system. The communication between the physician or other qualified health care professional and the patient should be commensurate with the same key components or requirements of those that would be required if the service had been rendered in a face-to-face setting.
- Codes 99315 and 99316 for nursing facility discharge services are appropriately assigned by the length of time devoted to performing the service (e.g., 99315 requires 30 minutes or less and 99316 requires more than 30 minutes).

99307

Documentation Requirements

Medical Decision Making: Straightforward

- Minimal number and complexity of problems addressed
- No or minimal amount and complexity of data reviewed and analyzed
- Minimal risk of complications and/or morbidity or mortality

History: Medically appropriate

Examination: Medically appropriate

Code Indicators (from the MDM table)

Number and Complexity of Problem(s)

- One self-limited or minor problem

Amount and/or Complexity of Data

- Minimal or none

Risk of Complications/Morbidity or Mortality

Minimal risk of morbidity from additional diagnostic tests or treatment

Time Spent on Date of the Encounter

- 10 minutes

Key Point

When determining the amount and/or complexity of data reviewed and analyzed, each unique test ordered is counted once; the review of that test is included within the order.

Key Point

Tests that are results only and are analyzed as part of MDM do not count as an independent interpretation but may count as one item when determining the amount/complexity of data reviewed and analyzed (e.g., dipstick UA, CBC, quick strep test).

Nursing Facility Services

99308

Documentation Requirements

Medical Decision Making: Low

- Low number and complexity of problems addressed
- Limited amount and complexity of data reviewed and analyzed
- Low risk of complications and/or morbidity or mortality

History: Medically appropriate

Examination: Medically appropriate

> **Key Point**
>
> **The nature and extent of the patient history and physical examination are determined by the treating provider reporting the service.**

Code Indicators (from the MDM table)

Number and Complexity of Problem(s)

- Two or more self-limited or minor problems
- One stable, chronic illness
- One acute, uncomplicated illness or injury
- One stable, acute illness
- One acute, uncomplicated illness or injury requiring hospital inpatient or observation level of care

Amount and/or Complexity of Data

**Each unique test, order, or document contributes to the combination of two or combination of three in Category 1 below.*

- Limited

(Must meet the requirements of at least one of the two categories.)

Category 1: Tests and documents

- Any combination of two from the following:
  - review of prior external note(s) from each unique source*
  - review of the result(s) of each unique test*
  - ordering of each unique test*

  or

Category 2: Assessment requiring an independent historian(s)

(For the categories of independent interpretation of tests and discussion of management or test interpretation, see moderate or high)

Risk of Complications/Morbidity or Mortality

Low risk of morbidity from additional diagnostic tests or treatment

Time Spent on Date of the Encounter

- 20 minutes

99309

Documentation Requirements

Medical Decision Making: Moderate
- Moderate number and complexity of problems addressed
- Moderate amount and complexity of data reviewed and analyzed
- Moderate risk of complications and/or morbidity or mortality

History: Medically appropriate

Examination: Medically appropriate

Code Indicators (from the MDM table)

Number and Complexity of Problem(s)
- One or more chronic illnesses with exacerbation, progression, or side effects of treatment
- Two or more stable chronic illnesses
- One undiagnosed new problem with uncertain prognosis
- One acute illness with systemic symptoms
- One acute, complicated injury

Amount and/or Complexity of Data
**Each unique test, order, or document contributes to the combination of two or combination of three in Category 1 below.*
- Moderate

(Must meet the requirements of at least one of the three categories.)

Category 1: Tests, documents, or independent historian(s)
- Any combination of three from the following:
  - review of prior external note(s) from each unique source*
  - review of the result(s) of each unique test*
  - ordering of each unique test*
  - assessment requiring an independent historian(s)

  or

Category 2: Independent interpretation of tests
- Independent interpretation of a test performed by another physician/other qualified health care professional (not separately reported)

  or

Category 3: Discussion of management or test interpretation
- Discussion of management or test interpretation with external physician/other qualified health care professional/appropriate source (not separately reported)

Risk of Complications/Morbidity or Mortality
Moderate risk of morbidity from additional diagnostic testing or treatment

Examples only:
- Prescription drug management
- Decision regarding minor surgery with identified patient or procedure risk factors
- Decision regarding elective major surgery without identified patient or procedure risk factors
- Diagnosis or treatment significantly limited by social determinants of health

Time Spent on Date of the Encounter
- 30 minutes

Quick Tip

These services require documentation that a face-to-face encounter with the patient was provided by the provider. "Chart rounds" are not covered services and should not be reported.

99310

Documentation Requirements

Medical Decision Making: High
- High number and complexity of problems addressed
- Extensive amount and complexity of data reviewed and analyzed
- High risk of complications and/or morbidity or mortality

History: Medically appropriate

Examination: Medically appropriate

Code Indicators (from the MDM table)

Number and Complexity of Problem(s)
- One or more chronic illnesses with severe exacerbation, progression, or side effects of treatment
- One acute or chronic illness or injury that poses a threat to life or bodily function

Amount and/or Complexity of Data
**Each unique test, order, or document contributes to the combination of two or combination of three in Category 1 below.*
- Extensive

(Must meet the requirements of at least two of the three categories.)

Category 1: Tests, documents, or independent historian(s)
- Any combination of three from the following:
  - review of prior external note(s) from each unique source*
  - review of the result(s) of each unique test*
  - ordering of each unique test*
  - assessment requiring an independent historian(s)

  or

Category 2: Independent interpretation of tests
- Independent interpretation of a test performed by another physician/other qualified health care professional (not separately reported)

  or

Category 3: Discussion of management or test interpretation
- Discussion of management or test interpretation with external physician/other qualified health care professional/appropriate source (not separately reported)

Risk of Complications/Morbidity or Mortality
High risk of morbidity from additional diagnostic testing or treatment

Examples only:
- Drug therapy requiring intensive monitoring for toxicity
- Decision regarding elective major surgery with identified patient or procedure risk factors
- Decision regarding emergency major surgery
- Decision regarding hospitalization or escalation of hospital-level care
- Decision not to resuscitate or to de-escalate care because of poor prognosis
- Parenteral controlled substances

Time Spent on Date of the Encounter
- 45 minutes

Nursing Facility Services

99315

Documentation Requirements

Nursing Facility Discharge Day Management

- 30 minutes or less
- Constitutes the total duration of time spent performing the discharge service, even if the time spent on that date was not continuous

Parameters

- Includes final physical examination
- Includes discussion regarding nursing facility stay and post-discharge patient care guidelines
- Includes preparation of discharge records, prescriptions, and referral forms, among other documents

Coding Exclusions

- Excludes services for patients admitted as a hospital inpatient
- Excludes annual nursing facility assessment

99316

Documentation requirements

Nursing Facility Discharge Day Management

- 31 minutes or more
- Constitutes the total duration of time spent performing the discharge service, even if the time spent on that date was not continuous

Key Point

To report this code, the provider must document that the time spent was more than 30 minutes.

Parameters

- Includes final physical examination
- Includes discussion regarding nursing facility stay and post-discharge patient care guidelines
- Includes preparation of discharge records, prescriptions, and referral forms, among other documents

Coding exclusions

- Excludes services for patients admitted as hospital inpatients
- Excludes annual nursing facility assessment

Knowledge Assessment Chapter 11

See chapter 21 for answers and rationale.

1. What level of history and exam are required to report 99305 or 99306?
   a. Detailed
   b. Detailed or comprehensive
   c. Comprehensive
   d. Medically appropriate
2. It is acceptable for a physician assistant to perform the initial nursing facility encounter as long as the physician reviews and signs the medical record.
   a. True
   b. False
3. What code would be assigned when the physician documents a subsequent nursing facility visit where the physician spent 25 minutes face-to-face with the patient and in non-face-to-face activities on the date of the encounter?
   a. 99309
   b. 99304
   c. 99315
   d. 99308
4. What code is reported when low complexity MDM is documented for a new patient in a psychiatric residential treatment facility?
   a. 99342
   b. 99304
   c. 99305
   d. 99308

Chapter 12. Home or Residence Services (99341–99350)

Home or Residence Services—New Patient (99341–99345)

E/M Code	Medical Decision Making	History	Exam	Time Spent on Date of Encounter
99341	Straightforward complexity	Medically appropriate	Medically appropriate	15 min.
99342	Low complexity	Medically appropriate	Medically appropriate	30 min.
99344	Moderate complexity	Medically appropriate	Medically appropriate	60 min.
99345	High complexity	Medically appropriate	Medically appropriate	75 min.

General Guidelines

- Use these CPT® codes to report any E/M services provided to a new patient in a private residence or temporary lodging. Short-term accommodation such as hotel, campground, hostel, or cruise ship are also included along with an assisted living facility, group home, custodial care facility, and residential substance abuse treatment facility.
- Do not confuse these codes with those for services provided by home care nurses or other home health providers.
- Code selection is based on MDM or total time, including face-to-face and non-face-to-face time spent on the date of the encounter.
- History and physical examination elements are not required for code level selection. However, a medically appropriate history and/or physical examination should still be documented. The nature and degree of the history and/or physical examination is determined by the treating physician or other qualified health care professional reporting the service.
- Total time for these services includes total face-to-face and non-face-to-face time personally spent by the physician or other qualified health care professional on the day of the encounter.
- Physician or other qualified health care professional time may include the following activities:
  - preparing to see the patient (e.g., review of tests)
  - obtaining and/or reviewing separately obtained history
  - performing a medically appropriate examination and/or evaluation
  - counseling and educating the patient/family/caregiver
  - ordering medications, tests, or procedures
  - referring and communicating with other health care professionals (when not separately reported)
  - documenting clinical information in the electronic or other health record
  - independently interpreting results (not separately reported) and communicating results to the patient/family/caregiver
  - care coordination (not separately reported)
- Comorbidities or other underlying conditions should not be considered when selecting the level of service unless they are addressed during the encounter and their presence increases the amount and/or complexity of data to be reviewed and analyzed or the risk of complications and/or morbidity or mortality.
- Do not include the time spent by any other staff (e.g., nurse, nurse practitioner or physician assistant) toward the time thresholds. Face-to-face and non-face-to-face time is the time the treating provider spent on the date of the encounter.
- Performance of diagnostic tests or studies during an encounter that require separate interpretation are not included when determining the level of E/M service when reported separately. A separate code(s) for the diagnostic tests or studies performed in addition to the E/M codes may be reported.
- Simple tests, such as UA, CBC, and quick strep, that are results only tests and do not require separate interpretation can be counted as ordered or reviewed as part of the Data element for MDM even if the test is reported by the provider performing the office E/M visit.
- A test/study that is independently interpreted by the provider that is not separately reported but is part of the E/M service is considered part of MDM.
- Report prolonged services code 99417 with 99345, when the service runs 15 minutes beyond the time specified in the CPT® code narrative. The time must be clearly documented in the medical record. For Medicare, report prolonged services code G0318 with 99345 when the service runs 15 or more minutes beyond the total time. See Chapter 19 for more information on G0318.
- For commercial payers, consider assigning the appropriate consultation code instead of these codes when an opinion or advice was provided about a patient for a specific problem at the request of another physician/qualified health care professional or other appropriate source.
- Use a case management code when coordination of care involved other providers or agencies but did not involve a patient encounter on that day.

- Assign modifier 24 to indicate that an E/M service performed during the postoperative period was not related to the prior procedure. The claim should show a different diagnosis from that for the surgery.
- Append modifier 25 to report that a separately identifiable E/M service was performed by the same physician/qualified health care professional on the same day as a procedure or service. Only the content of work associated with the separate E/M service should be considered when assigning the correct E/M code.
- User modifier 32 when the services were mandated, such as by a peer review organization, third-party payer, or as a result of a governmental, legislative, or regulatory requirement.

99341

Documentation Requirements

Medical Decision Making: Straightforward

- Minimal number and complexity of problems addressed
- No or minimal amount and complexity of data reviewed and analyzed
- Minimal risk of complications and/or morbidity or mortality

History: Medically appropriate

Examination: Medically appropriate

Code Indicators (from the MDM table)

Number and Complexity of Problem(s)

- One self-limited or minor problem

Amount and/or Complexity of Data

- Minimal or none

Risk of Complications/Morbidity or Mortality

Minimal risk of morbidity from additional diagnostic tests or treatment

Time Spent on Date of the Encounter

- 15 minutes

99342

Documentation Requirements

Medical Decision Making: Low

- Low number and complexity of problems addressed
- Limited amount and complexity of data reviewed and analyzed
- Low risk of complications and/or morbidity or mortality

History: Medically appropriate

Examination: Medically appropriate

Code Indicators (from the MDM table)

Number and Complexity of Problem(s)

- Two or more self-limited or minor problems
- One stable, chronic illness
- One acute, uncomplicated illness or injury
- One stable, acute illness
- One acute, uncomplicated illness or injury requiring hospital inpatient or observation level of care

Amount and/or Complexity of Data

**Each unique test, order, or document contributes to the combination of two or combination of three in Category 1 below.*

- Limited

(Must meet the requirements of at least one of the two categories.)

Category 1: Tests and documents

- Any combination of two from the following:
  - review of prior external note(s) from each unique source*
  - review of the result(s) of each unique test*
  - ordering of each unique test*

Key Point

When determining the amount and/or complexity of data reviewed and analyzed, each unique test ordered is counted once; the review of that test is included within the order.

or

Category 2: Assessment requiring an independent historian(s)

(For the categories of independent interpretation of tests and discussion of management or test interpretation, see moderate or high)

Risk of Complications/Morbidity or Mortality

Low risk of morbidity from additional diagnostic tests or treatment

Time Spent on Date of the Encounter

- 30 minutes

99344

Documentation Requirements

Medical Decision Making: Moderate

- Moderate number and complexity of problems addressed
- Moderate amount and complexity of data reviewed and analyzed
- Moderate risk of complications and/or morbidity or mortality

History: Medically appropriate

Examination: Medically appropriate

Key Point

The nature and extent of the patient history and physical examination are determined by the treating provider reporting the service.

Code Indicators (from the MDM table)

Number and Complexity of Problem(s)

- One or more chronic illnesses with exacerbation, progression, or side effects of treatment
- Two or more stable chronic illnesses
- One undiagnosed new problem with uncertain prognosis
- One acute illness with systemic symptoms
- One acute, complicated injury

Amount and/or Complexity of Data

**Each unique test, order, or document contributes to the combination of two or combination of three in Category 1 below.*

- Moderate

(Must meet the requirements of at least one of the three categories.)

Category 1: Tests, documents, or independent historian(s)

- Any combination of three from the following:
  - review of prior external note(s) from each unique source*
  - review of the result(s) of each unique test*
  - ordering of each unique test*
  - assessment requiring an independent historian(s)

  or

Category 2: Independent interpretation of tests

- Independent interpretation of a test performed by another physician/other qualified health care professional (not separately reported)

  or

Category 3: Discussion of management or test interpretation

- Discussion of management or test interpretation with external physician/other qualified health care professional/appropriate source (not separately reported)

Risk of Complications/Morbidity or Mortality

Moderate risk of morbidity from additional diagnostic testing or treatment

Examples only:

- Prescription drug management
- Decision regarding minor surgery with identified patient or procedure risk factors
- Decision regarding elective major surgery without identified patient or procedure risk factors
- Diagnosis or treatment significantly limited by social determinants of health

Time Spent on Date of the Encounter

- 60 minutes

99345

Documentation Requirements

Medical Decision Making: High

- High number and complexity of problems addressed
- Extensive amount and complexity of data reviewed and analyzed
- High risk of complications and/or morbidity or mortality

History: Medically appropriate

Examination: Medically appropriate

Quick Tip

Payers may require documentation indicating why the service was performed in the home setting.

Code Indicators (from the MDM table)

Number and Complexity of Problem(s)

- One or more chronic illnesses with severe exacerbation, progression, or side effects of treatment
- One acute or chronic illness or injury that poses a threat to life or bodily function

Amount and/or Complexity of Data

**Each unique test, order, or document contributes to the combination of two or combination of three in Category 1 below.*

- Extensive

(Must meet the requirements of at least two of the three categories.)

Category 1: Tests, documents, or independent historian(s)

- Any combination of three from the following:
  - review of prior external note(s) from each unique source*
  - review of the result(s) of each unique test*
  - ordering of each unique test*
  - assessment requiring an independent historian(s)

  or

Category 2: Independent interpretation of tests

- Independent interpretation of a test performed by another physician/other qualified health care professional (not separately reported)

  or

Category 3: Discussion of management or test interpretation

- Discussion of management or test interpretation with external physician/other qualified health care professional/appropriate source (not separately reported)

Risk of Complications/Morbidity or Mortality

High risk of morbidity from additional diagnostic testing or treatment

Examples only:

- Drug therapy requiring intensive monitoring for toxicity
- Decision regarding elective major surgery with identified patient or procedure risk factors
- Decision regarding emergency major surgery
- Decision regarding hospitalization or escalation of hospital-level care
- Decision not to resuscitate or to de-escalate care because of poor prognosis
- Parenteral controlled substances

Time Spent on Date of the Encounter

- 75 minutes

Home or Residence Services—Established Patient (99347–99350)

E/M Code	Medical Decision Making	History	Exam	Time Spent on Date of Encounter
99347	Straightforward complexity	Medically appropriate	Medically appropriate	20 min.
99348	Low complexity	Medically appropriate	Medically appropriate	30 min.
99349	Moderate complexity	Medically appropriate	Medically appropriate	40 min.
99350	High complexity	Medically appropriate	Medically appropriate	60 min.

General Guidelines

- Use these codes to report any E/M services provided to an established patient in a private residence or temporary lodging. Short-term accommodation such as hotel, campground, hostel, or cruise ship are also included along with an assisted living facility, group home, custodial care facility, and residential substance abuse treatment facility.
- Code selection is based on MDM or total time, including face-to-face and non-face-to-face time spent on the date of the encounter.
- History and physical examination elements are not required for code level selection. However, a medically appropriate history and/or physical examination should still be documented. The nature and degree of the history and/or physical examination is determined by the treating physician or other qualified health care professional reporting the service.
- Total time for these services includes total face-to-face and non-face-to-face time personally spent by the physician or other qualified health care professional on the day of the encounter.
- Physician or other qualified health care professional time may include the following activities:
  - preparing to see the patient (e.g., review of tests)
  - obtaining and/or reviewing separately obtained history
  - performing a medically appropriate examination and/or evaluation
  - counseling and educating the patient/family/caregiver
  - ordering medications, tests, or procedures
  - referring and communicating with other health care professionals (when not separately reported)
  - documenting clinical information in the electronic or other health record
  - independently interpreting results (not separately reported) and communicating results to the patient/family/caregiver
  - care coordination (not separately reported)
- Comorbidities or other underlying conditions should not be considered when selecting the level of service unless they are addressed during the encounter and their presence increases the amount and/or complexity of data to be reviewed and analyzed or the risk of complications and/or morbidity or mortality.
- Do not include the time spent by any other staff (e.g., nurse, nurse practitioner or physician assistant) toward the time thresholds. Face-to-face and non-face-to-face time is the time the treating provider spent on the date of the encounter.
- Performance of diagnostic tests or studies during an encounter that require separate interpretation are not included when determining the level of E/M service when reported separately. A separate code(s) for the diagnostic tests or studies performed in addition to the E/M codes may be reported.
- Simple tests, such as UA, CBC, and quick strep, that are results only tests and do not require separate interpretation can be counted as ordered or reviewed as part of the Data element for MDM even if the test is reported by the provider performing the office E/M visit.
- A test/study that is independently interpreted by the provider that is not separately reported but is part of the E/M service is considered part of MDM.
- Report prolonged services code 99417 with 99350, when the service runs 15 minutes beyond the time specified in the CPT® code narrative. The time must be clearly documented in the medical record. For Medicare, report prolonged services code G0318 with 99350 when the service runs 15 or more minutes beyond the total time. See Chapter 19 for more information on G0318.
- Consider assigning the appropriate consultation code instead of these codes when an opinion or advice was provided about a patient for a specific problem at the request of another physician/qualified health care professional or other appropriate source.
- Use a case management code when coordination of care involved other providers or agencies but did not involve a patient encounter on that day.
- Assign modifier 24 to indicate that an E/M service performed during the postoperative period was not related to the prior procedure. The claim should show a different diagnosis from that for the surgery.
- Append modifier 25 to report that a separately identifiable E/M service was performed by the same physician/qualified health care professional on the same day as a procedure or service. Only the content of work associated with the separate E/M service should be considered when assigning the correct E/M code.
- User modifier 32 when the services were mandated, such as by a third-party payer, or as a result of a governmental, legislative, or regulatory requirement.

99347

Documentation Requirements

Medical Decision Making: Straightforward

- Minimal number and complexity of problems addressed
- No or minimal amount and complexity of data reviewed and analyzed
- Minimal risk of complications and/or morbidity or mortality

History: Medically appropriate

Examination: Medically appropriate

Key Point

The nature and extent of the patient history and physical examination are determined by the treating provider reporting the service.

Code Indicators (from the MDM table)

Number and Complexity of Problem(s)

- One self-limited or minor problem

Amount and/or Complexity of Data

- Minimal or none

Risk of Complications/Morbidity or Mortality

Minimal risk of morbidity from additional diagnostic tests or treatment

Time Spent on Date of the Encounter

- 20 minutes

99348

Documentation Requirements

Medical Decision Making: Low

- Low number and complexity of problems addressed
- Limited amount and complexity of data reviewed and analyzed
- Low risk of complications and/or morbidity or mortality

History: Medically appropriate

Examination: Medically appropriate

Code Indicators (from the MDM table)

Number and Complexity of Problem(s)

- Two or more self-limited or minor problems
- One stable, chronic illness
- One acute, uncomplicated illness or injury
- One stable, acute illness
- One acute, uncomplicated illness or injury requiring hospital inpatient or observation level of care

Amount and/or Complexity of Data

**Each unique test, order, or document contributes to the combination of two or combination of three in Category 1 below.*

- Limited

(Must meet the requirements of at least one of the two categories.)

Category 1: Tests and documents

- Any combination of two from the following:
  - review of prior external note(s) from each unique source*
  - review of the result(s) of each unique test*
  - ordering of each unique test*

  or

Category 2: Assessment requiring an independent historian(s)

(For the categories of independent interpretation of tests and discussion of management or test interpretation, see moderate or high)

Risk of Complications/Morbidity or Mortality

Low risk of morbidity from additional diagnostic tests or treatment

Time Spent on Date of the Encounter

- 30 minutes

Quick Tip

Documentation examples may be found with codes 99242–99245.

99349

Documentation Requirements

Medical Decision Making: Moderate

- Moderate number and complexity of problems addressed
- Moderate amount and complexity of data reviewed and analyzed
- Moderate risk of complications and/or morbidity or mortality

History: Medically appropriate

Examination: Medically appropriate

Code Indicators (from the MDM table)

Number and Complexity of Problem(s)

- One or more chronic illnesses with exacerbation, progression, or side effects of treatment
- Two or more stable chronic illnesses
- One undiagnosed new problem with uncertain prognosis
- One acute illness with systemic symptoms
- One acute, complicated injury

Amount and/or Complexity of Data

**Each unique test, order, or document contributes to the combination of two or combination of three in Category 1 below.*

- Moderate

(Must meet the requirements of at least one of the three categories.)

Category 1: Tests, documents, or independent historian(s)

- Any combination of three from the following:
  - review of prior external note(s) from each unique source*
  - review of the result(s) of each unique test*
  - ordering of each unique test*
  - assessment requiring an independent historian(s)

or

Category 2: Independent interpretation of tests

- Independent interpretation of a test performed by another physician/other qualified health care professional (not separately reported)

Key Point

Tests that are results only and are analyzed as part of MDM do not count as an independent interpretation but may count as one item when determining the amount/complexity of data reviewed and analyzed (e.g., dipstick UA, CBC, quick strep test).

or

Category 3: Discussion of management or test interpretation

- Discussion of management or test interpretation with external physician/other qualified health care professional/appropriate source (not separately reported)

Risk of Complications/Morbidity or Mortality

Moderate risk of morbidity from additional diagnostic testing or treatment

Examples only:

- Prescription drug management
- Decision regarding minor surgery with identified patient or procedure risk factors
- Decision regarding elective major surgery without identified patient or procedure risk factors
- Diagnosis or treatment significantly limited by social determinants of health

Time Spent on Date of the Encounter

- 40 minutes

99350

Documentation Requirements

Medical Decision Making: High

- High number and complexity of problems addressed
- Extensive amount and complexity of data reviewed and analyzed
- High risk of complications and/or morbidity or mortality

History: Medically appropriate

Examination: Medically appropriate

Code Indicators (from the MDM table)

Number and Complexity of Problem(s)

- One or more chronic illnesses with severe exacerbation, progression, or side effects of treatment
- One acute or chronic illness or injury that poses a threat to life or bodily function

Amount and/or Complexity of Data

**Each unique test, order, or document contributes to the combination of two or combination of three in Category 1 below.*

- Extensive

(Must meet the requirements of at least two of the three categories.)

Category 1: Tests, documents, or independent historian(s)

- Any combination of three from the following:
  - review of prior external note(s) from each unique source*
  - review of the result(s) of each unique test*
  - ordering of each unique test*
  - assessment requiring an independent historian(s)

  or

Category 2: Independent interpretation of tests

- Independent interpretation of a test performed by another physician/other qualified health care professional (not separately reported)

  or

Category 3: Discussion of management or test interpretation

- Discussion of management or test interpretation with external physician/other qualified health care professional/appropriate source (not separately reported)

Risk of Complications/Morbidity or Mortality

High risk of morbidity from additional diagnostic testing or treatment

Examples only:

- Drug therapy requiring intensive monitoring for toxicity
- Decision regarding elective major surgery with identified patient or procedure risk factors
- Decision regarding emergency major surgery
- Decision regarding hospitalization or escalation of hospital-level care
- Decision not to resuscitate or to de-escalate care because of poor prognosis
- Parenteral controlled substances

Time Spent on Date of the Encounter

- 60 minutes

Quick Tip

The provider should document why the service was performed in the home and not the office or other outpatient setting.

Knowledge Assessment Chapter 12

See chapter 21 for answers and rationale.

1. What codes are used to report new patient encounters in the patient's home?
   a. 99341–99345
   b. 99241–99245
   c. 99347–99350
   d. 99202–99205
2. What home services code would be assigned for an established patient with moderate MDM?
   a. 99349
   b. 99350
   c. 99344
   d. None of the above
3. What modifier should be appended to codes 99341–99350 when services were mandated by a court order?
   a. 25
   b. 52
   c. 59
   d. 32
4. What home services code would be assigned for a new patient with moderate MDM?
   a. 99344
   b. 99343
   c. 99349
   d. None of the above

Chapter 13. Prolonged Physician Services (99358–99359, 99415–99416, 99417, 99418, 99360)

Prolonged Service Without Direct Patient Contact (99358–99359)

E/M Code	Office or Outpatient Facility	Inpatient Facility	Time Spent Before/After Direct Patient Care
99358	Yes	Yes	First 30–74 min.
99359	Yes	Yes	Each additional 30 min.

General Guidelines

- Use these codes when a physician or qualified health care professional provides a prolonged service on a date other than the date of a related face-to-face evaluation and management service with the patient and/or family or caregiver.
- These codes are reported in addition to the other evaluation and management service provided on a different date of service.
- For prolonged services in addition to office and other outpatient services on the same date of service with or without direct patient contact, see 99417.
- Services of less than 30 minutes beyond the usual service are not separately reported.
- These codes should not be used to report services that have more specific codes and no upper time limit, such as communication with other professionals and/or the patient family or review of extensive records and tests before and after direct patient care, such as care plan oversight services (99374–99380), chronic care management by a physician or other qualified health care professional (99437, 99491), home and outpatient INR monitoring (93792, 93793), medical team conferences (99366–99368), interprofessional telephone/Internet/electronic health record consultations (99446–99449, 99451–99452), online digital evaluation and management services (99421–99423) or principal care management services (99424–99427).
- Many third-party and commercial payers do not recognize these codes for payment.
- Prolonged services may be reported on a different date from the primary service to which they apply; however, they must relate to ongoing management of direct patient care on a separate service date.
- These codes report the total duration of non-face-to-face service time (including noncontiguous time) spent providing prolonged services.
- Codes 99358–99359 exclude other non-face-to-face services, which are reportable by more specific codes (e.g., online medical evaluations, anticoagulation management, and care plan oversight).

99358

Documentation Requirements

Intent of Service
- Extended evaluation of a patient's specific problem

Presence of Patient
- Not required

Time
- Document the time spent and content of services

Special Coding and Documentation Considerations
- Use this code only once per day.
- Time does not have to be continuous but should reflect the total time spent in providing prolonged service.
- Prolonged services of less than 15 minutes past the first hour or less than 15 minutes beyond the final 30 minutes are not reported separately.

Key Point

Do not report 99358 or 99359 on the same date of service as 99202-99215, 99221-99236, 99242-99255, 99281-99285, 99304-99310, 99341-99350, 99417-99418, or 99483.

Quick Tip

Note that some payers may not cover non-face-to-face prolonged services.

99359

Documentation Requirements

Intent of Service
- Extended evaluation of a patient's specific problem

Presence of Patient
- Not required

Time
- Document the time spent and content of services.

Special Coding and Documentation Considerations
- Time does not have to be continuous but should reflect the total time spent in providing prolonged service.
- Prolonged services of less than 15 minutes past the first hour or less than 15 minutes beyond the final 30 minutes are not reported separately.
- Never report this code alone—it should always be reported with 99358.

Prolonged Clinical Staff Services with Physician or Other Qualified Health Care Professional Supervision (99415–99416)

E/M Code	Office or Outpatient Facility	Inpatient Facility	Time Spent Face to Face (avg.)
99415	Yes	No	First 30–74 min.
99416	Yes	No	Each additional 30 min.

General Guidelines

- These CPT® codes are used when the clinical staff provides direct patient care for a prolonged period of time in an office or other outpatient setting beyond the highest total time stated in the E/M code description.
- These codes are reported in addition to the other evaluation and management service provided on the same date.
- A physician or other qualified health care professional (OQHP) must be available to provide direct supervision of the clinical staff.
- These codes are reported once per date for the total duration of face-to-face time (including noncontiguous time) spent with the patient.
- Services of less than 30 minutes beyond the usual service are not reported separately.
- Do not report codes 99415–99416 for more than two concurrent patients.
- Use code 99417 for face-to-face prolonged services provided by the physician or OQHP.

99415

Documentation Requirements

Intent of Service
- Extended evaluation and management of a patient's specific problem

Presence of Patient
- Required (direct, face-to-face contact)

Time Spent on Prolonged Service (average)
- First 30 to 74 minutes

Special Coding and Documentation Considerations
- Direct supervision of the clinical staff by the physician or other qualified health care professional is required.
- Use this code to report E/M services that exceed the highest total time defined in the code's narrative by 30 minutes. The service must be rendered in the office or outpatient setting.
- Time does not have to be continuous but should reflect the total time spent providing the prolonged service.
- Use this code only once per day.

Clinical Example

A patient presents with symptoms of clinical dehydration, the physician reports a 99203 and directs a member of his clinical staff to initiate IV hydration with normal saline. Prolonged clinical staff services would begin after 34 minutes, the typical service time included in 99203. Code 99415 would be reported when at least 64 minutes of total face-to-face time are provided by the clinical staff.

99416

Documentation Requirements

Intent of Service
- Extended evaluation and management of a patient's specific problem

Presence of Patient
- Required (direct, face-to-face contact)

Time Spent on Prolonged Service (average)
- Each additional 30 minutes

Special Coding and Documentation Considerations
- Never report this code alone—it should always be reported with 99415.
- Time does not have to be continuous but should reflect the total time spent providing the prolonged service.
- Prolonged services less than 15 minutes beyond the final 30 minutes are not reported.

Basic Service	Typical Time	Threshold for 99356	Threshold for 99416
99202	29 min.	59-103 min.	104 min.
99203	34 min.	64-108 min.	109 min.
99204	41 min.	71-115 min.	116 min.
99205	46 min.	76-120 min.	121 min.
99211	16 min.	46-90 min.	91 min.
99212	24 min.	54-98 min.	99 min.
99213	27 min.	57-101 min.	102 min.
99214	40 min.	70-114 min.	115 min.
99215	45 min.	75-119 min.	120 min.

Prolonged Service With or Without Direct Patient Contact (99417, 99418)

E/M Code	Office or Other Outpatient Facility	Inpatient or Observation Setting	Time Spent With and/or Without Patient Contact (Avg.)
99417	Yes	No	Each additional 15 min.
99418	No	Yes	Each additional 15 min.

General Guidelines

- Use 99417 to report each additional 15 minutes of outpatient E/M services beyond the time indicated in the code description. (Refer to the documentation requirements below for additional guidance on which time to use, since time is listed as a range in the descriptions for 99205 and 99215.)
- Code 99417 is used in addition to time-based evaluation and management services 98003, 98007, 98011, 98015, 99205, 99215, 99245, 99345, 99350, and 99483.
- Use 99418 to report each additional 15 minutes of inpatient or observation E/M services beyond the time indicated in the code description.
- Code 99418 is used only in addition to time-based evaluation and management services 99223, 99233, 99236, 99255, 99306, and 99310.
- These codes are used for prolonged services when time alone is used for code selection.
- Use of these codes is based on the total time the clinician spent on the day of the patient visit, including face-to-face and non-face-to-face activities.
- Other services provided during prolonged service periods may be reported separately. Time involved performing these activities should not count toward prolonged service times.
- Services of less than 15 minutes beyond the usual service are not reported separately.
- Code 99417 should not be reported with 90833, 90836, 90838, 99358–99359, or 99415–99416 on the same date of service.
- Code 99418 should not be reported with 90833, 90836, 90838, 99358, or 99359 on the same date of service.

99417

Documentation Requirements

Intent of Service

- Extended evaluation and management of a patient's specific problem

Presence of Patient

- Includes direct face-to-face contact and non-face-to-face activities

Time Spent on Prolonged Service (average)

- Each additional 15 minutes

Special Coding and Documentation Considerations

- This code is used to report total time spent on the date of the encounter, with or without direct patient contact, that extends beyond the time designated in the primary code description. **Note:** CPT states to report 99417 for services at least 15 minutes beyond the minimum time required to report the primary E/M code.
- In the CY 2021 PFS Final Rule, CMS finalized the creation and use of HCPCS code G2212 for prolonged office or other outpatient E/M services to be reported with 99205 and 99215 for Medicare beneficiaries. In the CY2023 PFS Final Rule, code G2212 may now be reported in addition to 99483. See Chapter 19 for more information on G2212.
- Document the total time (with and without direct patient contact) spent on the patient's case. Time does not have to be continuous but should reflect the total time spent on the day of the visit providing the prolonged service.
- Never report this code alone; it should be reported with 98003, 98007, 98011, 98015, 99205, 99215, 99245, 99345, 99350, or 99483.

99418

Documentation Requirements

Intent of Service
- Extended evaluation and management of a patient's specific problem

Presence of Patient
- Includes direct face-to-face contact and non-face-to-face activities

Time Spent on Prolonged Service (average)
- Each additional 15 minutes

Special Coding and Documentation Considerations
- This code is used to report total time spent on the date of the encounter, with or without direct patient contact, that extends beyond the time designated in the primary code description. **Note:** CPT states to report 99418 for services at least 15 minutes beyond the minimum time required to report the primary E/M code.
- In the CY2023 PFS Final Rule, CMS finalized the following prolonged E/M codes to use for Medicare beneficiary claims: 1) HCPCS code G0316 for prolonged hospital inpatient or observation services to be reported with 99223, 99233, and 99236; 2) HCPCS code G0317 for prolonged nursing facility services to be reported with 99306 and 99310; and 3) HCPCS code G0318 for prolonged home or residence services to be reported with 99345 and 99350. Refer to chapter 19 for more information on these new HCPCS codes.
- Document the total time (with and without direct patient contact) spent on the patient's case. Time does not have to be continuous but should reflect the total time spent on the day of the visit providing the prolonged service.
- Never report this code alone; it should be reported with 99223, 99233, 99236, 99255, 99306, or 99310.

Standby Services (99360)

E/M Code	Intent of Service	Face-to-Face Visits	Time Spent on Standby
99360	Standby services are provided by a clinician at the request of another clinician and include prolonged attendance without face-to-face contact with the patient (i.e., operative high-risk delivery standby, EEG monitoring)	No	Each 30 min.

Documentation Requirements

Intent of Service

- Professional services specifically requested by another clinician that involves extended attendance

Presence of Patient

- Not required

Time Spent on Prolonged Service (average)

- Each 30 minutes
- Report total duration of the standby time period; however, services of less than 30 minutes total duration should not be reported
- Report each additional 30 minutes of standby services beyond the initial time period only if a *full* 30-minute period was provided

Special Coding and Documentation Considerations

- Exclusive, no other care or services may be provided by the standby provider to other patients during this period.
- Do not use this code to report time spent proctoring another individual OR when the standby period ends with the performance of a global surgery package procedure by the same clinician who was on standby.

Knowledge Assessment Chapter 13

See chapter 21 for answers and rationale.

1. When coding prolonged services, what major element out of the following is the determining factor for when to use 99358–99359?
   a. New vs. established
   b. Office or outpatient facility
   c. With or without direct patient contact
   d. All of the above
2. Codes 99358 or 99415 may only be used once per date of service.
   a. True
   b. False
3. Codes 99359, 99415, 99416, 99417, and 99418 are all add-on codes and can be billed alone with sufficient documentation.
   a. True
   b. False
4. In order to bill prolonged services 99417–99418, the total time of the encounter must exceed the basic service by at least ______ minutes.
   a. 15
   b. 30
   c. 45
   d. 60
5. To report prolonged services provided by the clinical staff (99415–99416), direct supervision by a physician is required.
   a. True
   b. False
6. A clinician may not report standby services if the standby service period ends with the standby clinician performing a global surgery package procedure.
   a. True
   b. False

Chapter 14. Other E/M Services (99366–99459)

Medical Team Conferences (99366–99368)

E/M Code	Intent of Service	Provider	Presence of Patient	Time
99366	To plan and coordinate	Nonphysician member of interdisciplinary team	Patient and/or family present	30 min.
99367	To plan and coordinate	Physician member of interdisciplinary team	Patient and/or family not present	30 min.
99368	To plan and coordinate	Nonphysician member of interdisciplinary team	Patient and/or family not present	30 min.

General Guidelines

- A minimum of three health care professionals of different specialties or disciplines who provide direct care to the patient must participate.
- Participants must have performed a face-to-face evaluation or treatment of the patient in the prior 60 days.
- Physician's report team conferences with the patient present using the appropriate E/M code and time as the key controlling factor.
- Only one person per specialty may report participation in the team conference.
- Time is calculated based upon the review of the individual patient and ends at the conclusion of the review.
- Time does not include record keeping or generation of reports.
- Time is not reported concurrently with any other billable service.
- The services are reported as face-to-face if the patient is present for any part of the service.
- Team conference services of less than 30 minutes are not reported.
- Team conferences are not reported if part of a contractual agreement of a facility or organization.
- Each participant must document his or her participation and care recommendations.
- Code 99366 should not be reported for the same time reported for 99424–99427, 99437, 99439, 99487, 99489, or 99490–99491.
- Do not report 99367 or 99368 with 99437, 99439, 99487, or 99489–99491, during the same month.

Quick Tip

Health care professionals may include PT, OT, speech-language pathologists, social workers, dietitians, nurse practitioners, physician assistants, discharge coordinators, and other appropriate ancillary health care providers.

Care Plan Oversight Services (99374–99380)

Code	Intent of Service	Place of Service	Under Care of	Presence of Patient	Time
99374	Supervision of a patient requiring complex and multidisciplinary care modalities involving regular development and/or revision of care plans by that individual, review of subsequent reports of patient status, review of laboratory and other studies, communication (including telephone calls) for purposes of assessment or care decisions with health care professionals, family member(s), surrogate decision maker(s) (e.g., legal guardians) and/or key caregivers involved in the patient's care, integration of new information into the medical treatment plan and/or adjustment of medical therapy, within a calendar month	In home, a domiciliary or equivalent environment (e.g., Alzheimer's facility)	Home health agency	Patient not present	15–29 min.
99375	Supervision of a patient requiring complex and multidisciplinary care modalities involving regular development and/or revision of care plans by that individual, review of subsequent reports of patient status, review of laboratory and other studies, communication (including telephone calls) for purposes of assessment or care decisions with health care professionals, family member(s), surrogate decision maker(s) (e.g., legal guardians) and/or key caregivers involved in the patient's care, integration of new information into the medical treatment plan and/or adjustment of medical therapy, within a calendar month	In home, a domiciliary or equivalent environment (e.g., Alzheimer's facility)	Home health agency	Patient not present	30 min. or more
99377	Supervision of a patient requiring complex and multidisciplinary care modalities involving regular development and/or revision of care plans by that individual, review of subsequent reports of patient status, review of laboratory and other studies, communication (including telephone calls) for purposes of assessment or care decisions with health care professionals, family member(s), surrogate decision maker(s) (e.g., legal guardians) and/or key caregivers involved in the patient's care, integration of new information into the medical treatment plan and/or adjustment of medical therapy, within a calendar month	Hospice	Hospice	Patient not present	15–29 min.
99378	Supervision of a patient requiring complex and multidisciplinary care modalities involving regular development and/or revision of care plans by that individual, review of subsequent reports of patient status, review of laboratory and other studies, communication (including telephone calls) for purposes of assessment or care decisions with health care professionals, family member(s), surrogate decision maker(s) (e.g., legal guardians) and/or key caregivers involved in the patient's care, integration of new information into the medical treatment plan and/or adjustment of medical therapy, within a calendar month	Hospice	Hospice	Patient not present	30 min. or more
99379	Supervision of a patient requiring complex and multidisciplinary care modalities involving regular development and/or revision of care plans by that individual, review of subsequent reports of patient status, review of laboratory and other studies, communication (including telephone calls) for purposes of assessment or care decisions with health care professionals, family member(s), surrogate decision maker(s) (e.g., legal guardians) and/or key caregivers involved in the patient's care, integration of new information into the medical treatment plan and/or adjustment of medical therapy, within a calendar month	Nursing facility	Nursing facility	Patient not present	15–29 min.
99380	Supervision of a patient requiring complex and multidisciplinary care modalities involving regular development and/or revision of care plans by that individual, review of subsequent reports of patient status, review of laboratory and other studies, communication (including telephone calls) for purposes of assessment or care decisions with health care professionals, family member(s), surrogate decision maker(s) (e.g., legal guardians) and/or key caregivers involved in the patient's care, integration of new information into the medical treatment plan and/or adjustment of medical therapy, within a calendar month	Nursing facility	Nursing facility	Patient not present	30 min. or more

General Guidelines

- Care plan oversight (CPO) is physician, or other qualified health care provider, supervision of patients receiving either home health or hospice benefits where complex or multidisciplinary care modalities and the ongoing provider involvement are required.
- CMS extended Medicare coverage to allow separate payment for CPO services exceeding 30 minutes per month for patients who are receiving Medicare-covered home health or hospice benefits.
- Medicare does not pay for CPO services for nursing facility or skilled nursing facility patients.
- Code descriptors for these codes include communication with family member(s), surrogate decision maker(s) (e.g., legal guardians) and/or key caregivers as well as health care professionals. This broader definition is more consistent with current practice.
- These codes are reported separately from other E/M services.
- Total time for services provided within a 30-day period determine the code selection.
- Only one provider, per month, will be paid for CPO services for a patient.
- Care plan oversight for rest home (e.g., assisted living facility), or home care plan oversight services are reported with CPT® codes 99437, 99491, or principal care management 99424–99425.

Quick Tip

Providers must include their own documentation and may not rely on the orders or chart notes of the care giver to support care plan oversight. Each contact should be documented and include date, contact, orders given or changed, and time spent providing the remote care of the patient.

The following coverage requirements apply to CPO services:

- The patient must require complex or multidisciplinary care modalities requiring ongoing provider involvement in the plan of care
- The patient must be receiving Medicare covered home health or hospice services during the period in which the CPO services are furnished
- The provider who bills CPO must be the same individual who signed the home health or hospice plan of care
- The provider must have furnished a covered service that required face-to-face encounter with the patient within the six months immediately preceding the provision of the first CPO plan oversight service within that calendar month
- The provider must furnish at least 15 minutes of CPO within the calendar month for which payment is claimed and no other provider has been paid for CPO within that calendar month
- The CPO billed must not be routine postoperative care provided in the global surgical period of a surgical procedure billed by the provider
- For patients receiving Medicare-covered home health services, the provider must not have a significant financial or contractual interest in the home health agency (HHA)

Coding Axiom

The following are activities that count toward the requirement for care plan oversight:

- **Development or revision of care plans**
- **Review of subsequent charts, reports, treatment plans, or lab or study results**
- **Integration of new information into the treatment plan and/or therapy adjustment**
- **Communication with other health care professionals (not employed in the same practice) involved in the care of the patient**

Services that do not count towards the requirement for care plan oversight:

- **Time spent discussing treatment and medication adjustments with the patient, his or her family, or friends**
- **Time spent by staff getting or filing charts**
- **Travel time**
- **Provider time spent calling prescriptions into the pharmacist unless the telephone conversation involves a discussion of pharmaceutical therapies**

- For patients receiving Medicare hospice services, the provider must not be the medical director or an employee of the hospice or providing services under arrangements with the hospice
- CPO services must personally be furnished by the provider who bills them
- Services provided "incident-to" a physician's service do not qualify as CPO and do not count toward the time requirement for CPO
- The provider may not bill CPO during the same calendar month in which he or she bills the Medicare monthly capitation payment (end-stage renal disease benefit) for the same patient

- The provider billing for the CPO must document in the patient's medical record those services that were furnished, as well as the date and length of time associated with those services
- Do not report these codes for time reported with 98012-98016, 98966-98968, or 99421-99423

Inherent in the CPO concept is the expectation that the provider has coordinated some aspect of the patient's care with the home health agency or hospice during the month for which CPO services are billed. It is required that the provider who bills for CPO must be the same individual who signs the plan of care. As previously stated, only one provider, per month, will be paid for CPO for a patient. Other providers working with the individual who signed the plan of care are not permitted to bill for these services.

Sample Documentation

Meets Expected Requirements:
The managing physician documents all time spent over the past 30 days to supervise the care plan for the patient. The content and time spent on each phone call and conference as well as any test results, consultant reports, review of old records, etc., is documented. The managing physician documents the review of patient status reports and care plans, pertinent findings and the time spent. Documentation describes phone calls involving active management of a problem over the phone after hours, and telephone communication with a pharmacy, the outside reference lab, the patient's physical therapist, social worker, home care provider and consulting physicians. Documentation also indicates the time spent discussing and giving direction to office staff who interact with the patient and family in the patient's care. Total time spent over the past 30 days is calculated and noted in the documentation.

Does NOT Meet Expected Requirements:
The managing physician documents the date and time spent over the past 30 days to supervise the care plan for the patient, however, the content such as discussion of test results and pertient time is not documented.

Quick Tip

Care plan oversight services documentation should describe the care plan oversight services furnished, the dates and exact duration of time spent on these services

Guidelines for Nonphysician Practitioners

According to provisions of the Balanced Budget Act of 1997, nonphysician practitioners (NPP), nurse practitioners (NP), physician assistants (PA), and clinical nurse specialists (CNS) may bill for care plan oversight services as long as they are practicing within the scope of state law. These practitioners must be providing ongoing care through evaluation and management services. Although NPPs are not permitted to certify a patient for home health care services, NPPs can provide care plan oversight services only when the physician that signs the plan of care provides regular ongoing care under the same plan of care as the NPP billing for care plan oversight and either:

- The physician and NPP are part of the same group practice
- If the NPP is an NP or a CNS, the physician that signs the plan of care must also have a collaborative agreement with the NPP
- If the NPP is a PA, the physician signing the plan of care also provides general supervision of PA services for the practice

Billing may be made for care plan oversight services provided by an NPP when:

- The NPP providing care plan oversight services has seen and examined the patient
- The NPP providing care plan oversight services is not acting as a consultant with his or her participation limited to a single medical condition rather than multidisciplinary coordination of care
- The NPP providing care plan oversight services combines the care he or she provides with that provided by the physician who signed the plan of care

The attending physician or the nurse practitioner designated as the attending physician may bill for hospice CPO when they are acting in the capacity of an attending physician. An attending physician is defined as the one identified by an individual, at the time he or she elects hospice coverage, as having the most significant role in the determination and delivery of their medical care. Attending physicians are not employed or paid by the hospice.

Coding Axiom

No other service may be billed on the claim with CPO services. CPO should not be billed until after the end of the month in which the service is performed. Be sure the ICD-10-CM code is reported with the highest level of specificity and that the code used specifically identifies the reason for the service.

Special Instructions for CPO Services

Codes 99374–99378 are not covered under Medicare. For these services and for reporting physician certification and recertification for Medicare covered home health services, refer to "Chapter 19. HCPCS G Codes and Evaluation and Management Services."

Preventive Medicine Services (99381–99429)

Preventive Medicine Services—New Patient

E/M Code	Patient Status	Age	History	Exam	Medical Decision Making[1]
99381	No complaints	Under 1 year	Age and gender appropriate	Age and gender appropriate	Ordering lab/diagnostic procedures
99382	No complaints	1–4 years	Age and gender appropriate	Age and gender appropriate	Ordering lab/diagnostic procedures
99383	No complaints	5–11 years	Age and gender appropriate	Age and gender appropriate	Ordering lab/diagnostic procedures
99384	No complaints	12–17 years	Age and gender appropriate	Age and gender appropriate	Ordering lab/diagnostic procedures
99385	No complaints	18–39 years	Age and gender appropriate	Age and gender appropriate	Ordering lab/diagnostic procedures
99386	No complaints	40–64 years	Age and gender appropriate	Age and gender appropriate	Ordering lab/diagnostic procedures
99387	No complaints	65 and over	Age and gender appropriate	Age and gender appropriate	Ordering lab/diagnostic procedures

1 Includes age appropriate immunizations, laboratory/diagnostic procedures and age appropriate counseling/anticipatory guidance and risk factor reduction intervention(s).

Preventive Medicine Services—Established Patient

E/M Code	Patient Status	Age	History	Exam	Medical Decision Making[1]
99391	No complaints	Under 1 year	Age and gender appropriate	Age and gender appropriate	Ordering lab/diagnostic procedures
99392	No complaints	1–4 years	Age and gender appropriate	Age and gender appropriate	Ordering lab/diagnostic procedures
99393	No complaints	5–11 years	Age and gender appropriate	Age and gender appropriate	Ordering lab/diagnostic procedures
99394	No complaints	12–17 years	Age and gender appropriate	Age and gender appropriate	Ordering lab/diagnostic procedures
99395	No complaints	18–39 years	Age and gender appropriate	Age and gender appropriate	Ordering lab/diagnostic procedures
99396	No complaints	40–64 years	Age and gender appropriate	Age and gender appropriate	Ordering lab/diagnostic procedures
99397	No complaints	65 and over	Age and gender appropriate	Age and gender appropriate	Ordering lab/diagnostic procedures

1 Includes age appropriate immunizations, laboratory/diagnostic procedures, and age appropriate counseling/anticipatory guidance and risk factor reduction intervention(s).

Preventive Medicine Services—Counseling and/or Risk Factor Reduction Intervention

E/M Code	Patient Status	Intent of Service	Time
Individual Counseling			
99401	No complaints	Promote health, prevent illness or injury	15 min.
99402	No complaints	Promote health, prevent illness or injury	30 min.
99403	No complaints	Promote health, prevent illness or injury	45 min.
99404	No complaints	Promote health, prevent illness or injury	60 min.
Behavior Change Interventions, Individual			
99406	Smoking or tobacco history	Promote health, smoking or tobacco cessation counseling	3–10 min.
99407	Smoking or tobacco history	Promote health, smoking or tobacco cessation counseling	> 10 min.
99408	Alcohol or substance screening	Promote health, alcohol or substance abuse screening with brief intervention	15–30 min.
99409	Alcohol or substance screening	Promote health, alcohol or substance abuse screening with brief intervention	> 30 min.
Group Counseling			
99411	No complaints	Promote health	30 min.
99412	No complaints	Promote health	60 min.
Other Preventive Medicine Services			
99429		Unlisted preventive medicine service	

Other E/M Services

General Guidelines

- Select a code from the preventive medicine services category based on whether the patient is new or established, and the age of the patient.
- Report the appropriate problem-oriented E/M code (e.g., 99202–99215) if a significant problem is encountered or a pre-existing problem is addressed and requires additional work during the course of the preventive medicine E/M service. Do not report a problem-oriented E/M code if a problem is encountered during the preventive medicine service but does not require additional work.
- Append modifier 25 to report that a separately identifiable E/M service was performed by the same physician/qualified health care professional on the same day as a procedure or service. Only the content of work associated with the separate E/M service should be considered when assigning the correct E/M code.
- Assign only the appropriate preventive medicine service code when E/M service and preventive medicine counseling is provided during the same visit.
- Report the appropriate code from the subcategory for counseling and/or risk factor reduction intervention when this service is provided at an encounter separate from the preventive medicine examination (codes 99401–99404).
- Report the appropriate code from the subcategory behavior change interventions, individual (99406–99409), when the behavior itself is considered an illness and specific interventions are suggested as part of the treatment of the condition related to the behavior, or to change the behavior before it results in an illness. These behaviors include; tobacco addiction, substance abuse, or obesity.
- For codes 99406–99409, append modifier 95 to indicate that the E/M service was rendered to a patient at a distant site via a real-time interactive audio and video telecommunications system. The communication between the physician or other qualified health care professional and the patient should be commensurate with the same key components or requirements of those that would be required if the service had been rendered in a face-to-face setting.
- Use code 99078 when reporting group counseling of patients with symptoms or established illnesses.
- Report separately the codes for the diagnostic tests or studies performed, including screening tests identified by specific CPT codes.
- Immunizations and administrations, ancillary studies involving laboratory, radiology, other procedures, or screening tests (e.g., vision, hearing, developmental) identified by a separate CPT code are reported separately and part of the preventive medicine service.

Key Point

When a separate E/M service is reported with preventive medicine services, only the documentation specific to the separate problem may be considered when determining a separate E/M code. Usually, the additional E/M service is a low-level service as all other documentation is usually part of the comprehensive history and exam required for preventive medicine services.

Issues in This Code Range

- Although these codes were never the subject of specific documentation criteria from CMS (likely because they are not covered)—compliance auditors have long sought to ensure that these services were appropriately documented when performed. The definitions of comprehensive history and physical exam are not the same as for other E/M services.
- The CPT book indicates that the history and exam for preventive medicine services should be "age and gender appropriate."
- Check with other commercial or third-party payers to see if there is a protocol or method of reporting combined services of this nature. Many carriers will not pay for two such services on the same day, or their computer systems will routinely deny one of the codes. Bring the situation to their attention.
- Medicare does not cover preventive medicine visits listed in this section.
- Medicare does cover an initial preventive physical examination (IPPE) also commonly referred to as the welcome to Medicare examination. The IPPE is not a "routine physical checkup"; rather, the IPPE is more of an introduction to Medicare and enables new Medicare beneficiaries to receive important screenings and vaccinations. It also allows the providers to evaluate and review the patient's health. CMS also offers an annual wellness visit (AWV), which is an annual appointment for beneficiaries to discuss a plan for preventive care for the year ahead. While it is similar to the one-time only IPPE, the AWV is not a complete "head-to-toe" physical examination and the beneficiary cannot have an AWV during the first year of enrollment in the Medicare Program OR during the same year as an IPPE. There are also specific criteria associated with the AWV. **Note:** The IPPE and AWV services are represented with HCPCS Level II G codes and are further discussed in "Chapter 19: G Codes and Evaluation and Management Services."

Quick Tip

Pediatric practitioners may follow *Recommendations for Preventive Pediatric Healthcare/Bright Futures/American Academy of Pediatrics* when rendering preventive care services to their patients. For more information on the guidance and pocket guide, visit: https://brightfutures.aap.org/materials-and-tools/guidelines-and-pocket-guide/Pages/default.aspx.

Non-Face-to-Face Physician Services (99421–99423)

Online Digital Evaluation and Management Services (99421-99423)

E/M Code	Intent of Service	Type of Communication	Time
99421	Online E/M service at the request of established patient	Online digital	5–10 min.
99422	Online E/M service at the request of established patient	Online digital	11–20 min.
99423	Online E/M service at the request of established patient	Online digital	At least 21 min.

General Guidelines

- Care must be initiated through a HIPAA compliant platform by an established patient.
- The service cannot be reported if a related E/M service has been provided in the prior seven days.
- These services are for cumulative time over a seven-day period and include initial inquiry, records review, physician interaction with clinical staff regarding the patient's problem, development of management plans, generation of prescriptions, ordering tests, and subsequent communication with the patient online, via telephone, email, or other supported digital communication.
- Do not report cumulative services of less than five minutes.
- The service cannot be reported if it falls within the postoperative period of a previously performed procedure, even if more than seven days.
- Online digital E/M services require permanent storage of documentation (electronic or hard copy) of the encounter.
- When a separately reportable E/M service occurs within seven days of initiation of the online service, the work devoted to the online service is counted into the separately reportable E/M service.
- Online digital E/M services performed by nonphysician providers are reported with 98970–98972.
- These services are not reportable when performed concurrently with other billable services, such as anticoagulation management.
- When home and outpatient INR monitoring is evaluated during an online encounter, do not report these codes separately.
- Providers should not report these codes on the same day as E/M services codes 99202–99205, 99212–99215, or 99242–99245.

Interprofessional Telephone/Internet/Electronic Health Record Consultations (99446–99452)

E/M Code	Intent of Service	Time Spent
99446	Consultation, including verbal and written report, at the request of another provider via the telephone, internet, or EHR	5–10 min
99447	Consultation, including verbal and written report, at the request of another provider via the telephone, internet, or EHR	11–20 min.
99448	Consultation, including verbal and written report, at the request of another provider via the telephone, internet, or EHR	21–30 min.
99449	Consultation, including verbal and written report, at the request of another provider via the telephone, internet, or EHR	31 min. or more
99451	Consultation, including written report, at the request of another provider via the telephone, internet, or EHR	5 min. or more
99452	Interprofessional telephone, internet, or electronic health record referral services provided by a requesting or treating provider	30 min.

General Guidelines

In urgent or complex situations, an interprofessional telephone, internet, or electronic health record consultation (99446–99451) may be performed.

- Four levels, including a verbal and written report, are available depending on the time spent; time must be documented.
- Use code 99451 for consultation services of 5 minutes or more that include only a written report.
- In these consultations, a physician or other qualified health care provider requests an opinion from another provider who may have a specific specialty expertise.
- These codes do not require a face-to-face visit with the patient because the sole purpose is to help the treating physician diagnose or manage the patient's problem.
- As with other consultation codes, the verbal or written request and reason for the request must be documented in the patient chart. In addition, to report 99446–99449 the consultant must give a verbal opinion and written report back to the requesting provider. For 99451 only a written report is required.
- Additional time required to complete the consultation should be reported by adding together each segment of time spent in providing the service with the cumulative total used to determine the correct code assignment.
- The majority of time reported must be devoted to the verbal/internet discussion.
- Do not report 99446–99449 if more than 50 percent of the service time is spent reviewing and analyzing data.
- Do not report 99446–99451 more than once within a seven-day interval.
- There is no designation between new or established patient.
- These services include the review of records pertinent to the diagnosis in question, laboratory/pathology studies, radiology studies, and medication profile via mail or fax prior to the consultation.
- It is inappropriate for the consultant to report these codes if the patient has been seen 14 days prior to the consult or the consult leads to a transfer of the patient's care or other face-to-face service within 14 days.
- It is inappropriate for the consultant to report this service if it is less than 5 minutes.
- The physician consultant may report non-face-to-face direct communication with the patient and/or family via telephone with codes 98008-98016; for non-face-to-face, nonphysician services, see codes 98966–98968. Note: This time would not be included in the time spent providing the consultation with the requesting provider as reported with codes 99446–99451.
- When the consultation leads to an immediate transfer of patient care (e.g., surgery, hospital visit, scheduled face to face examination of the patient, etc), to the consulting provider within the next 14-day period, do not report these codes.
- Interprofessional telephone, internet, or electronic health record referral services provided by a requesting or treating provider (99452):
  - may be reported when 16 to 30 minutes is spent arranging a referral and/or communicating with the consultant.
  - can only be reported once in a 14-day period.
- In addition, if consultation exceeds 30 minutes beyond the typical time of the E/M service and the patient is physically present and available to the *requesting provider*, the provider may report prolonged services (99417–99418) for his/her time spent while on the telephone or internet with the consulting provider. If the patient is not present, the requesting provider may report non-face-to-face prolonged services (99358–99359).

Digitally Stored Data Services/Remote Physiologic Monitoring and Physiologic Monitoring Treatment Services (99453–99454, 99091, 99473–99474, 99457–99458)

E/M Code	Intent of Service	Face-to-Face Visit	Time Spent
99453	Setup and patient education on the use of remote monitoring equipment used by the patient that collects, monitors, and reports health-related data (e.g., weight, blood pressure, pulse oximetry) to the provider	No	N/A
99454	Daily recordings or program alert transmissions via the remote monitoring device, for each 30-day period	No	N/A
99091	Collection and interpretation of health-related data gathered via a remote patient monitoring system used to manage physiologic data (e.g., blood pressure, glucose), including education and training	No	At least 30 min.
99473	Patient education/training and device calibration for the patient to self-measure their blood pressure	Yes	N/A
99474	Collection of data reported to the provider of average systolic and diastolic pressures over a 30-day period (minimum of 12 readings) with subsequent treatment plan provided to the patient	No	N/A
99457	Remote patient monitoring by the provider/clinical staff utilizing data from an FDA-defined remote monitoring system to oversee the patient's treatment plan	No. Does require interactive communication with the patient	At least 20 min.
99458	Remote patient monitoring by the provider/clinical staff utilizing data from an FDA-defined remote monitoring system to oversee the patient's treatment plan	No. Does require interactive communication with the patient	Each additional 20 min.

Other E/M Services

General Guidelines

- Codes 99453, 99454, 99091, and 99457 are provided and reported once for each 30-day period. Code 99474 should be reported no more than once per calendar month.
- To report remote physiological monitoring, the device used must be a medical device as defined by the FDA.
- Services must be ordered by a physician or other qualified health care professional.
- Do not report 99453 or 99454 for monitoring services of less than 16 days.
- Time spent monitoring a more specific physiological condition, such as continuous glucose monitoring (95250), should not be included in time counted towards reporting 99453 or 99454.
- Do not report 99453 or 99454 in addition to codes for more specific physiologic conditions, such as 93296 (remote device monitoring of a pacemaker system).
- Report 99453 only once per episode of care.
- When the patient is seen for another E/M service, services provided in 99091 are included in that E/M service and should not be reported separately.
- Do not report 99091 in addition to 99374–99380, 99424–99427, 99437, 99457, 99487, or 99491 in the same calendar month.
- Report 99473 only once per device.
- Code 99457 requires live, interactive communication with the patient or caregiver and a minimum of 20 minutes of provider or staff time within a calendar month; report 99458 for each additional completed 20 minutes.
- Do not report remote physiologic monitoring treatment services (99457, 99458) of less than 20 minutes.
- Codes 99457 and 99458 may be reported in addition to 99424–99427, 99437, 99439, 99487–99491, 99495, 99496, 99484, and 99492–99494, when performed during the same reporting period. However, time spent performing those services should not be included in the time used to count toward 99457 and 99458.
- Only report 99457 and 99458 when requirements for a more specific treatment management service have not been met.
- Do not count the time toward 99457 or 99458 on days when other separate and distinct services are provided, including: 99202–99215, 99341–99350, 99221–99233, and 99252–99255.
- Do not report 99457 in addition to 93264 or 99091or in the same month as 99473 or 99474.

Special Evaluation and Management Services (99450–99456)

E/M Code	Intent of Service	Specific Data Provided
99450	Evaluation of patient prior to or after issuance of basic life policy or for determination of disability	Vital statistics, including blood pressure, height, weight Medical history completed as identified on life insurance pro forma Urine and blood samples collected and "chain of custody" protocols Complete documentation and certificates according to requester
99455	Evaluation of patient by treating physician for work related or medical disability examination	Medical history, including record review, completed as appropriate with patient condition. Examination appropriate to the patient condition and disability(ies) Identification of the diagnosis Assessment of patient stability, capabilities, and impairment calculation according to accepted guidelines (state or AMA impairment guidelines) Future treatment identified or developed Complete documentation, certificates and reports according to requester specifics
99456	Evaluation of patient by non treating physician for work-related or medical disability examination	Medical history, including record, review, completed as appropriate with patient condition Examination appropriate to the patient condition and disability(ies) Identification of the diagnosis Assessment of patient stability, capabilities, and impairment calculation according to accepted guidelines (state or AMA impairment guidelines) Future treatment identified or developed Complete documentation, certificates, and reports according to requester specifics

General Guidelines

- Select a code to report the evaluation of a patient and completion of the special forms based upon basic life/disability evaluation or work-related/medical disability evaluation.
- Report the appropriate problem-oriented E/M code (e.g., 99202–99215) if provided separate from the special evaluation. Do not report a problem-oriented E/M code if a problem is encountered during the service but does not require additional work.
- Append modifier 25 to report that a separately identifiable E/M service was performed by the same physician/qualified health care professional on the same day as a procedure or service. Only the content of work associated with the separate E/M service should be considered when assigning the correct E/M code.
- Report separately the codes for diagnostic tests or studies performed, including screening tests, identified by specific CPT codes.
- Work-related or medical disability evaluation services are selected based upon the provider being the treating or non treating physician.
- Codes 99455–99456 should **NOT** be reported with code 99080 Special reports such as insurance forms, or for completing workmens' compensation forms.

Quick Tip

Work-related or medical disability evaluation may require review of prior medical records to determine any pre-existing conditions when calculating disability.

Issues in This Code Range

- These services are not usually covered by government payers.
- Basic life and disability evaluation may be requested as a screening tool by special insurers (e.g., life, disability, long term care).
- Work-related or medical disability evaluations may be requested by workers' compensation carrier, state, or federal disability determination services.
- It is not appropriate to report a special report (99080) with these services.
- Special coverage of these services may require coordination with the requester prior to the services being rendered.
- Impairment guidelines are specified in state workers' compensation statute and may use the AMA impairment guidelines or state developed guidelines.

Quick Tip

Calculation of disability for some state workers' compensation carriers is based on state specific guidelines and others use the AMA impairment guidelines.

Other Evaluation and Management (99459)

E/M Code	Intent of Service	Face-to-Face Visit
99459	Pelvic examination performed at the time of an E/M service	Yes

General Guidelines

- Code 99459 is a practice-expense only code reported in addition to another evaluation and management (E/M) service provided in a non-facility setting and performed on the same date.
- Code 99459 is only used in addition to E/M services 99202-99205, 99212-99215, 99242-99245, 99383-99387, and 99393-99397.
- Medicare will only accept this code when reported in addition to 99202-99205 and 99212-99215.
- Report 99459 when the provider performing the E/M service deems it medically necessary to do a pelvic exam during the same visit.
- For a pelvic examination performed under anesthesia, report 57410.

Knowledge Assessment Chapter 14

See chapter 21 for answers and rationale.

1. How many health care professionals of different specialties must participate in order to bill for a medical team conference (99366–99368)?
   a. Two or more
   b. Four or more
   c. More than 10
   d. Three or more
2. Which of the following activities would not count toward total time when billing for care plan oversight services?
   a. Adding new information to the treatment plan
   b. Discussing treatment adjustments with the patient or a caregiver
   c. Revisions to the plan of care
   d. Reviewing treatment plans and lab results
3. What is the appropriate code for a well-visit/preventive service provided to a 20-year-old established patient?
   a. 99215
   b. 99385
   c. 99395
   d. 99396

Chapter 15. Newborn and Pediatric Services (99460–99486)

Newborn Care Services (99460–99465)

E/M Code	Patient Status	Site of Care	Intent of Service
99460	Normal newborn	Hospital or birthing room	Perform history and physical exam; initiate diagnostic and treatment programs; prepare records
99461	Normal newborn	Other than hospital or birthing room	Perform physical examination; confer with parents
99462	Normal newborn	Hospital	Provide E/M subsequent care service per day
99463	Normal newborn	Hospital or birthing room	Perform history and exam; prepare medical records. Use this code for newborns assessed and discharged on the same date
99464	Unstable newborn	Hospital or birthing room	Initial stabilization of newborn when requested by delivering physician
99465	High-risk newborn at delivery	Hospital or birthing room	Provide inhalation therapy, aspirate, administer medication for stabilization

General Guidelines

- These services are reported for the care of newborns in a variety of settings.
- Newborns are defined as birth through 28 days of age.
- Normal newborn services are to be used to report services to care of the newborn in the first days after birth.
- Review codes to determine the correct code based upon place of service.
- The provider should appropriately document newborn status and care required for unstable newborns and high-risk newborn infants.
- Initial stabilization codes may be reported the same date as initial evaluation of infant admitted to critical care.
- See codes 99468–99469 and 99477–99480 for newborns requiring additional care and supervision.
- For newborns seen for follow-up in the office or outpatient setting following discharge, refer to 99202–99215, 99381, or 99391.
- Codes 99464 and 99465 may be reported in addition to 99221–99223, 99291, 99460, 99468, and 99477.

Issues in This Code Range

- Newborns admitted and discharged in the hospital or birthing center on the same date should be reported with code 99463.
- Newborn care spanning more than one day should be reported with the appropriate codes, even if the patient was discharged before he or she was 24 hours old.
- Circumcision and other procedures are reported in addition to the admission and evaluation of the newborn.

Pediatric Critical Care Patient Transport (99466–99467 and 99485–99486)

E/M Code	Patient Status	Site of Care	Intent of Service
99466	Critically ill or critically injured, under 24 months	Constant during transport	First 30–74 min.
99467	Critically ill or critically injured, under 24 months	Constant during transport	Each additional 30 minutes beyond the first 74 min.
99485	Critically ill or critically injured, under 24 months	Two-way communication	First 16–45 min.
99486	Critically ill or critically injured, under 24 months	Two-way communication	Each additional 30 min.

General Guidelines

- Assign the appropriate outpatient visit or subsequent hospital care code if critical care services took less than 30 minutes on a given day.
- Record in the patient's record the time spent with the patient and the service provided.
- A critical illness or injury acutely impairs one or more vital organ systems such that there is a high probability of imminent or life-threatening deterioration in the patient's condition.
- Critical care involves high-complexity decision making to assess, manipulate, and support vital system functions to treat single or multiple vital organ system failure and/or to prevent further life-threatening deterioration of the patient's condition.
- Examples of vital organ system failure include but are not limited to central nervous system failure, circulatory failure, shock, and renal, hepatic, metabolic, and/or respiratory failure. Although critical care typically requires interpretation of multiple physiologic parameters and/or application of advanced technologies, critical care may be provided in life-threatening situations when these elements are not present.
- Codes 99466 and 99467 represent physician attendance for a critically ill or injured pediatric patient (less than 24 months of age) being transported to or from a facility or hospital. Codes 99291 and 99292 should be used for physician attendance during a transport of a critically ill patient older than 24 months.
- For total body and selective head cooling of neonates, use 99184.
- The first hour of critical care transport can be reported only once per day. Assign the correct code for critical care provided to a hospital inpatient according to the following guidelines:
  - less than 30 minutes assign appropriate E/M code
  - 30–74 minutes 99466 x 1
  - 75–104 minutes 99466 x 1 and 99467 x 1
  - 105–134 minutes 99466 x 1 and 99467 x 2
  - 135–164 minutes 99466 x 1 and 99467 x 3
  - 165–194 minutes 99466 x 1 and 99467 x 4
- Codes 99485–99486 represent the physician's role in interfacility transport of a critically ill or injured patient, (less than 24 months of age). These codes are for non-face-to-face contact; the physician is directing the transport services during an interfacility transport. The control physician uses a two-way radio to communicate treatment advice to the transport team providing the patient care. The first hour of critical care transport can be reported only once per day. Assign the correct code for critical care provided to a hospital inpatient according to the following guidelines:
  - less than 15 minutes assign appropriate E/M code
  - 16–45 minutes 99485 x 1
  - 46–75 minutes 99485 x 1 and 99486 x 1
  - 76–105 minutes 99485 x 1 and 99486 x 2
  - 106–135 minutes 99485 x 1 and 99486 x 3
  - 136–165 minutes 99485 x 1 and 99486 x 4
- There are no absolute limits on the amount of critical care transport time that can be reported per day or hospital stay as long as the medical records can support the need for all critical care services provided. However, time spent performing separately reportable procedures or services should not be included in the time reported as critical care transport time. The following services should not be reported separately when performed during the transport of a critical care pediatric patient:

36000	Introduction of needle or intracath, vein
36400	Venipuncture, younger than age 3 years, necessitating physician's skill, not to be used for routine venipuncture; femoral or jugular vein
36405	Venipuncture, younger than age 3 years, necessitating physician's skill, not to be used for routine venipuncture; scalp vein
36406	Venipuncture, younger than age 3 years, necessitating physician's skill, not to be used for routine venipuncture; other vein
36415	Venipuncture
36591	Collection of blood specimen from a completely implantable venous access device

36600	Arterial puncture
43752	Naso- or oro-gastric tube placement, necessitating physician's skill
43753	Therapeutic gastric intubation and aspiration(s), necessitating physician's skill
71045	Radiologic examination, chest; single view
71046	Radiologic examination, chest; 2 views
92953	Temporary transcutaneous pacing
93598	Cardiac output measurement(s), thermodilution or other indicator dilution method, performed during cardiac catheterization for the evaluation of congenital heart defects
94002	Ventilation assist and management, initiation of pressure or volume preset ventilators for assisted or controlled breathing; hospital inpatient/observation, initial day
94003	Ventilation assist and management, initiation of pressure or volume preset ventilators for assisted or controlled breathing; hospital inpatient/observation, each subsequent day
94660	Continuous positive airway pressure ventilation (CPAP) initiation and management
94662	Continuous negative pressure ventilation initiation and management
94760	Noninvasive ear or pulse oximetry for oxygen saturation; single determination
94761	Noninvasive ear or pulse oximetry for oxygen saturation; multiple determinations (e.g., during exercise)
94762	Noninvasive ear or pulse oximetry for oxygen saturation; by continuous overnight monitoring (separate procedure)

Inpatient Neonatal and Pediatric Critical Care (99468–99476)

E/M Code	Patient Status	Type of Visit
99468	Critically ill neonate, aged 28 days or less	Initial inpatient
99469	Critically ill neonate, aged 28 days or less	Subsequent inpatient
99471	Critically ill infant or young child, aged 29 days to 24 months	Initial inpatient
99472	Critically ill infant or young child, aged 29 days to 24 months	Subsequent inpatient
99475	Critically ill infant or young child, two to five years	Initial inpatient
99476	Critically ill infant or young child, two to five years	Subsequent inpatient

General Guidelines

- The same definitions for critical care services apply, regardless of the age of the patient. See "General Guidelines" for codes 99291–99292 for additional information. Note that codes 99291–99292 should not be reported by the same provider or different provider of the same specialty and group when neonatal or pediatric critical care services are reported for the same patient on the same date of service; however, these codes may be reported when the services are reported by a provider of a different specialty whether that provider is part of the same group or not, on the same date of service as neonatal or pediatric critical care services were reported.
- Critical care face-to-face transport or supervisory services may be reported by the same or different provider on the same date of service as neonatal or pediatric critical care services are reported for the same patient.
- Critical care services provided to a pediatric patient who is six years of age or older are reported using the time-based, critical care codes 99291–99292.
- Unlike the adult critical care codes, these codes are not measured in time but by day. Report "initial" care for the first day of services and "subsequent" care for the following day or days.
- Codes 99468–99476 include the following management, monitoring, and treatment services, which cannot be billed separately:
  - respiratory
  - pharmacologic control of the circulatory system
  - enteral and parenteral nutrition
  - metabolic and hematologic maintenance
  - parent/family counseling
  - case management services

Key Point

Use 99184 to report selective head or total body hypothermia in critically ill neonates.

- Codes 99468 and 99469 are used to represent care starting with the date of admission (99468) to a critical care unit and subsequent day(s) (99469) that the neonate or infant remains critical. They may only be reported by one physician and only once per day, per patient.
- If a neonate or infant is readmitted to the critical care unit during the same day or same stay, report the subsequent day code 99469 for the first day of readmission, and 99469 for each subsequent day following readmission.
- Codes 99471–99476 may only be reported by one physician and only once per day, per patient. If readmitted to the pediatric critical care unit during the same day or same stay, report the subsequent day code, 99472 or 99476, for the first day of readmission and for each subsequent day following readmission.
- Report codes 99468, 99471, and 99475 only once per hospital stay.
- For a critically ill neonate or pediatric patient transferred to another provider in a different group and to a lower level of care within the same facility, the transferring provider should report a subsequent hospital care code 99231–99233 or time-based critical service 99291–99292. The provider taking over care reports subsequent intensive care services 99478–99480 or a subsequent hospital care code 99231–99233, as appropriate.
- Personal direct supervision of the health care team in the performance of cognitive and procedural activities.
- In addition to the services included in critical care codes 99291–99292, these codes include the following procedures:

31500	Intubation, endotracheal, emergency procedure
36000	Introduction of needle or intracatheter, vein
36140	Introduction of needle or intracatheter; extremity artery
36400	Venipuncture, younger than age 3 years, necessitating physician's skill, not to be used for routine venipuncture; femoral or jugular vein
36405	Venipuncture, younger than age 3 years, necessitating physician's skill, not to be used for routine venipuncture; scalp vein

36406	Venipuncture, younger than age 3 years, necessitating physician's skill, not to be used for routine venipuncture; other vein
36420	Venipuncture, cutdown; under age 1 year
36430	Transfusion, blood or blood components
36440	Push transfusion, blood, 2 years or under
36510	Catheterization of umbilical vein for diagnosis and therapy, newborn
36555	Insertion of non-tunneled centrally inserted central venous catheter; younger than 5 years of age
36600	Arterial puncture, withdrawal of blood for diagnosis
36620	Arterial catheterization or cannulation for sampling, monitoring, or transfusion; percutaneous
36660	Catheterization, umbilical artery, newborn, for diagnosis or therapy
43752	Naso or orogastric tube placement, necessitating physician's skill
51100	Aspiration of bladder by needle
51701	Insertion of non indwelling bladder catheter
51702	Insertion of temporary indwelling bladder catheter; simple
62270	Spinal puncture, lumbar, diagnostic
94002	Ventilation assist and management, initiation of pressure or volume preset ventilators for assisted or controlled breathing; hospital inpatient/observation, initial day
94003	Ventilation assist and management, initiation of pressure or volume preset ventilators for assisted or controlled breathing; hospital inpatient/observation, each subsequent day
94004	Ventilation assist and management, initiation of pressure or volume preset ventilators for assisted or controlled breathing; nursing facility, per day
94375	Respiratory flow volume loop
94610	Intrapulmonary surfactant administration by a physician through endotracheal tube
94660	Continuous positive airway pressure ventilation (CPAP), initiation and management
94760	Noninvasive ear or pulse oximetry for oxygen saturation; single determination
94761	Noninvasive ear or pulse oximetry for oxygen saturation; multiple determinations
94762	Noninvasive ear or pulse oximetry for oxygen saturation; by continuous overnight monitoring
94780	Car seat/bed testing for airway integrity, neonate, with continual nursing observation and continuous recording of pulse oximetry, heart rate and respiratory rate, with interpretation and report; 60 minutes
94781	each additional full 30 minutes (List separately in additional to code for primary procedure)

These services are considered bundled into codes 99468–99476 and are therefore not separately billable:

- Any services performed that are not shown in the above listings should be reported separately.
- Unlike codes 99291 and 99292, Medicare considers codes 99468–99476 as "inpatient only" codes, and no APC payment will be made for them in an outpatient setting.
- For initiation of selective head or total body hypothermia in a critically ill neonate, report 99184. Included services may be reported separately by the facility.

Newborn and Pediatric Services

Initial and Continuing intensive Care Services (99477–99480)

E/M Code	Patient Status	Type of Visit
99477	Neonate, aged 28 days or less	Initial inpatient care for the neonate requiring intensive observation, frequent interventions, and other intensive care services who is not critically ill
99478	Infant with present body weight of less than 1500 grams, no longer critically ill	Subsequent inpatient
99479	Infant with present body weight of 1500 - 2500 grams, no longer critically ill	Subsequent inpatient
99480	Infant with present body weight of 2501-5000 grams, no longer critically ill	Subsequent inpatient

General Guidelines

- These services are not used to report the care of a normal newborn.
- These services are not used to report the care of a critically ill neonate.
- Inpatient care of a neonate not requiring intensive observation, interventions, or other services, weighing more than 5,000 grams, is reported with the inpatient treatment codes 99221–99233.
- Do not use 99477 to report services for an infant older than 28 days.
- Subsequent intensive care codes are reported based upon patient weight.
- These patients may require:
  - cardiac monitoring
  - respiratory monitoring
  - vital sign monitoring
  - heat maintenance
  - nutritional management
  - oxygen monitoring
  - laboratory evaluations
  - constant observations
- These codes include the same procedures that are listed under the critical codes (99291–99292) and the neonatal and pediatric inpatient critical care codes (99468–99476).

Newborn and Pediatric Services

Knowledge Assessment Chapter 15

See chapter 21 for answers and rationale.

1. Patients from birth to 28 days of age are considered newborns when assigning codes 99460–99486.
   a. True
   b. False
2. What codes would be used to report physician attendance of a critically ill infant less than 24 months of age being transported to the hospital?
   a. 99485–99486
   b. 99466–99467
   c. 99291–99292
   d. None of the above
3. What codes are used to report critical care services of a 3-year-old patient?
   a. 99291 and 99292
   b. 99468 and 99469
   c. 99475 and 99476
   d. 99471 and 99472
4. Subsequent *intensive* critical care codes (99478–99480), are determined based on the patient's body weight.
   a. True
   b. False
5. What code is reported when a newborn is admitted and discharged in the hospital or birthing center on the same date of service?
   a. 99460
   b. 99461
   c. 99462
   d. 99463
6. Adult critical care codes are reported based on the amount of time spent with the patient. What factors determine which neonatal or pediatric critical care code is appropriate?
   a. Type of visit (initial or subsequent)
   b. Time
   c. Age
   d. a and c

Chapter 16. Care Plan and Care Management Services (99483–99494)

Cognitive Assessment and Care Plan Services (99483)

E/M Code	Intent of Service	Face-to-Face Visit	Time Spent
99483	Assessment of and care planning for a patient with cognitive impairment, requiring an independent historian, in the office or other outpatient, home or domiciliary or rest home, with several required elements	Patient and/or family/caregiver	60 min. on average

General Guidelines

- These services are provided for new or existing patients that display signs of cognitive impairment that require a comprehensive assessment to determine a specific diagnosis, etiology, and severity of the impairment.
- All of the following elements must be performed in order to report this code.
  - cognition-focused evaluation that includes a relevant history and physical exam
  - medical decision making of moderate to high complexity
  - assessment of performance of activities of daily living, including decision-making capabilities
  - use of standardized tests (e.g., FAST, CDR) to determine the stage of dementia
  - medication reconciliation and review of high-risk medications
  - evaluation, including standardized tests, for neuropsychiatric and behavioral symptoms, such as depression
  - evaluation of patient safety in the home and operating a motor vehicle
  - identification of caregiver, the caregivers abilities, needs, support, and willingness to take on caregiving tasks
  - review, develop, update, or revise an advance care plan
  - creation of a written care plan that includes:
    - initial plans to address neuropsychiatric issues, neurocognitive issues, and functional limitations
    - referral to community resources as needed
    - initial education and support provided to the patient and/or caregiver
- Provider typically spends 60 minutes face to face with the patient and/or caregiver.
- A single provider can only report 99483 once every 180 days for a given patient.
- This service includes assessment of medical and psychosocial issues that may contribute to increased morbidity.
- This code further defines what cognition-relevant history may be considered, as well as other factors contributing to the patient's cognitive impairment that this service includes:
  - psychoactive medication
  - infection
  - chronic pain syndromes
  - depression
  - tumor
  - stroke
  - normal pressure hydrocephalus
  - other brain disease
- Report prolonged services code 99417 when the service runs 15 minutes beyond the time specified in the CPT® code narrative. The time must be clearly documented in the medical record. For Medicare, report prolonged services code G2212 when the service runs 15 or more minutes beyond the total time.
- Code 99483 should not be reported on the same date of service as the following services: 99202–99205, 99211–99215, 99242–99245, 99341–99345, 99347–99350, 99366–99368, 99497–99498, 90785, 90791–90792, 96127, 96146, 96160–96161, or 99605–99607.

Issues in This Code Range

- This code should not be reported if all of the required elements listed above are not performed or are considered unnecessary to assess the patient's condition. In these circumstances, an appropriate evaluation and management service should be reported instead.

Chronic and Complex Care Management Services (99490, 99439, 99491, 99437, 99487, 99489, 99424–99427)

E/M Code	Intent of Service	Face-to-Face Visit	Time Spent
99490	Chronic care management services, first 20 minutes of clinical staff time directed by a physician or other qualified health care professional, per calendar month	No	20 min.
99439	Chronic care management services, each additional 20 minutes of clinical staff time directed by a physician or other qualified health care professional, per calendar month	No	Each additional 20 min.
99491	Chronic care management services, first 30 minutes provided personally by a physician or other qualified health care professional, per calendar month	No	30 min.
99437	Chronic care management services, each additional 30 minutes by a physician or other qualified health care professional, per calendar month	No	Each additional 30 min.
99487	Complex chronic care management services directed by a physician or other qualified health care professional, per calendar month	No	60–89 min.
99489	Complex chronic care management services directed by a physician or other qualified health care professional, per calendar month	n/a	Each additional 30 min.
99424	Principal care management services, for a single high-risk disease, first 30 minutes provided personally by a physician or other qualified health care professional, per calendar month	No	30 min.
99425	Principal care management services, for a single high-risk disease, each additional 30 minutes provided personally by a physician or other qualified health care professional, per calendar month	No	Each additional 30 min.
99426	Principal care management services, for a single high-risk disease, first 30 minutes of clinical staff time directed by a physician or other qualified health care professional, per calendar month	No	30 min.
99427	Principal care management services, for a single high-risk disease, each additional 30 minutes of clinical staff time directed by a physician or other qualified health care professional, per calendar month	No	Each additional 30 min.

General Guidelines

- These services are generally provided for chronically ill patients with continuous or episodic health conditions.
- These patients live at home or in an assisted living facility, domiciliary, or rest home. The services are not reported by location like other coordination services and are in part performed by clinical staff.
- To report face-to-face visits by the physician that are performed in the same month as 99487, use the appropriate E/M code(s).
- For 99426, 99427, 99490, 99439, 99487, and 99489, the clinical staff develops, implements, and many times substantially revises and monitors the care plan under the direction of the physician or other qualified health care professional.
- Use 99491 and 99437 to report chronic care management services provided directly by the physician or other qualified health care professional.
- Complex chronic care management (CCCM) patients require coordination of multiple medical specialties and services and moderate or high medical decision making (MDM). In addition, they have multiple illnesses and medications, are unable to perform daily activities, require a caregiver, and have repeat visits to the emergency room and hospital admissions.
- CCCM codes further define what a typical adult patient and a pediatric patient would require to support the use of these codes.
- An adult patient:
  - takes or receives three or more prescription medications
  - may receive therapeutic interventions such as physical or occupational therapy
  - has two or more chronic continuous or episodic health conditions. The duration of their conditions is expected to be at least 12 months or until the death of the patient, or the conditions place the patient at a significant risk of death, acute exacerbation/decompensation, or functional decline.
- A pediatric patient:
  - takes or receives three or more prescription medications or therapeutic interventions (e.g., medications, nutritional support, respiratory therapy)
  - has two or more chronic continuous or episodic health conditions. The duration of their conditions is expected to be at least 12 months or until the death of the patient, or the conditions place the patient at a significant risk of death, acute exacerbation/decompensation, or functional decline.

- Principal care management services require one complex chronic condition that is expected to last at least three months, places the patient at significant risk of acute exacerbation, hospitalization, functional decline, or death. Requires development, monitoring, and/or revision of a care plan, including frequent medication adjustments and/or management of the condition is extremely complex due to comorbidities.
- Care management services are provided by a physician, other qualified health care professional, or clinical staff when directed by a physician or other qualified health care professional.
- Services that may be provided by the clinical staff include:
  - assessment and support for treatment regimen adherence and medication management
  - collection of health outcomes data and registry documentation
  - communication with home health agencies and other community services the patient may utilize
  - communication and engagement with patient, family members, caretaker or guardian, surrogate decision makers, and/or other professionals regarding aspects of care
  - development, communication and maintenance of a comprehensive care plan
  - facilitating access to care and services needed by the patient and/or family
  - identification of available community and health resources
  - patient and/or family/caretaker education to support self-management, independent living, and activities of daily living
  - ongoing review of patient status, including review of laboratory and other studies not reported as part of an E/M service
  - management of care transitions not reported separately with transitional care management codes 99495 or 99496
- A care plan should be designed around the physical, mental, cognitive, social, functional, and environmental needs of the patient after an assessment or reassessment as well as an inventory of resources and supports available.
- Care plan elements should be addressed when applicable for the patient, these include, but are not limited to, the following:
  - problem list
  - prognosis
  - expected outcome
  - measurable treatment objectives
  - management of patient symptoms
  - medical management
  - planned interventions
  - cognitive assessment
  - functional assessment
  - advance directives summary
  - environmental evaluation
  - assessment of caregivers
  - interaction and coordination with outside resources and health care professionals and others
  - summary of advance directives
- The following services may not be reported in addition to 99437, 99439, 99487, 99489, 99490 or 99491 in the same 30-day period by a physician or other qualified health care professional:
  - care plan oversight (99374–99380)
  - ESRD related services (90951–90970)
  - principal care management (99424–99427)
  - medication therapy management (99605–99607)
- Code 99439, 99490, 99437, and 99491 should not be reported together or with 99487 or 99489 in the same calendar month.
- The following services may not be reported in addition to 99424, 99425, 99426, or 99427 in the same 30-day period by a physician or other qualified health care professional:
  - care plan oversight (99374-99380)
  - ESRD related services (90951-90970)
  - medication therapy management (99605-99607)
- Do not report 99424 or 99425 with 99426, 99427, 99437, 99439, 99487, 99489, 99490, or 99491.
- A care management office or practice is required to have the following capabilities:
  - 24/7 access for physicians or other qualified health care professionals or clinical staff to provide patients and/or caregivers the ability to connect with health care professionals in order to address immediate needs, regardless of the time of day or day of the week
  - continuing care with a specified care team member with whom the patient can schedule consecutive, routine appointments
  - timely access and management for follow-up care upon discharge from an emergency department or facility
  - electronic health record system usage to ensure timely access to clinical information
  - ability to engage and educate patients and caregivers in addition to coordinating care among all appropriate service professionals for each patient
  - reporting provider to supervise activities of the care team
  - clinical integration of all care team members that provide services to the patient
- Care management services codes factor in both face-to-face and non-face-to-face time spent by the clinical staff in communicating with the patient and/or the patient's family, caregiver, as well as other professionals and agencies to

determine the total amount of time. Additionally, documentation and implementation of the care plan and the teaching of self-management, when appropriate are also required components to report these services.

- Report these services once per calendar month. Only count the time of one clinical staff member when two or more clinical staff members are discussing the patient. Do not count any clinical staff time for a particular day if the physician or other qualified health care professional reports an E/M service.
- It is not appropriate to report these services when the care plan remains unchanged or required only minimal revisions such as a change in medication.
- If the physician or other qualified health care professional provides face-to-face visits in the month, these visits should be reported with the appropriate E/M code.
- These codes should not be reported by the surgeon if the services he or she rendered are within a global surgery period of the surgical procedure performed.
- In the event that a physician or qualified health care professional performs any of the clinical staff activities described in these codes, his/her time may be counted towards the clinical staff time to meet the requirements of the elements of the code.
- For chronic care management provided by clinical staff, assign the correct code according to the following guidelines:
  - less than 20 minutes not reported separately
  - 20–39 minutes 99490
  - 40–59 minutes 99490 and 99439 x 1
  - 60 minutes or more 99490 and 99439 x 2
- For chronic care management provided by the physician or other qualified health care professional, assign the correct code according to the following guidelines:
  - less than 30 minutes not reported separately
  - 30-59 minutes 99491
  - 60-89 minutes 99491 and 99437 x 1
  - 90 minutes or more 99491 and 99437 x 2 or more for each additional 30 minutes
- For complex chronic care management assign the correct code according to the following guidelines:
  - less than 60 minutes not reported separately
  - 60–89 minutes 99487
  - 90–119 minutes 99487 and 99489 x 1
  - 120 minutes or more 99487 and 99489 x 2 or more for each additional 30 minutes
- For principal care management provided by the clinical staff, assign the correct code according to the following guidelines:
  - less than 30 minutes not reported separately
  - 30-59 minutes 99426
  - 60-89 minutes 99426 and 99427 x 1
  - 90-119 minutes 99426 and 99427 x 2
  - 120 minutes or more 99426 and 99427 x 3 or more for each additional 30 minutes
- For principal care management provided by the physician or other qualified health care professional, assign the correct code according to the following guidelines:
  - less than 30 minutes not reported separately
  - 30-59 minutes 99424
  - 60-89 minutes 99424 and 99425 x 1
  - 90-119 minutes 99424 and 99425 x 2
  - 120 minutes or more 99424 and 99425 x 3 or more for each additional 30 minutes
- Code 99490 is reported for the first 20 minutes of clinical staff time spent in care coordination activities during the calendar month.
- Code 99439 is reported for each additional 20 minutes of clinical staff time spent in care coordination activities during the calendar month.
- Code 99439 or 99427 should not be reported more than twice per calendar month.
- Code 99491 is reported for the first 30 minutes of physician or other qualified health care professional time is spent in care coordination activities during the calendar month.
- Code 99437 is reported for each additional 30 minutes spent by a physician or other qualified health care professional on chronic care management services during the calendar month.
- Chronic care coordination services of less than 20 minutes, in a calendar month, are not reported separately.
- Care management services are reportable in any month when clinical staff time requirements have been satisfied.
- Care management services which restart following a discharge during a *new* month begin a new period or the provider may use the transitional care management codes (99495–99496), as appropriate.
- For a discharge that occurs in the *same* month, continue the reporting period or use the transitional care management codes (99495–99496).

Behavioral Health Intervention Services (99492–99494, 99484)

E/M Code	Intent of Service	Face-to-Face Visit	Time Spent
99492	Initial psychiatric collaborative care management, first 70 minutes in the first calendar month of behavioral health care manager activities, in consultation with a psychiatric consultant, and directed by the treating provider	No	36–85 min.
99493	Subsequent psychiatric collaborative care management, first 60 minutes in a subsequent month of behavioral health care manager activities, in consultation with a psychiatric consultant, and directed by the treating provider	No	31–75 min.
99494	Initial or subsequent psychiatric collaborative care management, each additional 30 minutes in a calendar month of behavioral health care manager activities, in consultation with a psychiatric consultant, and directed by the treating provider	N/A	Each additional 30 min.
99484	Care management services for behavioral health conditions, at least 20 minutes of clinical staff time, directed by a physician or other qualified health care professional, per calendar month	Face to face or non-face-to-face	A minimum of 20 min.

General Guidelines

- Codes 99492, 99493, and 99494 are used for patients with common psychiatric conditions, such as depression, anxiety disorders, post-traumatic stress disorders, and substance use disorders, that are treated in a primary care or other specialty setting by a care team.
- Codes 99492, 99493, and 99494 are reported by the treating provider for a calendar month and include the services of the treating physician or other qualified health care professional, a behavioral care manager and a psychiatric consultant.
- The initiating encounter must be performed face to face by the treating provider and the behavioral health care manager must be available to provide face-to-face visits if necessary. There are no other requirements for in-person encounters.
- The behavioral health care manager is a designated individual with formal education or specialized training in behavioral health that provides coordination services, assesses needs, develops a plan of care, maintains the registry, must be available to provide face-to-face services with the patient, and has a collaborative, integrated relationship with the treating physician and psychiatric consultant.
- The psychiatric consultant must be trained in psychiatry or behavioral health and be qualified to prescribe the full range of medication. The psychiatric consultant advises and makes treatment recommendations to the behavioral health care manager and/or the treating provider, including:
  - referrals to specialty services
  - psychiatric and other medical diagnoses
  - medical management of complications due to treatment of psychiatric disorders
  - medication management
- To report 99492, the following services must be performed:
  - outreach to and engagement in treatment of a patient directed by the treating provider
  - initial patient assessment, including administration of validated rating scales, with the development of an individualized treatment plan
  - review by a psychiatric consultant with plan changes if recommended
  - entering the patient in a registry and using the registry to track the patient's progress and follow-up, with appropriate documentation, and participation in weekly caseload consultation with the psychiatric consultant
  - providing brief interventions using evidence-based methods such as behavioral activation, motivational interviewing, and other focused treatment plans
- To report 99493, the following services must be performed:
  - using the registry to track patient progress and follow-up, with appropriate documentation
  - participation in weekly caseload consultation with the psychiatric consultant
  - ongoing collaboration and coordination of the patient's mental wellbeing with the treating provider and any other treating mental health providers
  - additional review of progress and recommendations of changes in treatment, as necessary, including medication changes, based on recommendations provided by the psychiatric consultant
  - using validated rating scales to monitor patient outcomes
  - providing brief interventions using evidence-based methods, such as behavioral activation, motivational interviewing, and other focused treatment plans
  - relapse prevention planning with patients who achieve remission of symptoms or other treatment goals and are ready for discharge from active treatment
- The time thresholds are based on total time over a calendar month.

- For psychiatric collaborative care coordination services, assign the correct code according to the following guidelines:
  - initial services less than 36 minutes are not reported separately
  - initial services 36–85 minutes — 99492
  - initial services 86–115 minutes — 99492 and 99494 x 1
  - subsequent services less than 31 minutes are not reported separately
  - subsequent services 31–75 minutes — 99493
  - subsequent services 76–105 minutes — 99493 and 99494 x 1
  - report 99494 for each additional increment up to 30 minutes for initial and subsequent services
- The treating provider supervises the patient's care, including referring the patient to specialty care when applicable, prescribing medication, and providing treatment for medical conditions.
- The treating provider may report evaluation and management (E/M) and other services separately within the same calendar month.
- Do not report 99492 and 99493 in the same calendar month.
- Typically 99492–99494 would not be reported by a psychiatrist because the psychiatrist's work is defined as a subcomponent of these behavioral services codes.
- Code 99484 is used to report general behavioral health integration (BHI) care coordination services reported by the supervising physician or other qualified health care professional.
- The supervising/reporting provider for the BHI service must perform the initial evaluation and management service.
- BHI services are typically performed by the clinical staff but may be provided solely by the reporting provider. Services require face-to-face and non-face-to-face care coordination services that must total 20 minutes or more in a calendar month.
- To report 99484, the following services must be performed:
  - initial assessment or follow-up monitoring, including the use of applicable validated rating scales
  - behavioral health care planning in relation to behavioral/ psychiatric health problems, including revising plans for patients who are not improving or whose status change
  - facilitating and coordinating treatment such as psychotherapy, pharmacotherapy, counseling, and/or psychiatric consultation
  - continuity of care with a designated member of the care team
- Code 99484 is reported when at least 20 minutes of clinical staff time is spent in general behavioral health care coordination activities during the calendar month.
- General behavioral health integration care coordination activities of less than 20 minutes in a calendar month are not reported separately.
- Code 99484 may be used in any outpatient setting, as long as the clinical staff is available for face-to-face encounters with the patient, and the reporting provider has an ongoing relationship with the patient and clinical staff.
- The same provider should not report 99484 in addition to 99492, 99493, and 99494 in the same calendar month.
- All bulleted items listed for 99484, 99492, and 99493 must be performed and documented and the specific time thresholds met in order to report these codes.
- Time spent in the emergency department coordinating care may be counted toward the time elements for 99484, 99492, 99493, and 99494. However, time spent while the patient is an inpatient or admitted to observation status may not be reported using 99484, 99492, 99493, and 99494.
- When the treating/supervising provider performs the activities of the behavioral health care manager and is not counting these activities toward another service, this time may be added to the total time thresholds used to report 99484, 99492, 99493, and 99494.

Knowledge Assessment Chapter 16

See chapter 21 for answers and rationale.

1. A patient's chart indicates that 15 minutes of chronic care management services were provided for the month. What code would be reported for this service?
   a. 99490
   b. 99487
   c. 99489
   d. The service is not reportable
2. Care management services include both face-to-face and non-face-to-face time spent by clinical staff with the patient, caregiver, or other professionals and agencies involved in the patient's care.
   a. True
   b. False
3. Which of the following would be included in the care plan documentation for chronic care management?
   a. Expected outcomes
   b. Medication management
   c. Planned interventions
   d. All of the above
4. Care management services may only be provided by a physician or other qualified health care professional.
   a. True
   b. False
5. There are 10 required elements listed in the description for code 99483. For this patient only eight were performed. What code should be reported for the services provided?
   a. 99483-52
   b. 99483
   c. Another appropriate E/M code
   d. None of the above
6. Behavioral health intervention codes 99484, 99492, and 99493, may only be reported once by the same provider in a calendar month.
   a. True
   b. False
7. A patient's chart indicates that a total of 1 hour and 30 minutes of subsequent psychiatric collaborative care management services was provided for the calendar month. Which code(s) would be reported for these services?
   a. 99492 and 99494 x 1
   b. 99493
   c. 99492 and 99493
   d. 99493 and 99494 x 1
8. Psychiatric collaborative care management services are provided by a care team that includes a treating provider, a behavioral health care manager, and a psychiatric consultant. Which care team member reports codes 99492, 99493, and 99494 for the services provided?
   a. Behavioral health care manager
   b. Treating provider
   c. Psychiatric consultant
   d. Each provider reports his or her own services
9. General behavioral health integration management services of less than 20 minutes are not reportable.
   a. True
   b. False

Chapter 17. Transitional Care Management Services (99495–99496)

E/M Code	Medical Decision Making	Intent of Service	Patient Presence	Medical Decision Making	Face-to-Face Visit Within 7 Days	Face-to-Face Visit Within 8 to 14 Days
99495	Moderate complexity	Transitional care management services with these required elements: communication (direct contact, telephone, electronic), within 2 business days of discharge	Patient or caregiver present	Moderate complexity	99495	99495
99496	High complexity	Transitional care management services with these required elements: communication (direct contact, telephone, electronic), within 2 business days of discharge	Patient or caregiver present	High complexity	99496	99495

Coding Axiom

The Centers for Medicare and Medicaid Services (CMS) established a facility and nonfacility payment for transitional care management services. Practitioners should report these services with the appropriate place of service code for the face-to-face visit.

General Guidelines

- Transitional care management (TCM) services are provided to new and established patients that are transitioning from an inpatient facility, partial hospital, observation status, or skilled nursing facility to an assisted living facility, home, domiciliary, or a rest home. The medical and psychological issues these patients may have necessitate a moderate or high level of medical decision making.
- TCM requires a face-to-face visit (first visit is included in the TCM service and is not reported separately), initial patient contact, and medication reconciliation within a specific time frame.
- The services are provided by a physician, other qualified health care professional, or clinical staff when directed by a physician or other qualified health care professional.
- Code 99495 requires one face-to-face visit within 14 calendar days of discharge.
- Code 99496 requires one face-to-face visit within seven calendar days of discharge.
- The required face-to-face visit must be performed by the physician or other qualified health care professional.
- The 30-day transitional care management (TCM) period begins on the date the beneficiary is discharged from the inpatient hospital setting and continues for the next 29 days. During the 30-day period, the following three TCM components must be furnished, per CMS:
  - interactive contact—The provider is required to make an interactive contact with the beneficiary and/or caregiver, as appropriate, within two business days following the patient's discharge. The contact may be via telephone, email, or face to face. If two or more separate attempts to communicate with the patient or caregiver are made but are unsuccessful and all other criteria for TCM codes are met, the service may be reported. Per CMS guidelines, providers may not bill the TCM codes if there was not a successful communication within the 30-day period between the facility discharge and the date of service for the post-discharge TCM code.
  - non-face-to-face services—The provider must furnish non-face-to-face services to the patient unless the services are determined to be not medically indicated or necessary. Certain non-face-to-face services may be furnished by licensed clinical staff under the provider's direction.
  - face-to-face visit—One face-to-face visit must be furnished within certain timeframes as described by codes 99495 (14 days) and 99496 (7 days)
- If the physician or other qualified health care professional provides more than one face-to-face visit in a month, additional visits should be reported with the appropriate E/M code.
- Services that may be provided by the physician or other qualified health care professional include:
  - assistance in scheduling any required follow-up with community providers and services
  - education of the patient, family, caregiver, and/or guardian.
  - establishment or re-establishment of referrals and arranging for needed community resources
  - interaction with other providers who will assume or reassume care of the patient's system-specific problems
  - obtaining and reviewing the discharge information (discharge summary or continuity of care documents)
  - reviewing the need for or follow-up on pending diagnostic tests and treatments
- Services that may be provided by the clinical staff include:

- assessment and support for treatment regimen adherence and medication management
- communication with home health agencies and other community services the patient may use
- communication with patient, family members, caretaker or guardian, surrogate decision makers, and/or other professionals regarding aspects of care
- facilitating access to care and services needed by the patient and/or family
- identification of available community and health resources
- patient and/or family/caretaker education to support self-management, independent living, and activities of daily living (ADL)

- Do not report these services with 99421–99423 for the same time period.
- These codes should not be reported by the surgeon if the services he or she rendered are within a global surgery period of the surgical procedure performed.
- If another provider reports these services during a postoperative period of a surgical procedure, modifier 54 is not required.
- Append modifier 95 to indicate that the E/M service was rendered to a patient at a distant site via a real-time interactive audio and video telecommunications system. The communication between the physician or other qualified health care professional and the patient should be commensurate with the same key components or requirements of those that would be required if the service had been rendered in a face-to-face setting.
- These services may be reported only one time within 30 days of discharge and by only one provider.

Knowledge Assessment Chapter 17

See chapter 21 for answers and rationale.

1. Transitional care services may only be reported when a face-to-face visit by a physician or other qualified health care professional has been performed.
   a. True
   b. False
2. When does the 30-day transitional care management period begin?
   a. The day after the patient is discharged from the inpatient setting
   b. The day the patient is discharged from the inpatient setting
   c. The day the physician performs the face-to-face visit
   d. The first Monday following discharge
3. If the physician or other qualified health care professional provides more than one face-to-face visit in a month, these services are included in the transitional care codes and are not separately reportable.
   a. True
   b. False
4. Transitional care management services require interactive contact with the patient or caregiver within how many business days of discharge?
   a. Seven
   b. Two
   c. One
   d. Five
5. Which of the following are acceptable methods of communication for the required interactive contact? Select all that apply.
   a. Telephone
   b. Mail
   c. Face to face
   d. E-mail

Transitional Care Service

Chapter 18. Advance Care Planning (99497–99498)

E/M Code	Intent of Service	Health Care Face-to-Face Visit	Time Spent
99497	Advance care planning including the explanation and discussion of advance directives such as standard forms (with completion of such forms, when performed), by the physician or other qualified health care professional	Yes	Initial 30 min.
99498	Advance care planning including the explanation and discussion of advance directives such as standard forms (with completion of such forms, when performed), by the physician or other qualified health care professional	Yes	Each additional 30 min.

General Guidelines

- These codes describe counseling and discussion of advance care directives with the patient, family members, and/or surrogate that may or may not include completion of pertinent legal documents.
- No active management of the patient's problems is undertaken for the time period reported when these codes are used.
- Codes 99497–99498 should not be reported on the same date of service as the following E/M services: 99291–99292, 99468–99469, 99471–99472, 99475–99480, and 99483. However, these codes may be separately reported when performed on the same date of service in conjunction with the following E/M services: 99202–99215, 99221–99223, 99231–99236, 99238–99239, 99242–99245, 99252–99255, 99281–99285, 99304–99310, 99315–99316, 99341–99345, 99347–99350, 99381–99397, and 99495–99496.
- An advance directive is described as a written document that the patient uses to appoint a representative as well as to record his or her wishes as they relate to future medical treatment in the event the patient is incapacitated and unable to make decisions on his or her own.
- Types of written advance directives include, but are not limited to:
  - health care proxy
  - durable power of attorney for health care
  - living will
  - medical orders for life-sustaining treatment (MOLST)

Effective January 1, 2016, CMS made voluntary advance care planning (ACP) services separately payable by Medicare when the ACP is provided on the same date of service and by the same provider that performs the annual wellness visit (AWV). When the ACP and the AWV are provided on the same day, the ACP is considered a preventive service and the coinsurance and deductible are waived. Providers would report code 99497 and 99498, if applicable, for the advance care planning, along with code G0438 or G0439 for the annual wellness visit. Both services must be reported on the same claim with modifier 33 appended to the ACP service. **Note:** When the ACP is performed on a different date of service than the AWV or by a different provider, the coinsurance and deductible would apply. For more information on HCPCS Level II G codes, see chapter 19.

Information pertaining to the ACP change may be found at:
https://www.cms.gov/Regulations-and-Guidance/Guidance/Transmittals/Downloads/R216BP.pdf.

Knowledge Assessment Chapter 18

See chapter 21 for answers and rationale.

1. Which range of E/M codes should not be reported with 99497–99498 on the same date of service?
   a. 99202–99215
   b. 99304–99310
   c. 99381–99397
   d. 99475–99480
2. The physician provides active management of the patient's problems as part of the advance care planning.
   a. True
   b. False

Chapter 19. HCPCS G Codes and Evaluation and Management Services

Medicare Covered Care Plan Oversight Services (G0179–G0182)

HCPCS Code	Medicare Covered CPO Services	Place of Service	Under Care of	Presence of Patient	Time
G0179	Physician recertification for Medicare-covered home health services under a home health plan of care (patient not present), including contacts with home health agency and review of reports of patient status required by physicians to affirm the initial implementation of the plan of care that meets patient's needs, per recertification period	In home, a domiciliary or equivalent environment (e.g., Alzheimer's facility)	Home health agency	Patient not present	N/A
G0180	Physician certification for Medicare-covered home health services under a home health plan of care (patient not present), including contacts with home health agency and review of reports of patient status required by physicians to affirm the initial implementation of the plan of care that meets patient's needs, per recertification period	In home, a domiciliary or equivalent environment (e.g., Alzheimer's facility)	Home health agency	Patient not present	N/A
G0181	Physician supervision of a patient receiving Medicare-covered services provided by a participating home health agency (patient not present) requiring complex and multidisciplinary care modalities involving regular physician development and/or revision of care plans, review of subsequent reports of patient status, review of laboratory and other studies, communication (including telephone calls) with other health care professionals involved in the patient's care, integration of new information into the medical treatment plan and/or adjustment of medical therapy, within a calendar month, 30 minutes or more	In home, a domiciliary or equivalent environment (e.g., Alzheimer's facility)	Home health agency	Patient not present	30 min. or more
G0182	Physician supervision of a patient under a Medicare-approved hospice (patient not present) requiring complex and multidisciplinary care modalities involving regular physician development and/or revision of care plans, review of subsequent reports of patient status, review of laboratory and other studies, communication (including telephone calls) with other health care professionals involved in the patient's care, integration of new information into the medical treatment plan and/or adjustment of medical therapy, within a calendar month, 30 minutes or more	Hospice	Hospice	Patient not present	30 min. or more

General Guidelines

- Care plan oversight (CPO) is physician, or other qualified health care provider, supervision of patients receiving either home health or hospice benefits where complex or multidisciplinary care modalities and ongoing provider involvement are required.
- CMS extended Medicare coverage to allow separate payment for CPO services of or exceeding 30 minutes per month for patients who are receiving Medicare-covered home health or hospice benefits.
- Medicare does not pay for CPO services for nursing facility or skilled nursing facility patients.
- Code descriptors for these codes include communication with family member(s), surrogate decision maker(s) (e.g., legal guardians) and/or key caregivers as well as health care professionals.
- Only one provider, per month, will be paid for CPO services for a patient.
- Codes 99374–99378 are not covered under Medicare. These services should be reported to Medicare with codes G0181 and G0182.
- Care plan oversight provided to Medicare patient's for home health or hospice care plan oversight services are reported with HCPCS Level II codes G0181–G0182.
- Care plan oversight for certification and recertification of home health services are reported with HCPCS Level II codes G0179–G0180.
- Home health certification includes creation of a plan of care and verification that the home health agency complies with the written plan of care.
- The physician must maintain awareness of a patient's ongoing needs and of changes in the patient's condition or medications.

- Code G0180 can only be reported when the patient has not received any Medicare covered home health services for a period of at least 60 days.
- The recertification code G0179 can be reported only when a patient has received services for at least 60 days.
- Code G0179 is to be reported only once every 60 days except in the rare instance whereby a patient starts a new episode of care prior to the end of 60 days and a new plan of care is needed to start the new episode of care.
- Codes G0179–G0182 are reported separately from other E/M services.

Quick Tip

Providers must include their own documentation and may not rely on the orders or chart notes of the care giver to support care plan oversight. Each contact should be documented and include date, contact, orders given or changed, and time spent providing the remote care of the patient.

The following coverage requirements apply to CPO services G0181 and G0182:

- The patient must require complex or multidisciplinary care modalities requiring ongoing provider involvement in the plan of care.
- The provider will review subsequent reports regarding patient status, labs, and other studies during the calendar month, as well as communicate with other health care professionals involved in the patient's care.
- The patient must be receiving Medicare-covered home health or hospice services during the period in which the CPO services are furnished.
- The provider who bills CPO must be the same individual who signed the home health or hospice plan of care.
- CPO services should be reported after the end of the month in which the services were provided.
- No other services should be reported on the same claim form with the CPO service.
- The provider must furnish at least 30 minutes of CPO within the calendar month for which payment is claimed.
- For patients receiving Medicare-covered home health services, the provider must not have a significant financial or contractual interest in the home health agency (HHA).
- For patients receiving Medicare hospice services, the provider must not be the medical director or an employee of the hospice or providing services under arrangements with the hospice.
- The provider billing for the CPO must document in the patient's medical record those services that were furnished, as well as the date and length of time associated with those services.

Coding Axiom

Services that do not count towards the 30-minute required threshold include:

- **Time spent discussing treatment and medication adjustments with the patient, his or her family, or friends**
- **Time spent by staff getting or filing charts**
- **Travel time**
- **Provider time spent calling prescriptions into the pharmacist unless the telephone conversation involves a discussion of pharmaceutical therapies**

Preventive Medicine Services (G0402, G0438–G0439)

E/M Code	Patient Status	Intent of Service	Time
G0402	No complaints	Welcome to Medicare evaluation and management service	Preventive-within first 12 months of coverage effective date
G0438	No complaints	Annual wellness visit with prevention plan services	Initial visit
G0439	No complaints	Annual wellness visit with prevention plan services	Subsequent visit

General Guidelines

- Code G0402 initial preventive physical exam (IPPE) is a preventive evaluation and management service provided to Medicare beneficiaries within the first 12 months of their coverage effective date. If a patient does not receive an IPPE within the first 12 months from their effective date, the patient may receive an annual wellness visit (AWV) with personalized prevention plan services (PPPS) instead.
- Medicare does not cover routine physicals. The IPPE is provided as an introduction to Medicare and enables new beneficiaries to receive important screenings and vaccinations.
- Physicians may measure the patient's body mass index (BMI) and discuss end-of-life planning when necessary.
- Neither the IPPE or AWV are subject to a deductible; however, the IPPE is subject to coinsurance.
- The IPPE face-to-face exam comprises nine individual components:
  - review the patient's medical and social history
  - review the patient's potential risk factors for depression and other mood disorders
  - review the patient's functional ability and level of safety
  - physical examination that includes height, weight, BP, visual acuity, BMI, and other factors as applicable depending on the patient's medical and social history and current clinical standards
  - end-of-life planning
  - review of current prescriptions of opioids
  - screening for potential substance use disorders
  - education, counseling, and referral based on the results of the review and evaluation services described above
  - education, counseling, and referral, including a brief written plan or checklist, for obtaining the appropriate screening or other Part B preventive services

Key Point

Reporting G0402 more than once in a lifetime, or after the initial 12 months or 12 months after the beneficiary's effective date of their first part B coverage period will be denied. Likewise, the initial annual wellness visit (G0438) should only be reported once in a lifetime.

Note: Each component must be provided or referred to another physician in order to appropriately submit this benefit to Medicare.

- HCPCS Level II code G0438 Annual wellness visit; includes a personalized prevention plan of service (PPPS), initial visit
- HCPCS Level II code G0439 Annual wellness visit, includes a personalized prevention plan of service (PPPS), subsequent visit

The AWV can be performed by a physician, physician's assistant, nurse practitioner, or clinical nurse specialist other medical professional as defined by CMS regulations and consists of the following services for the first AWV:

- Health risk assessment
- Establishment of the patient's health history, including family history
- Establishment of the patient's current list of providers and suppliers routinely providing care to the individual
- Measurement of the patient's height, weight, BMI, blood pressure, and other routine measurements as appropriate
- Detection of any cognitive impairment
- Review of any potential risk factors for depression, including current or past experiences with depression or other mood disorders, based on the use of an appropriate screening instrument for persons without a current diagnosis of depression
- Review of the patient's functional ability and level of safety based on direct observation or the use of an appropriate screening questionnaire
- Establishment of a written screening schedule for the individual; i.e., a checklist for the next 5–10 years, as appropriate, based on recommendations of the United States Preventive Services Task Force (USPSTF) and the Advisory Committee on Immunization Practices (ACIP) as well as the patient's health history, screening history, and age appropriate preventive services covered by Medicare

- Establishment of a list of risk factors and conditions for which primary, secondary, or tertiary interventions are recommended or are underway for the patient; including any mental health conditions, or any such risk factors that have been identified through an IPPE, and a list of treatment options and their associated risks and benefits
- Furnishing personalized health advice to the patient and referrals, as appropriate, to health education or preventive counseling services or programs aimed at reducing identified risk factors and improving self-management or community based lifestyle interventions to reduce health risks, encourage self-management and wellness, including weight loss, increasing physical activity, smoking cessation, preventing falls, and good nutrition
- Review of current prescriptions of opioids including identifying risk factors for opioid use disorder, evaluating the severity of pain and the current treatment plan, providing alternative treatment options, and referral to a specialist when necessary
- Screening for potential substance use disorders to identify any need for treatment and a referral if necessary
- Advance care planning services at the patient's discretion to discuss future health care decisions, identify potential caregivers, and explain advance directives such as a living will, health care proxy, or health care power of attorney
- Other service element(s) as determined appropriate by the HHS secretary through national coverage determinations (NCD)

The following are elements to be included in a subsequent AWV:

- Update of Health Risk Assessment
- Update of medical and family history
- Measurement of the patient's height, weight, BMI, blood pressure, and other routine measurements, as appropriate
- Update to the patient's current list of providers and suppliers routinely providing care to the individual
- Detection of any cognitive impairment
- Update of the list of risk factors and conditions for which primary, secondary, or tertiary interventions are recommended or are underway for the patient
- Personalized health advice furnished to the patient and a referral, as applicable, to health education or preventive counseling services or programs
- Update of the written screening schedule for the patient
- Review of current prescriptions of opioids including identifying risk factors for opioid use disorder, evaluating the severity of pain and the current treatment plan, providing alternative treatment options, and referral to a specialist when necessary
- Screening for potential substance use disorders to identify any need for treatment and a referral if necessary
- Advance care planning services at the patient's discretion to discuss future health care decisions, identify potential caregivers, and explain advance directives such as a living will, health care proxy, or health care power of attorney

CMS created "quick reference" tools that function as a checklist for providers to ensure that all of the details of the specific elements of each visit type are documented appropriately. Copies of these documents can be downloaded from the following URLS: https://www.cms.gov/Outreach-and-Education/Medicare-Learning-Network-MLN/MLNProducts/preventive-services/medicare-wellness-visits.html.

Additional information on both the IPPE and AWV can be found at: https://www.cms.gov/Medicare/Prevention/PrevntionGenInfo/ProviderResources.html.

For prolonged preventive services provided to Medicare beneficiaries, G0513 may be reported separately for the first 30 minutes beyond the usual service time and G0514 may be reported for each additional 30 minutes of service.

Telehealth Follow-up Inpatient Consultation Services (G0406–G0408)

HCPCS Code	Medical Decision Making	History	Exam	Counseling and/or Coordination of Care	Time Spent Communicating with the Patient via Telehealth
G0406	Straightforward or low complexity	Problem-focused interval history	Problem-focused exam	Consistent with problems and patient's or family's needs	15 min.
G0407	Moderate complexity	Expanded interval history	Expanded problem-focused exam	Consistent with problems and patient's or family's needs	25 min.
G0408	High complexity	Detailed interval history	Detailed	Consistent with problems and patient's or family's needs	35 min.

General Guidelines

- Note that the general guidelines described in the next section for codes G0425–G0427 up to and including the Special Note on Coverage Criteria are also applicable to follow-up telehealth consultative services.
- A follow-up telehealth consultation is one requested by the attending physician and subsequent to an initial inpatient consultation whether provided in person or via telehealth.
- Follow-up inpatient telehealth consultations are defined by CMS as when a provider requests the opinion or advice of another physician or qualified health care provider to evaluate and/or manage a specific problem in the hospital or skilled nursing facility to follow up on an initial consultation or subsequent consultative visit requested by the attending physician and includes the following services:
  - monitoring progress
  - recommending management modifications
  - advising on a new plan of care based upon the patient's response to changes in status or no changes on the consulted health matter
- These consultations include monitoring the patient's progress, as well as making recommendations and/or modifications to the patient's management or instituting a new plan of care based on changes in the patient's condition including no changes on the health issue for which the provider was consulted. Any counseling or coordination of care with other health care providers or agencies consistent with the nature of the problem and the patient's needs is also included in the follow-up consultation service.
- As with the emergency department and initial inpatient consultations, all consultation-related services rendered before, during, and after communicating with the patient are included in the payment. This may include, but is not limited to, review of patient diagnostic and/or imaging studies and interim lab work, as well as communications with family members or other health care professionals, completing medical records, and documentation or communication of results and care plans to the requesting provider.
- Initial inpatient consult may have been provided in person or via telehealth.
- The follow-up telehealth consultation would be distinct from the follow-up care provided by the physician of record or the attending physician.
- When the consultation has been provided, the consultant prepares a written report containing his or her findings and recommendations to the referring provider.
- When counseling and coordination of care with other providers are included, consistent with the nature of the presenting problem, as well as the patient's needs.
- Beginning January 1, 2024, CMS requires the use of place of service (POS) 02 or 10 for telehealth services. POS 02 is used to report professional telehealth services when the originating site is other than the patient's home. POS 10 is used to report telehealth services when the patient is in their home.

Telehealth ED or Initial Inpatient Consultation Services (G0425–G0427)

HCPCS Code	Medical Decision Making	History	Exam	Counseling and/or Coordination of Care	Time Spent Communicating with the Patient via Telehealth
G0425	Straightforward	Problem-focused	Problem-focused	Consistent with problems and patient's or family's needs	30 min.
G0426	Moderate complexity	Detailed	Detailed	Consistent with problems and patient's or family's needs	50 min.
G0427	High Complexity	Comprehensive	Comprehensive	Consistent with problems and patient's or family's needs	70 min.

General Guidelines

- Teleconsultations most often involve a primary care practitioner with a patient at a remote, rural (spoke) site and a consulting medical specialist at an urban or referral (hub) facility with the primary care practitioner requesting advice from the consulting physician about the patient's condition or treatment.
- As a result of the Balanced Budget Act (BBA) of 1997, physicians and other appropriate practitioners providing professional consultations via telecommunication systems to Medicare beneficiaries residing in rural areas that have been designated as health professional shortage areas can receive payment for their services. The Benefits Improvement and Protection Act (BIPA) of 2000 greatly expanded many aspects of coverage and billing of telehealth services. In addition to coverage for teleconsultations, the legislation mandates coverage of many services using telecommunications systems including office visits, psychotherapy, and drug management. Telehealth services have also been extended to Medicare beneficiaries beyond the boundaries of HPSAs.
- The following are approved origination sites for telehealth services:
  - physician or practitioner offices
  - hospitals
  - community access hospitals (CAH)
  - rural health centers (RHC)
  - federally qualified health centers (FQHC)
  - hospital-based or critical access hospital-based renal dialysis centers (including satellites)
  - skilled nursing facilities (SNF)
  - community mental health centers (CMHC)

The following list identifies approved telehealth services:

  - ED or initial inpatient consultations
  - follow-up inpatient consultations
  - office or other outpatient visits
  - subsequent hospital care services (limit to one telehealth visit every three days)
  - subsequent inpatient nursing facility visits
  - individual and group kidney disease education services
  - individual and group diabetes self-management training services (minimum of 1 hour in-person instruction furnished within the initial year training period to ensure effective injection training)
  - individual psychotherapy
  - pharmacologic management
  - psychiatric diagnostic interview examination
  - end stage renal disease (ESRD) related services
  - individual and group medical nutrition therapy (MNT)
  - neurobehavioral status exam
  - individual and group health and behavior assessment and intervention (HBAI)
  - smoking cessation services
  - alcohol and/or substance (other than tobacco) abuse assessment and intervention services

- The following list identifies approved distant site practitioners:
  - physician
  - physician assistant (PA)
  - nurse practitioner (NP)
  - clinical nurse specialist (CNS)
  - nurse midwife
  - clinical psychologist
  - clinical social worker
  - certified registered nurse anesthetists
  - registered dietitian or nutrition professional
- It is also important to note that current deductible and coinsurance policies apply to these services.
- The originating site should report services with Q3014 Telehealth originating site facility fee. Submission of a claim with Q3014 attests that the originating site is a rural HPSA or non-MSA county or an entity that participates in a federal telemedicine demonstration project.
- Professional services commonly furnished remotely using telecommunications technology, but that do not require the patient to be present in person with the practitioner when they are furnished, are covered and paid in the same way as services delivered without the use of telecommunications technology when the practitioner is in-person at the medical facility furnishing care to the patient.

Special Instructions Regarding Coverage Criteria

To qualify as a teleconsultation, the patient encounter must meet criteria for a consultation service as defined by CPT code descriptors, as well as include the following requirements:

- Clinical assessment is performed via medical examination directed by the consultant (specialist)
- Audiovisual communications equipment is used that allows real-time communication between the beneficiary, primary care practitioner, and the specialist; this does not include the use of telephones, electronic mail, or facsimile machines
- If a practitioner other than the referring practitioner presents the patient, he or she is an employee of the referring practitioner
- The presenting practitioner's participation is appropriate for the needs of the patient and for providing information to the consultant and at the consultant's direction
- Feedback of the consultation is provided to the referring practitioner

In the majority of cases, it is expected that the referring practitioner will be present for the teleconsultation to satisfy the face-to-face examination requirement that is a prerequisite of a consultation under Medicare. The teleconsultation is subject to review if the referring practitioner is not present.

Physicians and other practitioners are instructed by CMS to report new or established patient office/other outpatient services codes, nursing facility care codes, or initial hospital visit codes. The first inpatient encounter by any physician is reported with initial hospital care codes 99221–99223, and subsequent inpatient encounters using codes 99231–99233. Knowing that only one physician may be the admitting physician, CMS created HCPCS Level II modifier AI Principal physician of record, that is to be reported with the initial hospital care code by the attending physician.

CMS also redistributed the value of the consultation codes across the other E/M codes for Medicare services. CMS retained values for codes 99242–99255 in the Medicare physician fee schedule for those private payers who use the data for reimbursement. Note that private payers may choose to follow CMS or CPT guidelines and the use of consultation codes should be verified with the individual payers.

Medicare requires the use of interactive audio and video telecommunications that allow for real-time communication between the physician or other practitioner at the distant site and the beneficiary. This may include x-rays, EKGs, MRIs, laboratory results, audio clips, photographs specific to the patient's condition that are capable of rendering or supporting a diagnosis, and text. It does not include telephone calls, electronic mail, or images transmitted via facsimile. CMS developed modifier GQ Via asynchronous telecommunications system, to identify the use of store-and-forward technology.

The following criteria necessitate the use of a telehealth consultation code for the emergency department or an initial inpatient consultative service:

- When a provider requests the opinion or advice of another physician or qualified health care provider to evaluate and/or manage a specific problem in the emergency department or as an inpatient service.
- When the reason for the telehealth consultation is clearly documented in the patient's medical record and included in the requesting provider's plan of care for the patient.
- When the consultation has been provided, the consultant prepares a written report containing his or her findings and recommendations to the referring provider.
- When counseling and coordination of care with other providers is included, consistent with the nature of the presenting problem as well as the patient's needs.
- All consultation related services rendered before, during, and after communicating with the patient is included in the payment. This may include but is not limited to review of patient diagnostic and/or imaging studies and interim lab work, as well as communications with family members or other health care professionals, completing medical records, and documenting or communicating results and care plans to the requesting provider.
- Beginning January 1, 2024, CMS requires the use of place of service (POS) 02 or 10 for telehealth services. POS 02 is used to report professional telehealth services when the originating site is other than the patient's home. POS 10 is used to report telehealth services when the patient is in their home.

Behavioral Screenings and Intervention (G0442–G0444)

E/M Code	Patient Status	Intent of Service	Time
G0442	Alcohol screening	Promote health, alcohol misuse screening	15 min.
G0443	Alcohol use	Promote health, alcohol misuse counseling	15 min.
G0444	Depression screening	Promote health, depression screening	15 min.

General Guidelines

- Medicare covers annual alcohol screening and up to four, brief face-to-face behavioral counseling sessions per year to reduce alcohol misuse.
- Deductible and coinsurance do not apply to these services.
- Counseling must be furnished by a qualified primary care physician or other primary care practitioner in a primary care setting.
- Medicare does not require use of a specific alcohol misuse screening tool. The provider in the primary care setting may choose the specific screening tool(s) he or she prefers.
- Counseling is covered for those patients that misuse alcohol, but do not meet the criteria for alcohol dependence, and are competent and alert when the counseling is provided.
- Annual screening and counseling for alcohol misuse in adults is recommended with a grade of B by the U.S. Preventive Services Task Force (USPSTF)
- The behavioral counseling intervention should follow the 5A's approach adopted by the USPSTF: assess, advise, agree, assist, and arrange.
- Medicare will cover a screening for depression provided in a primary care setting that has staff-assisted support in place to help ensure accurate diagnosis, as well as effective treatment plans, and patient follow-up.
- Staff-assisted support should at least consist of clinical staff that can advise the provider of screening results and who can coordinate referrals to mental health treatment when necessary.
- Medicare does not require use of a specific depression screening tool. The provider in the primary care setting may choose the specific screening tool(s) he or she prefers.
- Coverage for G0444 includes a screening service only it does not include treatment options for depression.
- Medicare covers an annual depression screening up to 15 minutes.

Key Point

For reporting and payment for alcohol and substance abuse not provided as a screening service but performed in the context of diagnosis and treatment of illness or injury, CMS created HCPCS Level II codes G0396 and G0397.

Issues in This Code Range

- Alcohol screening (G0442) is only covered one time in a 12-month period.
- Brief face-to-face behavioral counseling interventions (G0443) are only covered once per day.
- Brief face-to-face behavioral counseling interventions (G0443) are only covered four times in a 12-month period.
- Screening for depression (G0444) is only covered one time in a 12-month period.

Care Management Services (G0506)

E/M Code	Intent of Service	Face-to-Face Visit
G0506	Add-on code for reporting comprehensive assessment of and care planning for patients that require chronic care management services	Yes

General Guidelines

- HCPCS Level II code G0506 is an add-on code and must be reported with a primary E/M service.
- This code may be applicable when the billing provider initiating CCM services personally performs extensive assessment and care planning outside the usual effort described by the primary procedure.
- Initial chronic care management (CCM) services including, the IPPE, AWV, and other qualifying face-to-face E/M services, are primary E/M services that may be reported with G0506. These include:
  - G0402
  - G0438
  - G0439
  - 99202–99205
  - 99212–99215
  - 99495–99496
- Code G0506 cannot be used as an add-on code for behavioral health initiative services.
- The provider must create a written care plan centered on physical, mental, cognitive, psychosocial, functional, and environmental assessment, and the patient's available resources and support.
- Work and time used to report G0506 should not also be counted toward any other reported services, including CCM services.
- Code G0506 is only billable once, at the time of the CCM services.

Critical Care Telehealth Consultations (G0508–G0509)

E/M Code	Type of Visit	Intent of Service	Time Spent Communicating with the Patient via Telehealth
G0508	Initial	Critical care consultation provided using telehealth technology	60 min.
G0509	Subsequent	Critical care consultation provided using telehealth technology	50 min.

General Guidelines

- HCPCS Level II codes G0508 and G0509 represent critical care consultations furnished via an interactive real-time telecommunication system.
- Report G0508 for the initial consultation requiring critical care services, such as stroke.
- Report G0509 for subsequent consultations requiring critical care services.
- The provider may communicate with either the patient or the patient's caregiver.
- Do not report these services more than one time per day.
- As a condition of Medicare payment for telehealth services, the provider at the distant site must be licensed to provide the services.
- The following list identifies approved distant site practitioners:
  - physician
  - physician assistant (PA)
  - nurse practitioner (NP)
  - clinical nurse specialist (CNS)
  - nurse midwife
  - clinical psychologist
  - clinical social worker
  - registered dietitian or nutrition professional
  - certified registered nurse anesthetists
- Beginning January 1, 2024, CMS requires the use of place of service (POS) 02 or 10 for telehealth services. POS 02 is used to report professional telehealth services when the originating site is other than the patient's home. POS 10 is used to report telehealth services when the patient is in their home.

Prolonged Service With or Without Direct Patient Contact (G0316, G0317, G0318, G2212)

E/M Code	Location of Service(s)	Time Spent With or Without Direct Patient Contact
G2212	Office or Other Outpatient Facility	Each additional 15 minutes
G0316	Hospital Inpatient or Observation Care	Each additional 15 minutes
G0317	Nursing Facility Services	Each additional 15 minutes
G0318	Home or Residence Services	Each additional 15 minutes

General Guidelines

- Use these codes to report each additional 15 minutes of E/M services beyond the time indicated in the code description.
- Code G2212 is only used in addition to time-based evaluation and management services 99205, 99215, and 99483.
- Code G0316 is only used in addition to time-based evaluation and management services codes 99223, 99233, and 99236.
- Code G0317 is only used in addition to time-based evaluation and management services codes 99306 and 99310.
- Code G0318 is only used in addition to time-based evaluation and management services codes 99345 and 99350.
- Use of these codes is based on the total time the clinician spent on the day of the patient visit, including face-to-face and non-face-to-face activities.
- Other services provided during prolonged service periods may be reported separately. Time involved performing these activities should not count toward prolonged service times.
- Services of less than 15 minutes beyond the maximum required time are not reported separately.

For additional information and reporting guidelines for G0316, G0317, and G0318, refer to the MLN006764 Evaluation and Management Services Guide at https://www.cms.gov/outreach-and-education/medicare-learning-network-mln/mlnproducts/downloads/eval-mgmt-serv-guide-icn006764.pdf. For time thresholds to report these prolonged services, refer to Table 3 of the MLN.

G0316

Documentation Requirements

Intent of Service
- Extended evaluation and management of a patient's specific problem

Presence of Patient
- Includes direct face-to-face contact and non-face-to-face activities

Time Spent on Prolonged Service
- Each additional 15 minutes

Special Coding and Documentation Considerations
- This code is used to report time spent on the date of the encounter, with or without direct patient contact, that extends beyond the total time designated in the primary code description.
- Document the total time (with and without direct patient contact) spent on the patient's case. Time does not have to be continuous but should reflect the total time spent on the day of the visit providing the prolonged service.
- Never report this code alone—it should be reported with 99223, 99233, and 99236.
- Do not report with 99358, 99359, 99415, 99416, or 99418 for the same date of service.
- The prolonged service starts 15 minutes after the total time for the primary service, and the entire 15-minutes increment must be completed. See table below.
- Codes 99223 and 99233 are based on time spent on the date of the encounter. Code 99236 is based on time spent on the same date or within three subsequent calendar days.

Prolonged Services Time Threshold Table

Primary E/M Service Prolonged	Code	Time Threshold to Report One Unit of Prolonged Service	Count physician/NPP time spent within this time period
99223 Initial Inpatient/ Observation visit	G0316	**105**	Date of visit
99223 Subsequent Inpatient/ Observation visit	G0316	**80**	Date of visit
99236 Initial/Discharge same date	G0316	**125**	Date of visit to 3 days after

Note: CMS published a table in the MLN006764 Evaluation and Management Services Guide indicating the time thresholds that need to be documented to report one additional unit of prolonged services. This table reflects the total physician time used to determine the work RVU for the indicated code plus the 15 minutes of prolonged services. Note that the times vary from code to code and are in excess of the time listed in the CPT code description. For additional information and reporting guidelines for G0316, G0317, and G0318, refer to the MLN006764 Evaluation and Management Services Guide at https://www.cms.gov/outreach-and-education/medicare-learning-network-mln/mlnproducts/downloads/eval-mgmt-serv-guide-icn006764.pdf.

G0317

Documentation Requirements

Intent of Service
- Extended evaluation and management of a patient's specific problem

Presence of Patient
- Includes direct face-to-face contact and non-face-to-face activities

Time Spent on Prolonged Service
- Each additional 15 minutes

Special Coding and Documentation Considerations
- This code is used to report time spent on the date of the encounter, with or without direct patient contact, that extends beyond the typical time designated in the primary code description.
- Document the total time (with and without direct patient contact) spent on the patient's case. Time does not have to be continuous but should reflect the total time spent on the day of the visit providing the prolonged service.
- Never report this code alone—it should be reported with 99306 or 99310.
- Do not report with 99358, 99359, or 99418 for the same date of service.
- The prolonged service starts 15 minutes after the total time for the primary service, and the entire 15-minutes increment must be completed. See table below.

Prolonged Services Time Threshold Table

Primary E/M Service Prolonged	Code	Time Threshold to Report One Unit of Prolonged Service	Count physician/NPP time spent within this time period
99306 Initial nursing facility visit	G0317	**95**	Date of visit plus 1 day prior & 3 days after
99310 Subsequent nursing facility visit	G0317	**85**	Date of visit plus 1 day prior & 3 days after

Note: CMS published a table in the MLN006764 Evaluation and Management Services Guide indicating the time thresholds that need to be documented to report one additional unit of prolonged services. This table reflects the total physician time used to determine the work RVU for the indicated code plus the 15 minutes of prolonged services. Note that the times vary from code to code and are in excess of the time listed in the CPT code description. For additional information and reporting guidelines for G0316, G0317, and G0318, refer to the MLN006764 Evaluation and Management Services Guide at: https://www.cms.gov/outreach-and-education/medicare-learning-network-mln/mlnproducts/downloads/eval-mgmt-serv-guide-icn006764.pdf.

G0318

Documentation Requirements

Intent of Service
- Extended evaluation and management of a patient's specific problem

Presence of Patient
- Includes direct face-to-face contact and non-face-to-face activities

Time Spent on Prolonged Service
- Each additional 15 minutes

Special Coding and Documentation Considerations
- This code is used to report time spent on the date of the encounter, with or without direct patient contact, that extends beyond the typical time designated in the primary code description.
- Document the total time (with and without direct patient contact) spent on the patient's case. Time does not have to be continuous but should reflect the total time spent on the day of the visit providing the prolonged service.
- Never report this code alone—it should be reported with 99345 or 99350.
- Do not report with 99358, 99359, or 99417 for the same date of service.
- The prolonged service starts 15 minutes after the total time for the primary service, and the entire 15-minutes increment must be completed. See table below.

Prolonged Services Time Threshold Table

Primary E/M Service Prolonged	Code	Time Threshold to Report One Unit of Prolonged Service	Count physician/NPP time spent within this time period
99345 New home/residence visit	G0318	**140**	Date of visit plus 3 days prior & 7 days after
99350 Established home/ residence visit	G0318	**110**	Date of visit plus 3 days prior & 7 days after

Note: CMS published a table in the MLN006764 Evaluation and Management Services Guide indicating the time thresholds that need to be documented to report one additional unit of prolonged services. This table reflects the total physician time used to determine the work RVU for the indicated code plus the 15 minutes of prolonged services. Note that the times vary from code to code and are in excess of the time listed in the CPT code description. For additional information and reporting guidelines for G0316, G0317, and G0318, refer to the MLN006764 Evaluation and Management Services Guide at: https://www.cms.gov/outreach-and-education/medicare-learning-network-mln/mlnproducts/downloads/eval-mgmt-serv-guide-icn006764.pdf.

G2212

Documentation Requirements

Intent of Service
- Extended evaluation and management of a patient's specific problem

Presence of Patient
- Includes direct face-to-face contact and non-face-to-face activities

Time Spent on Prolonged Service
- Each additional 15 minutes

Special Coding and Documentation Considerations
- This code is used to report time spent on the date of the encounter, with or without direct patient contact, that extends beyond the typical time designated in the primary code description. **Note:** CPT states to report 99417 for prolonged services at least 15 minutes beyond the time required to report the highest level of primary service. CMS stated in the CY 2021 PFS Final Rule to report G2212 for prolonged services when the *maximum* required time for 99205, 99215, or 99483 is exceeded.
- Document the total time (with and without direct patient contact) spent on the patient's case. Time does not have to be continuous but should reflect the total time spent on the day of the visit providing the prolonged service.
- Never report this code alone—it should be reported with 99205, 99215, or 99483.
- Do not report G2212 with 99358, 99359, 99415, or 99416 for the same date of service.

Office/Outpatient E/M Visit Complexity Add-On (G2211)

E/M Code	Office or Other Outpatient Facility	Inpatient or Observation Setting	Type of Visit
G2211	Yes	No	New or Established

General Guidelines

- Described as an add-on code for visit complexity inherent to evaluation and management associated with medical care services that serve as the continuing focal point for all necessary health care services and/or with medical care services that are part of ongoing care related to a patient's single, serious, or complex condition.
- Services for all patients that allow providers to address a patient's health care needs with consistency over longer periods of time, including providing services on an ongoing basis that result in personalized, comprehensive care of the patient, and involve delivery of team-based care that is accessible and coordinated through multiple providers.
- Should only be reported with office and outpatient E/M visits 99202–99205 and 99211–99215.
- Not restricted to a specific specialty and may be reported with any visit level.
- Do not report G2211 with a primary office/outpatient E/M visit that is reported with payment modifiers 24, 25, or 53.
- May not be applicable when comorbidities are either not addressed or not present, when the provider has not taken responsibility for, or does not plan on taking responsibility for ongoing medical care for a particular patient with consistency and continuity over time (e.g., treatment of a simple virus, fracture treatment, counseling regarding seasonal allergies).
- When using time to report the primary service, reviewers will use the medical record documentation to determine medical necessity of the service.
- Do not report this code if the provider does not assume responsibility for ongoing care of the patient.

Medicare created HCPCS Level II code G2211 to be effective January 1, 2021; however, the Consolidated Appropriations Act (CAA), 2021, delayed PFS payment for G2211 until January 1, 2024, or later. In the CY 2025 physician fee schedule proposed rule, CMS proposes to expand the guidelines to allow payment for G2211 on the same day as an annual wellness visit, vaccine administration, or other preventive service provided in an office or outpatient setting.

Knowledge Assessment Chapter 19

See chapter 21 for answers and rationale.

1. What code is reported for a Medicare patient who received 30 minutes of physician supervised care plan oversight services in the calendar month under a Medicare-approved hospice program?
   a. G0181
   b. G0182
   c. 99378
   d. The service is not reportable

2. Code G0180 for physician certification for Medicare-covered, home health services can only be reported if the patient has not received any Medicare-covered, home health services for a period of at least 31 days.
   a. True
   b. False

3. Medicare does not cover preventive medicine services (99381–99429); however, the agency does cover a welcome to Medicare visit or initial preventive physical exam (IPPE). What code is used to report this visit?
   a. G0402
   b. 99387
   c. 99397
   d. G0438

4. How do providers reporting telehealth services to Medicare administrative contractors (MAC) indicate that the service was provided via telehealth real-time telecommunication systems?
   a. Report only the G code if the word telehealth is part of the code description
   b. Append modifier GT to the G code
   c. Submit using place of service (POS) code 02 or 10
   d. Both b and c

5. Which of the following are approved distant site telehealth practitioners?
   a. Nurse practitioner
   b. Clinical psychologist
   c. Nurse midwife
   d. All of the above

6. Codes G0425–G0427 and G0406–G0408 are only used to report telehealth consultations provided to Medicare beneficiaries.
   a. True
   b. False

Chapter 20. Coding and Compliance

Ongoing Compliance Investigations

E/M Service	Compliance Issue	Investigating Agency
E/M codes reported during the global period	E/M services bundled into the global surgical package not provided	Office of Inspector General (OIG), recovery audit contractors (RAC)
Use of modifiers during the global surgery period	Modifiers used inappropriately to report E/M services that are bundled into the global surgical package	Office of Inspector General (OIG),
Initial preventive physical examination (IPPE)	Misuse due to the likelihood that non-Medicare patients may have already received the preventive services listed under the IPPE	Office of Inspector General (OIG), recovery audit contractors (RAC)
Assigning new patient E/M codes	More than one new patient E/M service reported for the same beneficiary within a three-year period	Recovery audit contractors (RAC)
High level subsequent nursing facility care codes	Higher levels of care reported but not supported by documentation	Centers for Medicare and Medicaid Services (CMS), Medicare Administrative Contractor (MAC)—National Government Services (NGS)
Anesthesia care package and billing E/M codes separately	Unbundling of E/M services in anesthesia claims	Recovery audit contractors (RAC)
Critical care and emergency department (ED) services	Inappropriate use of critical care codes	Office of Inspector General (OIG), Recovery audit contractors (RAC)
Pulmonary diagnostic procedures with E/M services	Overpayments associated with E/M services and diagnostic pulmonary procedures	Recovery audit contractors (RAC)

E/M Codes Reported During the Global Period

General Guidelines

- CMS established a national definition for a global surgical package to ensure consistent payment for the same services across all carrier regions.
- CMS defined the global surgical package to include:
  - preoperative visits
  - intraoperative services
  - complications following surgery
    - does not require a return trip to the operating room
  - postoperative visits related to recovery
  - postsurgical pain management provided by the surgeon
  - certain supplies
  - miscellaneous services, including:
    - dressing changes
    - local incisional wound care
    - removal of packing material
    - removal of sutures, staples, wires, lines, tubes, drains, casts, and splints
    - insertion, irrigation, and removal of urinary catheters, routine peripheral intravenous lines, nasogastric and rectal tubes
    - changes and removal of tracheostomy tubes
- In determining global surgery fees, CMS estimates the number of E/M services a physician provides to a typical beneficiary during the surgery period; physicians are compensated for the surgical service and related E/M services regardless of the number of E/M services actually provided during the global surgery period.
- Postoperative periods that apply to each surgical procedure are provided in the Medicare Physician Fee Schedule Data Base (MPFSDB). Payment rules for surgical procedures apply to codes with postoperative periods of 000, 010, 090, and sometimes YYY.
- Major surgeries include one day preceding the day of surgery, the day of surgery, and the 90 days immediately following the day of surgery.
- Minor surgeries include the day of surgery and the appropriate number of days immediately following the day of surgery.

Explanation of Investigation

- OIG has sought to determine whether payments were made to physicians for E/M services not provided during the global surgery period.
- One study showed the number of office visits were counted and compared to the number of E/M services included in the global surgery fee. Out of 300 claims reviewed, 201 of the surgeries performed showed that physicians provided fewer visits than those included in the global surgery fee.
  - OIG concluded that Medicare paid almost $98 million for E/M services bundled in to global surgery fees that were never provided.
- OIG recommendations to CMS included making an adjustment to the estimated number of E/M services included in the global surgery fee for surgeries that would reflect the actual number of services being provided, OR update the annual Medicare physician fee schedule (MPFS) to apply the audit results and other information.
  - CMS would not make changes to the codes in the MPFS stating the changes would simply end up being redistributed to all services and not result in savings to the Medicare program due to a requirement in the Medicare statute that mandated all changes must be done in a budget-neutral manner.
  - CMS did indicate the agency would work with the AMA Relative Value Scale Update Committee (RUC) and relevant physician specialty societies to identify and change services where the number of E/M services provided in the global period has changed.

Strategies for Risk Prevention

- Educate staff members on National Correct Coding Initiative (CCI) edits and demonstrate how to look up codes and determine the global period associated with the procedure code.
- Understand what is—and is not—included in the Medicare global surgery package vs. a commercial carrier global surgery fee. Many commercial carriers use CMS guidelines, but not all; therefore, it is important to note any differences. One example of differences in the global surgery package description is often reflected in complications. Medicare includes all complications except those requiring a return trip to the operating room in the global fee for the surgery; however, many commercial carriers pay for procedures such as incision and drainage performed in the physician office.
- Implement a process or mechanism, manual or automated, to indicate the start and stop dates for the global surgery period. This is helpful in knowing whether the type of visit is a preoperative visit and also to track the number of postoperative visits.
  - If the patient is being seen for reasons other than those related to the surgical service reminders should be given to the billing staff that a modifier may be appropriate and should be appended to the applicable E/M or other service; such as:
    - Modifier 24 Significant, Separately Identifiable E/M Service during a Postoperative Period
    - Modifier 79 Unrelated Procedure or Service by the Same Physician or Other Qualified Health Care Professional during the Postoperative Period in cases where the patient is scheduled for an unrelated procedure during the postoperative period of another procedure
    - Modifier 58 Staged or Related Procedure or Service by the Same Physician or Other Qualified Health Care Professional during the Postoperative Period

    Note: Modifier 24 is used to bypass carrier edits and, as such, should be used only when appropriate. The inappropriate use of any modifier to receive payment without following the necessary guidelines and documentation requirements can subject the provider to scrutiny and possible audits. In addition, as previously stated, append modifier 24 only to the evaluation and management service, not to the surgical procedure. Modifiers 58 and 79 may be used in conjunction with the procedure or other service codes.
- Download or print out a copy of the MPFS. Each surgery code shows the global period associated with it. Knowing whether the surgery has a 0-, 10-, or 90-day postoperative period can ensure that the proper number of visits are provided.
- Implement periodic spot checks of surgical claims to verify that any services reported during the global period have been reported in compliance with the carrier guidelines.
  - In many cases, when an E/M service is related to the surgery and inappropriately reported, carrier edits reject the claim.
  - Proactive review of claims prior to submission, as well as processed claims, allows identification of any recurrent errors or issues and provides an opportunity for corrections.
- Address billing issues with all staff members and providers as an educational tool to ensure that the problem has been remedied for future claims.

Quick Tip

Regular and ongoing review of the CMS Pub. 100-04, *Medicare Claims Processing Manual* sections on global surgery guidelines and commercial payer contract requirements will help ensure that coding staff members are informed and aware of any revisions or changes to current policies.

Use of Modifiers During the Global Surgery Period

General Guidelines

- CMS established a national definition for a global surgical package to ensure consistent payment for the same services across all carrier regions.
- CMS defined the global surgical package to include:
  - preoperative visits
  - intraoperative services
  - complications following surgery
    - does not require a return trip to the operating room
  - postoperative visits related to recovery
  - postsurgical pain management provided by the surgeon
  - certain supplies
  - miscellaneous services, including:
    - dressing changes
    - local incisional wound care
    - removal of packing material
    - removal of sutures, staples, wires, lines, tubes, drains, casts, and splints
    - insertion, irrigation, and removal of urinary catheters, routine peripheral intravenous lines, nasogastric and rectal tubes
    - changes and removal of tracheostomy tubes
- Major surgeries include one day preceding the day of surgery, the day of surgery, and the 90 days immediately following the day of surgery.
- Minor surgeries include the day of surgery and the appropriate number of days immediately following the day of surgery.
- Modifier 24 allows for an E/M service to be reported if the service was provided during the postoperative period of a surgical procedure by the same physician or other qualified health care professional who performed the procedure.
  - Documentation must support that the evaluation and management service is not related to the postoperative care of the procedure.
- Modifier 25 is used when the E/M service is separate from a procedure performed at the same encounter and signifies a clearly documented, distinct, and significantly identifiable service was rendered.
- Medicare and other payers require modifier 57 to be appended to the E/M service code only when the decision for surgery was made during the preoperative period of a surgical procedure with a 90-day postoperative period (i.e., major surgery). The preoperative period is defined as the day before and the day of the surgical procedure.

Explanation of Investigation

- The OIG has previously reported that inappropriate use of modifiers during the global surgical period has resulted in erroneous payments.
- Reporting E/M services related to the surgical procedure during the global period is a form of unbundling.

Strategies for Risk Prevention

- Maintain the most current version of the CCI edits; integrate these edits directly into the practice management system, if possible.
- Educate staff members on CCI edits and demonstrate how to look up codes and determine the global period associated with the procedure code.
- Understand what is—and is not—included in the Medicare global surgery package vs. a commercial carrier global surgery fee.
  - Many commercial carriers use CMS guidelines, but not all; therefore, it is important to note any differences.
  - One example of differences in the global surgery package description is often reflected in complications. Medicare includes ALL complications, except those requiring a return trip to the operating room in the global fee for the surgery. However, many commercial carriers pay for procedures such as incision and drainage performed in the physician office.
- Implement a process or mechanism, manual or automated, to indicate the start and stop dates for the global surgery period. This is helpful in knowing whether the type of visit is a preoperative visit and also to track the number of postoperative visits.

- Educate staff and clinicians on the appropriate use of E/M modifiers:
  - Modifier 24 permits an E/M service to be reported (other than inpatient hospital care before discharge from the hospital following surgery) if the service was provided during the postoperative period of a surgical procedure by the same physician or other qualified health care professional who performed the procedure. Documentation must support that the evaluation and management service is not related to the postoperative care of the procedure.
  - Modifier 25 should only be appended to codes describing E/M services and only when the services are provided by the same physician (or same qualified nonphysician practitioner) to the same patient on the same day as another procedure or service. It is not necessary to have a different diagnosis when reporting the E/M service on the same date as the procedure or other service.
    - Append modifier 25 to the E/M code only.
    - Both the E/M service and the procedure must be appropriately and sufficiently documented by the physician (or qualified nonphysician practitioner) in the patient's medical record demonstrating the medical necessity of the services reported; however, documentation is not required to be submitted with the claim.
  - Modifier 57 indicates an evaluation and management service provided on the day of or the day before surgery for codes assigned a 90-day global surgical period.
    - Modifier 57 indicates the E/M service provided resulted in the decision for surgery
    - It is not appropriate to report E/M services with a 0- or 10-day global surgical period with modifier 57.
      Note: The modifiers discussed above are reported to bypass carrier edits; therefore, it is very important to only use when appropriate. Inappropriate use of any modifier to receive payment without following the necessary guidelines and documentation requirements can subject the provider to scrutiny and possible audits.
- Download or print out a copy of the Medicare physician fee schedule (MPFS).
  - Each surgery code shows the global period associated with it. Knowing whether the surgery has a 0-, 10-, or 90-day postoperative period can ensure that the proper number of visits are provided.
- Review regularly the CMS IOM Pub.100-04 sections on global surgery guidelines and commercial payer contract requirements to ensure staff and clinicians remain informed and aware of any revisions or changes to policies.
- Implement periodic spot checks of surgical claims to verify that any services reported during the global period have been reported in compliance with the carrier guidelines.
  - In many cases, when an E/M service is related to the surgery and inappropriately reported, carrier edits reject the claim, but not always.
  - Proactive review of claims prior to submission, as well as processed claims, allows identification of any recurrent errors or issues and provides an opportunity for corrections.
- Address billing issues with all staff members and providers as an educational tool to ensure that the problem has been remedied for future claims.

Initial Preventive Physical Exam (IPPE)

General Guidelines

- The IPPE is a preventive evaluation and management service first allowed under section 611 of the Medicare Prescription Drug Improvement and Modernization Act (MMA) of 2003
- Considered to be an introduction to Medicare and covered benefits.
- The IPPE is not a "routine physical checkup" that seniors may receive every one to two years from their provider as Medicare does not cover routine physical exams.
- This is a one-time benefit and beneficiaries have 12 months from their effective date to receive this, as it's commonly referred to, Welcome to Medicare visit.
- Each component of the IPPE must be provided or referred to another physician in order to appropriately submit this benefit to Medicare. The IPPE face-to-face exam consists of the following nine distinct components:
  - review of patient's medical and social history
  - review the patient's potential risk factors for depression
  - review the patient's functional ability and level of safety
  - physical examination that includes height, weight, blood pressure, visual acuity, and BMI
  - end-of-life planning
  - review of any current opioid prescriptions
  - review of potential risk factors for substance use disorders with referral for treatment when appropriate
  - education, counseling, and referral based on the results of the review and evaluation services described above
  - education, counseling, and referral, including a brief written plan or checklist, for obtaining the appropriate screening or other Part B preventive services
- Providers must use the appropriate screening tools typically used in routine physician practices and document all pertinent clinical information in the medical record, including any referrals and a medical plan.

Explanation of Investigation

- The OIG reviews claims and evaluates billing practices and payments as they relate to the initial preventive physician examination (IPPE).
- Some of the services included in the IPPE may have already been performed in a previous evaluation and management service previously reported yet the full IPPE service is billed by the provider.
- The OIG has focused on the IPPE as an area of possible fraud and abuse due to the higher reimbursement for this service and due to the likelihood that non-Medicare patients may have already received preventive services similar to those listed under the IPPE.

Strategies for Risk Prevention

- Have a well-designed compliance program in place.
- Ensure all seven components of the IPPE are provided or referred to another physician and that these preventive services were not provided before the patient became Medicare eligible.
- Refer to the CMS quick reference checklist that details the specific elements that must be documented for each of the seven components within the IPPE.

Assigning New Patient E/M Codes

General Guidelines

- A new patient is defined by the American Medical Association (AMA) as a patient who is receiving face-to-face care from the provider or other qualified health care professional of the exact same specialty/subspecialty within the same practice for the first time in three years.
  - new patient examples include:
    - a patient sees the physician/qualified health care professional for the first time
    - a patient previously seen by a cardiologist 18 months prior sees an endocrinologist in the same group practice
    - a patient who has not seen the physician/qualified health care professional for 40 months returns complaining of abdominal pain
- Providers should not report a new patient E/M service for the same beneficiary more than once in a three-year period.
- For many of the E/M codes, correct code assignment is dependent upon whether the patient is new or established.

Explanation of Investigation

- The 2023 Medicare Improper Payment Report indicated that 9.4 percent of new patient office visits were paid erroneously, resulting in $319,432,777 in projected improper payments.
  - This number included established patients billed with a new patient E/M code and incorrect level of new patient visits reported.

Strategies for Risk Prevention

- Ensure appropriate administrative and clinical staff members understand the guidelines for reporting new patient E/M codes.
- Perform provider and staff education.
- Develop a policy and procedure for determining patient status and include the policy as part of the compliance manual.
- Perform internal pre- and postprovider education audits to determine the prevalence, if any, of inappropriately reporting a patient's status.
- Develop a short questionnaire that the appointment clerk can use to help determine if a patient may be billed with a new patient status at the time the appointment is made.
- Use a decision tree to determine new vs. established patient status.

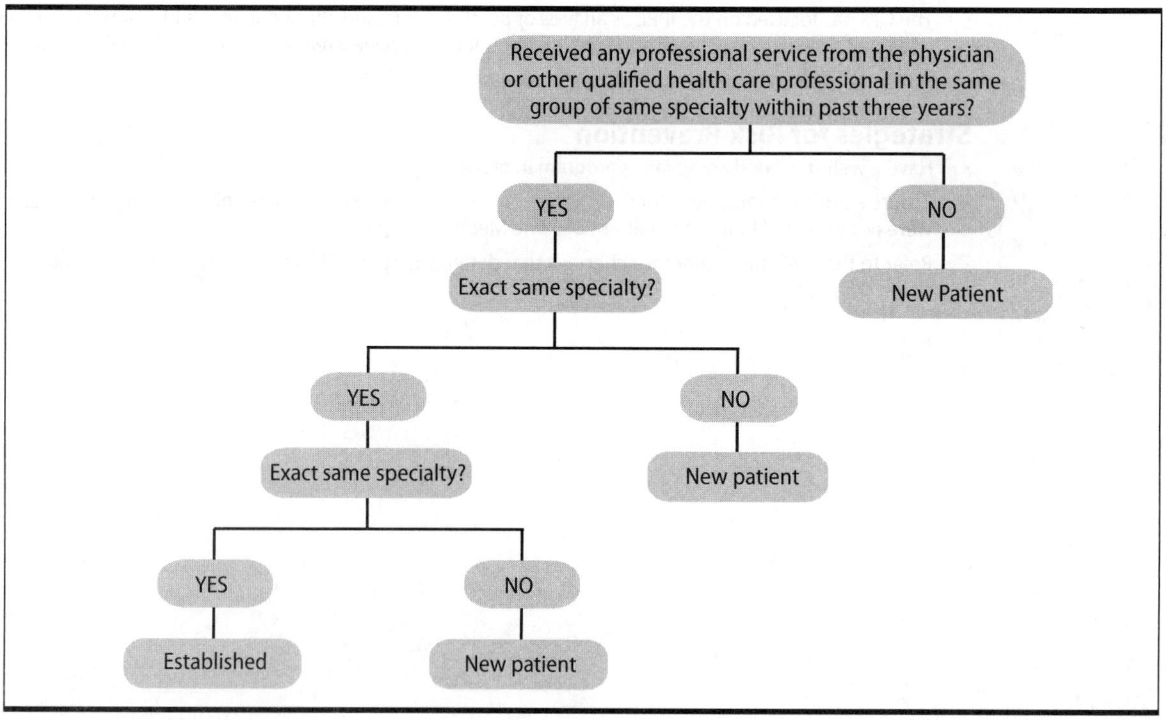

High-Level Subsequent Nursing Facility Care Codes

General Guidelines

- Codes 99309–99310 represent per day, subsequent nursing facility care that requires a detailed to comprehensive history, detailed to comprehensive exam, and/or moderate to high complexity medical decision making.
- Reporting of these codes typically indicates the patient:
  - will have developed a significant complication or significant new problem
  - be unstable
  - require immediate physician attention
- It is not appropriate to bill a higher level of evaluation and management service when a lower level of service is warranted.

Explanation of Investigation

- A prepayment review of claims reported with codes 99309 and 99310.
- On average, 44 percent of claims were reported with a higher level of care than was supported by medical record documentation.

Strategies for Risk Prevention

- Ensure all coding staff is appropriately trained in the use of the documentation guidelines for accurate coding of E/M services.
- Ongoing audits of E/M services and sharing results with staff. (See appendix A for sample physician E/M audit forms.)
- Continued training and educational opportunities in E/M coding.

Anesthesia Care Package and Billing E/M Codes Separately

General Guidelines

- The CMS and American Society of Anesthesiologists (ASA) base unit value (BUV) represents all of the usual anesthesia services, with the exception of the time actually spent in anesthesia care, as well as any modifying factors that may occur.
- The following are included in the BUV:
  - pre- and postoperative visits
  - administration of fluids and/or blood as incident to the anesthesia care
  - interpretation of noninvasive monitoring such as electrocardiogram, temperature, blood pressure, oximetry, capnography, and mass spectrometry
- The basic documentation requirements include the preoperative evaluation, presurgery review, patient question and answer discussion, attendance during surgery, postanesthesia care unit evaluation, and attendance, as necessary.
- Pre-anesthesia examination and evaluation include a review of the patient's past medical, family, and social history; medications; and adverse reactions to previous anesthesia.
- To bill an anesthesia service AND an E/M service, review medical record documentation to determine that the E/M service performed was a significant, separately identifiable service that was not related to the condition for which anesthesia was performed.

Explanation of Investigation

- Review of anesthesia claims to determine if E/M services have been unbundled.

Strategies for Risk Prevention

- Inform and educate providers regarding services and procedures that are considered standards of anesthesia care, including pre- and postexamination of the patient.
- Review anesthesia coding and billing guidelines with clinicians.
- Determine if any claims have been billed with both anesthesia and E/M codes.
- Review documentation for these claims to verify the medical necessity of both services.
- Educate staff on CCI edits as they pertain to anesthesia services.

Coding Axiom

Per CCI, E/M services (99202–99499) related to the anesthesia service (i.e., pre-anesthesia examination and evaluation) are bundled into the anesthesia codes.

Coding and Compliance

Critical Care and Emergency Department (ED) Services

General Guidelines

- CMS defines critical care services as medical care directly delivered by a physician to a critically ill or injured patient.
- For a patient to be deemed critically ill or injured, the illness or injury should represent grave harm to one or more vital organ systems and thereby present a worsening of the patient's condition including a strong likelihood of death.
- CMS guidance clearly states that providers should not report both critical care services and emergency department services on the same date of service. When both services are provided, only the critical care services may be billed.
- When an inpatient hospital service or office or other outpatient service is provided to the patient who subsequently requires critical care on the same date of service, both the critical care and the E/M service may be reimbursed.
- Physicians should submit documentation to substantiate the use of critical care services and separate E/M services on the same date of service by the same physician or physicians of the same specialty in the same group practice.
- For group practices, critical care services can be provided by providers of different specialties as long as those services are not duplicated by other members of the same specialty in the same group practice.
- Providers delivering critical care services to the same patient on the same date of service representing the same specialty and group practice are required to report their services as a single provider.
- Initial critical care time reported with code 99291 must be reached by a single provider, either in a single period of time or cumulatively on the same date.
- Subsequent critical care beyond the initial time period may be reported by a single provider or multiple providers of the same specialty in the same group practice in order to meet the total number of minutes required by code 99292.

For More Information

To review Medicare guidance regarding the use of critical care services see *Medicare Claims Processing Manual*, **Pub. 100-04, chapter 12, section 30.6.12.**

Explanation of Investigation

- RAC auditors investigated whether critical care services were billed and paid when rendered to the same patient, by the same physician, on the same day as emergency department services.
- RAC auditors also sought to determine whether physicians of the same specialty, in the same group practice, were billing for services separately. By doing so, physicians would have clearly been in violation of Medicare policy that required physicians representing the same specialty and group practice to function as a single physician for the purposes of billing and reimbursement.

Strategies for Risk Prevention

- Providers and staff should be made aware of CMS policies regarding appropriate reporting of critical care services in conjunction with other evaluation and management services.
- Particular emphasis should be made to advise providers that emergency department services are not reportable with critical care services despite these codes being categorized in the E/M section of the CPT® code book.
- Providers within the same group of the same specialty offering call service should be counseled as to appropriate billing of critical care codes to ensure reporting services as a single provider representing the entire group rather than individual providers as per Medicare payment policy.
- Implementing a review of services prior to billing may be one way to ensure compliance and understanding of CMS guidelines:
  - Conduct a random review of claims containing critical care services to ensure that emergency department service codes were not also inadvertently submitted for the same date of service.
  - Consider checking with the practice management vendor to determine if it is possible to program the practice management system to provide a flag or alert when critical care codes are billed on the same patient claim with the same date of service as an emergency department service code, thereby allowing billing and coding staff to make the appropriate corrections prior to claims submission.
- Upon determining that a claim containing both critical care services and an emergency department service code was paid inappropriately, take the following steps:
  - Inform the Medicare administrative contractor (MAC) that processed the claim of the error.
  - Remit payment for the incorrectly paid ED service.
    - appropriate adjustments should be made in the practice management system
  - Ensure appropriate education is provided to staff members responsible for submitting the claim.
  - Proactively run a report to identify claims submitted with both critical care codes and ED codes to identify any further outstanding claims.
    - if more claims have been submitted, contact the MAC to see if the claims can be denied or pended for a corrected claim

- Discuss all identified claims with providers and staff.
- Implement a review of claims containing critical care services prior to billing.

Pulmonary Diagnostic Procedures with E/M Services

General Guidelines

- The *National Correct Coding Initiative Policy Manual*, chapter 11, section J.2 states that if "the physician in attendance during the course of a pulmonary function study obtains a limited history and performs a limited physical examination related to the pulmonary function testing, it is *not* appropriate to report a separate E/M service as this would be considered part of the service." Clearly, an unrelated E/M service performed can and should be reported separately with modifier 25 appended.
- Documentation for the E/M service must meet the requirements for the appropriate level selected and should be unrelated to the pulmonary diagnostic procedure performed.
- Laboratory procedures performed during the course of diagnostic pulmonary testing, as well as the provider's interpretation of results from those laboratory services, is included in the description of those codes.
  - It would not be appropriate to further factor in the results from those tests during the medical decision making process when the lab services were both ordered and performed by the same provider.
  - Note that in the event the lab services were performed at a different laboratory and the results were then delivered to the treating provider, any information obtained as a result of reviewing the laboratory values could be used as a determining factor while deciding the level of medical decision making.

Explanation of Investigation

- Recovery audit contractors initiated an automated review to identify overpayments associated with E/M services billed without modifier 25 on the same date of service as a pulmonary diagnostic procedure reported with CPT codes 94010–94799.

Strategies for Risk Prevention

- Identify all billed services in code range 94010–94799.
  - If the practice management system being used permits, runs a report that also identifies additional services billed with the aforementioned code range, particularly E/M service codes 99211–99215.
  - Note whether modifier 25 was appended to the E/M service.
  - Review the medical record documentation supporting the medical necessity of the two services for accuracy and appropriateness.
  - Ensure that any E/M service reported with the pulmonary diagnostic procedure is separate and distinct.
- Updates to the *National Correct Coding Initiative Policy Manual* should be downloaded quarterly.
  - Ensure the updates have been reviewed by all staff members each quarter.
  - Specific policies that relate to the specialty of the practice, such as those relating to pulmonary services should be printed and all staff members should sign off on that policy indicating an understanding of, and agreement to comply with, the guidelines.
  - Designate a specific individual, perhaps a coding or billing representative, to check for updates to the *National Correct Coding Initiative Policy Manual* and ensure each staff member has been made aware of any new versions released.
  - Some of the commercial payers with which the practice is in network may have specific language within the contract or terms that does not permit an E/M service on the same date as a pulmonary diagnostic procedure, regardless of whether modifier 25 was appended. Always know which contracts the provider is under and the terms of those contracts. In addition, determine the circumstances as to when an E/M service can be reported in conjunction with this type of procedure.
- Verify the patient's insurance coverage prior to the procedure being performed and determine the circumstances as to when an E/M service can be reported in conjunction with diagnostic pulmonary procedures.
- Ensure that policies are enacted and implemented regarding appropriate use of modifier 25 for an E/M billed in conjunction with diagnostic pulmonary procedures.

Knowledge Assessment Chapter 20

See chapter 21 for answers and rationale.

1. Out of the following, which are considered part of a global surgery package?
   a. Postoperative visits
   b. Postsurgical pain management
   c. Preoperative visits
   d. All postoperative complications not requiring a return to the operating room
   e. All of the above
2. Where is Medicare's official list of the number of postoperative days included in each surgical procedure found?
   a. *Medicare Claims Processing Manual*
   b. Medicare Physician Fee Schedule Database
   c. *Medicare Program Integrity Manual*
   d. National Correct Coding Initiative
3. Preoperative visits for major procedures begin the day before a major procedure.
   a. True
   b. False
4. How many distinct components must be provided or referred to another physician, in order to bill for Medicare's initial preventive physician examination (IPPE)?
   a. Four
   b. Nine
   c. The number varies based on preventive services already provided to the patient
   d. 10
5. How should providers delivering critical care services to the same patient on the same date of service representing the same specialty and group practice report their services?
   a. As a single provider
   b. One provider would report 99291 and the other providers would report 99292 for each additional 30 minutes of critical care time provided
   c. Each provider reports services separately
   d. None of the above

Chapter 21. Knowledge Assessments with Answers

Chapter 2 Questions and Answers

1. How is using a documentation method beneficial?
   a. Using a standardized documentation format expedites the revenue cycle process
   b. Using a standardized documentation format ensures a lower medical malpractice premium
   c. Using a standardized documentation format can help decrease audit liability
   d. Using a standardized documentation format has not been proven to be beneficial

   Rationale: Standardized documentation formats not only decrease audit liability by consistently and uniformly establishing medical necessity and ensuring that all of the appropriate elements are documented but they also help to promote continuity of care and quality of care. When all elements are regularly and reliably documented, the likelihood of omissions and errors greatly diminish and, furthermore, clinicians become more confident and comfortable in their documentation. More detailed, consistent, thorough documentation ensures more appropriate, accurate, and timely billing.

2. Why are E/M services considered the dominant source of revenue for most providers?
   a. They are among the most frequently billed services
   b. They have high reimbursement values
   c. Providers can bill all high levels of care
   d. These services are not monitored

   Rationale: Although the reimbursement amount for E/M services is considered relatively low in comparison to surgical services, the volume of E/M services performed makes them a significant source of revenue for most providers.

3. What can providers use to assess overall coding patterns?
   a. Reimbursement rates from payers
   b. Coder productivity
   c. Payer requests for documentation
   d. Benchmark data

   Rationale: Using E/M benchmark data can help providers analyze patterns of use for specific E/M codes.

4. Which modifier should be reported to indicate to a payer that service was provided via synchronous telemedicine?
   a. 25
   b. 57
   c. 95
   d. 97

   Rationale: CPT® modifier 95, effective January 1, 2017, is to be appended to certain CPT codes designated as synchronous telemedicine services, identified in the CPT book with a star symbol [★]. A list of applicable CPT codes for reporting real time telehealth services with modifier 95 can be found in appendix P of the CPT book.

Knowledge Assessments

Chapter 3 Questions and Answers

1. Tests that are results only and are reviewed (e.g., quick strep test) do not count when determining the amount/complexity of data reviewed?
   a. True
   b. <u>False</u>

   Rationale: Results only tests that are reviewed as part of MDM count as one item when determining amount of data reviewed. Results only tests analyzed do not count as independent interpretation.

2. Using the MDM table included in the CPT E/M guidelines section, level of MDM is based on how many elements?
   a. One out of three
   b. <u>Two out of three</u>
   c. Three out of three

   Rationale: Levels of E/M codes selected using MDM are based on two out of three elements. For example, If a patient presents with one undiagnosed new problem with uncertain prognosis (moderate) and is given a prescription (moderate) as part of the treatment plan, the visit qualifies as moderate level of complexity. The amount and/or complexity of data does not have to be counted as two of three elements have been met.

3. When using time to determine the level of E/M service, which of the following count towards total time?
   a. Reviewing a separately obtained history
   b. Documenting information regarding the patient in an electronic health record
   c. Ordering medication or tests
   d. <u>All of the above</u>
   e. None of the above

   Rationale: When using total time to report office or other outpatient services, hospital inpatient and observation care, consultations, emergency department services, nursing facility, and home or residence services, total time includes face-to-face and non-face-to-face time personally spent by the provider on the date of the encounter.

4. Which is an example of additional information to determine ICD-10-CM code selection for the chief complaint of "my foot hurts?"
   a. What caused the pain?
   b. Do other body parts hurt?
   c. <u>Which foot?</u>
   d. Is the injury weather related?

   Rationale: In the ICD-10-CM coding system, laterality is required for proper code assignment, as shown below:

   - M79.67 Pain in foot and toes
   - M79.671 Pain in right foot
   - M79.672 Pain in left foot
   - M79.673 Pain in unspecified foot
   - M79.674 Pain in right toe(s)
   - M79.675 Pain in left toe(s)
   - M79.676 Pain in unspecified toe(s)

5. Of all the body areas/organ systems reviewed during an E/M encounter, which body system requires the greatest level of specificity in terms of documentation as it relates to ICD-10-CM?
   a. Neurological
   b. Respiratory
   c. Ears, nose, throat
   d. <u>Musculoskeletal</u>

   Rationale: The musculoskeletal system requires the most documentation in regard to specificity. The American Health Information Management Association (AHIMA) and other specialty societies note two factors that call for enhanced specificity when documenting conditions involving the musculoskeletal system. First, the musculoskeletal system contains a large number of codes because it includes both muscles and bones. Further, these codes are expanded in ICD-10-CM to accommodate laterality. The result is that the documentation for the musculoskeletal system requires significantly more specificity as compared to other body systems.

Chapter 4 Questions and Answers

1. Abbreviations can have multiple meanings and can confuse those who need to review the medical record documentation.
   a. True
   b. False

   Rationale: From a medico-legal standpoint, it is extremely important to have standardization in the use of abbreviations in medical records. Everyone who accesses the patient's record, from the clinicians to clinical staff, coders and even to auditors, must come to the same conclusion when reading an abbreviation to ensure that everyone infers the same meaning from the abbreviations used. Without consistency and uniformity, patient care and the meaning of what happened with the patient is compromised.

2. Why is legibility a key requirement of documentation?
   a. Patient care and treatment may be delayed and/or compromised
   b. If the handwriting of the provider cannot be read, Medicare auditors, as well as other payers, consider the service as not billable or reimbursable
   c. Legibility is not a key requirement of documentation at the present time
   d. None of the above

   Rationale: In a similar way to abbreviations, it is imperative for the provider's handwriting to be legible in order to correctly interpret the information in the patient's record. This is vitally important from a billing and reimbursement standpoint but also from a quality of care and continuity of care standpoint.

3. The benefits of the SOAP formats of documentation are that the SOAP format is a sequential record of how information is obtained, analyzed, and acted upon during the encounter.
   a. True
   b. False

   Rationale: See chapter 4 for more information on the benefits of these two formats.

4. What is a common reason a provider might over-document an encounter?
   a. Using a template as a documentation mandate and completing all fields regardless of the presenting problem and misinterpretation of the Table of Risk
   b. Using a template as a prompter to record the history and exam completed
   c. Using nursing and ancillary staff as scribes
   d. Using the Table of Risk for the final level of E/M service

   Rationale: Providers that have not been properly trained in the use of EHR templates may consider the list of check boxes to be mandatory documentation requirements rather than prompts. Misinterpretation of the table of risk can also cause providers to unintentionally increase the level of medical decision making.

5. What is an advantage to using templates with an electronic health record?
   a. Templates are used to document all necessary elements for a specific level of E/M service
   b Templates help provide consistent format and tools for electronic documentation
   c. Templates allow other staff to fill in blank data
   d. Templates are mandated by the EHR legislation

   Rationale: Templates serve as documentation prompts and do not mandate specific elements of history, exam, or testing. Documentation should reflect the provider's history, exam, and decision making based on the patient's presenting problems. A template should never be used to direct a provider to a specific level of E/M.

6. Why should billing patterns be evaluated after implementing an EHR?
   a. To penalize providers not using an EHR
   b. To verify any shift in coding patterns
   c. To keep the coders busy
   d. Both a and b

   Rationale: One of the largest concerns when adopting an EHR system, especially one with an encoder, is that the level of services reported suddenly increases. This can be due to a misunderstanding of how to use a template and providers feeling that they need to complete every check box or blank on the template.

Chapter 5 Questions and Answers

1. Medical necessity is a critical element to medical record documentation because without it claims may be rejected or outright denied.
   a. True
   b. False

   Rationale: Section 1862(a)(1)(A) of the Social Security Act states that Medicare will not cover services that "are not reasonable and necessary for the diagnosis or treatment of illness or injury or to improve the functioning of a malformed body member."

   In addition, the CMS Pub. 100-04, *Medicare Claims Processing Manual* says that medical necessity is the "overarching criterion for payment in addition to the individual requirements of a CPT code. It would not be medically necessary or appropriate to bill a higher level of evaluation and management service when a lower level of service is warranted. The volume of documentation should not be the primary influence upon which a specific level of service is billed. Documentation should support the level of service reported."

   Simply put, medical necessity becomes the main factor considered during an audit or claim review, even over the history, examination, and medical decision making. Therefore, a claim determined to be lacking in medical necessity may end up rejected or denied and subsequently not paid.

2. What is the description of "incident-to" services?
   a. Services provided by auxiliary personnel of a facility for a physician
   b. Services provided by a nurse practitioner using their own provider identification number
   c. Services provided by auxiliary personal under the supervision of and billed by the physician
   d. Services provided directly by the physician for secondary conditions

   Rationale: Incident-to services and supplies are furnished as an integral, although incidental, part of the physician's personal professional services in the course of diagnosis or treatment of an illness or injury. Auxiliary personnel performing these services must be employed by the physician or clinic and services must be performed under the direct supervision of the physician and billed by the physician.

3. What are the disadvantages of using documentation templates?
   a. They can be abused by providing "stock" or comprehensive prerecorded, histories or exams
   b. No disadvantages; they are designed to replace provider work
   c. May not be used solely as a prompt to document elements performed
   d. Both a and c

   Rationale: See rationale for question 4 in chapter 4.

4. The teaching physician does not need to be present for the key portion of an encounter if the resident relays all pertinent information in chart notes.
   a. True
   b. False

   Rationale: Guidelines state that in order for teaching physicians to bill for services, they must be present during the key portion of the exam and document appropriately.

5. Which of the following is acceptable teaching physician documentation?
   a. Seen and agreed
   b. No changes
   c. Patient evaluated, care plan reviewed with resident and agreed with findings, no additional changes
   d. Signature and date

   Rationale: Teaching physician documentation does not need to restate the resident notes but it must demonstrate that the teaching physician has seen the patient, reviewed the care plan with the resident, including changes to treatment, testing, and medications, and agreed with the findings.

6. What is the responsibility of the teaching physician in a primary care exception program?
   a. Supervise residents in providing all E/M services
   b. Supervise up to four residents providing primary responsibility for the patient's care and review each case with the resident during or immediately after the encounter
   c. Have a full schedule of patients concurrent with the residents
   d. Cosign all resident notes

   Rationale: See complete guidelines under the subheading "Exception: E/M Services Furnished in Certain Primary Care Centers" in chapter 5.

7. What is conveyed with modifier GC?
   a. The teaching physician completed the service without resident participation
   b. The teaching physician and the resident provided the service
   c. The resident provided the service under the primary care exception
   d. The resident acted as scribe for the teaching physician

   Rationale: Modifier GC, (this service has been performed, in part, by a resident under the direction of a teaching physician), is to be reported with all services provided by a teaching physician except in circumstances where modifier GE, which certifies that the physician was present during the key portion of the service and was immediately available during the other parts of the services, is applicable.

8. What special criteria must a teaching physician utilize for psychiatric services?
   a. The resident service is concurrently monitored using one-way mirrors or video equipment and audio transmission
   b. The teaching physician records the audio transmission for review
   c. The teaching physician is not required to participate in the service due to patient privacy
   d. The teaching physician is only required to review medication changes

   Rationale: For psychiatry services furnished under an approved GME program, the requirement that the teaching physician be present during the service may be met by concurrent observation of the service using one-way mirror or video equipment. Audio-only equipment does not suffice.

Chapter 6 Questions and Answers

1. History and physical examination elements are no longer used in selection of the level of office or other outpatient visit and therefore don't have to be documented in the medical record.
   a. True
   b. False

   Rationale: These elements must still be documented for continuity of patient care. The change based on the new guideline is that they will no longer be factors in code level selection for office or other outpatient E/M services. The nature and extent of history and physical examination is determined by the treating provider and per CMS must be "medically appropriate."

2. Total time on the date of the encounter includes non-face-to-face time. Which of the following activities personally performed by the treating provider may count toward the total time reported for purposes of code level selection? Select all that apply.
   a. Reviewing tests or other records
   b. Documenting clinical information in the medical record
   c. Ordering tests/procedures or medications
   d. Counseling and educating the patient or caregiver

   Rationale: Per the 2021 CPT guidelines, all of these count toward the total time personally spent by the provider on the date of the encounter. Refer to the General Guidelines sections in Chapter 6 for the complete list.

3. Based on the time documented at the end of the sample documentation for 99205 that starts on page 54, code 99205 could be reported based on time alone.
   a. True
   b. False

   Rationale: In the sample, a total of 70 minutes is documented. The new time range listed in the code descriptor for 99205 is 60–74 minutes.

4. A new patient presents to the office with two stable chronic illnesses. Limited data is reviewed, and changes are made to the patient's prescription drug regimen. Based on MDM elements, what level of service would be reported?
   a. 99203
   b. 99204
   c. 99214
   d. 99205

   Rationale: Levels of MDM, based on the redefined table published by the AMA and adopted by CMS, are based on two out of three elements. In this example, there is moderate complexity of problems (two stable chronic illnesses), limited data reviewed, and moderate risk based on the prescription drug management. Two out of three elements of MDM are moderate, which equates to a moderate level of MDM or a level four.

Chapter 7 Questions and Answers

1. An established patient is evaluated in real-time, using an interactive audio-video system. The patient is complaining of headache and ear pain. The provider documents that a total of 35 minutes was spent on the date of the encounter reviewing records, documenting the visit, ordering a prescription, and visiting with the patient. Using time to report the service, what telemedicine service should be reported?
   a. 98001
   b. 98006
   c. 98009
   d. 98014

   Rationale: Synchronous, real-time, audio-video services for established patients are reported using codes 98004-98007. Using time for code selection, a service of 35 minutes is reported with 98006, which is specified as meeting or exceeding 30 minutes of time on the date of the encounter.
2. Codes 98000-98015 require a specific time interval from the last in-person visit or telemedicine visit of at least seven days.
   a.True
   b.False

   Rationale: According to section guidelines, codes 98000-98015 do not require a specific time interval from the last in-person visit or telemedicine visit. However, code 98016 should not be reported if a related E/M service has been provided in the prior seven days or leads to an E/M service within the next 24 hours.
3. How many minutes of medical discussion are required to report new and established synchronous audio-only services (98008-98015)?
   a. Five to 10 minutes
   b. At least 5 minutes
   c. 10 minutes
   d. More than 10 minutes

   Rationale: The section guidelines indicate that 10 minutes of medical discussion must be exceeded to report the audio-only services.
4. 4.Which of the following components are applicable to code 98016 *Brief communication technology-based service*? Select all that apply.
   a. Patient-initiated service
   b. Five to 10 minutes of medical discussion
   c. Requires video technology
   d. MDM does not apply

   Rationale: Code 98016 may be reported for audio-only services of five to 10 minutes of medical discussion provided to an established patient. The service is patient-initiated and intended to determine if a more extensive visit may be required. Code 98016 is based solely on time; MDM does not apply.

Knowledge Assessments

Chapter 8 Questions and Answers

1. Codes 99234–99236 are used to report E/M services provided to an observation patient or inpatient admitted and discharged on the same day.
   a. True
   b. False

   Rationale: See the general guidelines section in this chapter for "Subsequent Hospital Care and Hospital Discharge Services (99231–99239)" for more information on this code range.

2. What code is used to report a patient admitted to observation with a history, exam, and moderate MDM documented?
   a. 99221
   b. 99222
   c. 99231
   d. 99232

   Rationale: Revised E/M guidelines state that if the patient is only seen once and is admitted and discharged on the same date only the documented admission code is reported. When the MDM level is moderate, the hospital initial or observation code level 99222 would be reported.

3. What codes are used to report a patient who is admitted and discharged the same date and the provider had two encounters documented with the patient?
   a. 99221–99223
   b. 99231–99233
   c. 99234–99236
   d. 99238–99239

   Rationale: Revised E/M guidelines state the patient who is admitted and discharged from inpatient or observation on the same date must have two separate encounters documented by the provider. If the provider does the admitting encounter but does not see the patient a second time only the documented code for the initial inpatient or observation E/M service (99221–99223) may be reported.

Chapter 9 Questions and Answers

1. Which of the following are appropriate places of service for use of office or other outpatient consultation codes (99241–99245)?
   a. Physician office
   b. Patient's home
   c. Hospital inpatient
   d. Emergency department

   Rationale: In addition to the above places of service, these may also be performed in outpatient or other ambulatory facilities, a hospital observation unit, rest home, or custodial care facility.

2. Codes 99241–99255 may be used to report consults initiated by a physician or the patient themselves.
   a. True
   b. False

   Rationale: Consults cannot be initiated by the patient, they must be requested by a physician who is seeking the opinion or advice of another physician regarding a specific problem.

3. Medicare no longer recognizes consultation codes but they are still used and reimbursable by some carriers.
   a. True
   b. False

   Rationale: Although Medicare no longer recognizes 99241–99255 as viable codes, other carriers may still reimburse for these codes. Check with the specific carrier to determine use.

4. Based on the documentation for code 99243, what is the level for number and complexity of problems addressed?
   a. Straightforward
   b. Low
   c. Moderate
   d. High

   Rationale: The consulting physician is evaluating the patients' retinopathy. Documentation states that her diabetes is stable but the ophthalmologist in this case is not addressing or managing the diabetes, only the minimal nonproliferative retinopathy. The ophthalmologist is managing one stable, chronic illness which qualifies as Low complexity.

Chapter 10 Questions and Answers

1. To qualify as an emergency department service, the encounter must be performed in a hospital-based facility that is open 24 hours a day.
   a. True
   b. False

   Rationale: Per the guidelines, the service must be provided in a hospital-based facility open 24 hours a day and is reported regardless if the patient is new or established.

2. What code would be reported when a physician or other qualified health professional at the hospital is in two-way communication with rescue workers on site at a major traffic accident?
   a. This is not a billable service
   b. 99288
   c. 99285
   d. 99291

   Rationale: Although 99288 is a valid code, typically these communications are bundled in to the emergency department physicians E/M service and are not separately reported.

3. The physician documented that 75 minutes was spent monitoring a critical patient who was given fluids and pressors after becoming hypoxic and hypotensive. What critical care code(s) would be reported?
   a. 99291 and 99292
   b. 99291
   c. 99292
   d. 99291, 99292 x 2

   Rationale: Using the table for critical services provided in this chapter, the table indicates that 75 to 104 minutes of critical-care time would be reported with 99291x1 and 99292x1.

4. When additional procedures are performed by the same physician on the same date as critical care services, the time spent performing the additional procedures is counted toward the total critical-care time.
   a. True
   b. False

   Rationale: Per the *Medicare Claims Processing Manual*, Pub. 100-04, chapter 12, 30.6.12, time spent performing procedures not bundled in to the critical care service may not be factored into the total critical care time.

5. What code is assigned for 25 minutes of total critical-care time?
   a. 99291
   b. 99292
   c. Not reportable
   d. Another appropriate level of E/M but not a critical-care code

   Rationale: Guidelines in the *Medicare Claims Processing Manual*, Pub. 100-04, state that a minimum of 30 minutes must be spent providing critical care services in order to report a critical care code. If at least 15 minutes but less than 30 minutes of critical care services are provided, another appropriate level of E/M service may be reported. Critical care services of less than 15 minutes are not reported separately.

Chapter 11 Questions and Answers

1. What level of history and exam are required to report 99305 or 99306?
   a. Detailed
   b. Detailed or comprehensive
   c. Comprehensive
   d. Medically appropriate

   Rationale: Effective January 1, 2023, nursing facility services require a medically appropriate history and physical exam as determined by the treating provider or other qualified health care provider. These elements are no longer used in selection of these E/M codes.

2. It is acceptable for a physician assistant to perform the initial nursing facility encounter as long as the physician reviews and signs the medical record.
   a. True
   b. False

   Rationale: Per the guidelines, the physician must perform the first assessment in the nursing facility.

3. What code would be assigned when the physician documents a subsequent nursing facility visit where the physician spent 25 minutes face-to-face with the patient and in non-face-to-face activities on the date of the encounter?
   a. 99309
   b. 99304
   c. 99315
   d. 99308

   Rationale: When time is used to report the E/M service code, it includes total time personally spent by the provider on the date of the encounter, including face-to-face and non-face-to-face time. For nursing facility codes, the times listed in the code descriptions must be met or exceeded. In this case 99308 (20 minutes) is the correct code for 25 minutes, as 99309 must be at least 30 minutes.

4. What code is reported when low complexity MDM is documented for a new patient in a psychiatric residential treatment facility?
   a. 99342
   b. 99304
   c. 99305
   d. 99308

   Rationale: Per the AMA guidelines nursing facility care codes are also used to report E/M services provided in psychiatric residential treatment centers and immediate care facilities for patients with intellectual disabilities. Low complexity MDM for a new patient is reported with 99304.

Chapter 12 Questions and Answers

1. What codes are used to report new patient encounters in the patient's home?
   a. 99341–99345
   b. 99241–99245
   c. 99347–99350
   d. 99202–99205

   Rationale: Codes 99341–993445 are used to report new patient encounters and codes 99347–99350 are used to report established patient encounters.

2. What home services code would be assigned for an established patient with moderate MDM?
   a. 99349
   b. 99350
   c. 99344
   d. None of the above

   Rationale: Code 99349 is reported for moderate complexity MDM.

3. What modifier should be appended to codes 99341–99350 when services were mandated by a court order?
   a. 25
   b. 52
   c. 59
   d. 32

   Rationale: Modifier 32 is appended to a service formally ordered by a court or other superior official.

4. What home services code would be assigned for a new patient with moderate MDM?
   a. 99344
   b. 99342
   c. 99349
   d. None of the above

   Rationale: Code 99344 requires a moderate level of MDM and medically appropriate history and examination. As the MDM met the requirements for 99344 it would be the correct code to report.

Chapter 13 Questions and Answers

1. When coding prolonged services, what major element out of the following is the determining factor for when to use 99358–99359?
   a. New vs. established
   b. Office or outpatient facility
   c. With or without direct patient contact
   d. All of the above

   Rationale: A close look at this code range in this chapter and in the CPT book include "without direct" patient contact in the description and should be the first consideration when assigning the correct code for these services.

2. Codes 99358 or 99415 may only be used once per date of service.
   a. True
   b. False

   Rationale: These codes constitute the first 30 to 74 minutes of prolonged service time and may only be billed once for a given date of service. Codes 99359 and 99416 report each additional 30 minutes and may be billed as many times as necessary to report the total amount of time spent providing prolonged services. See the documentation requirements in this chapter for more detail on properly billing these codes.

3. Codes 99359 and 99415–99418 are all add-on codes and can be billed alone with sufficient documentation.
   a. True
   b. False

   Rationale: Add-on codes should never be billed as stand-alone codes. They are always billed with a primary code.

4. In order to bill prolonged services 99417–99418, the total time of the encounter must exceed the basic service by at least ______ minutes.
   a. 15
   b. 30
   c. 45
   d. 60

   Rationale: Per the E/M guidelines, prolonged services of less than 15 minutes are not reported separately.

5. To report prolonged services provided by the clinical staff (99415–99416), direct supervision by a physician is required.
   a. True
   b. False

   Rationale: A physician or other qualified health care professional must be available to provide direct supervision to the clinical staff in order to report codes 99415 and 99416. See the general guidelines section under 99415–99416 for more information.

6. A clinician may not report standby services if the standby service period ends with the standby clinician performing a global surgery package procedure.
   a. True
   b. False

   Rationale: If the standby period ends with the standby clinician performing a procedure that is subject to the surgical package, this code is not reported separately.

Chapter 14 Questions and Answers

1. How many health care professionals of different specialties must participate in order to bill for a medical team conference (99366–99368)?
   a. Two or more
   b. Four or more
   c. More than 10
   d. Three or more

   Rationale: At least three health care professionals of different specialties who provide direct care to the patient must participate in order to report the team conference codes. Each provider must document his or her participation and care recommendations.

2. Which of the following activities would not count toward total time when billing for care plan oversight services?
   a. Adding new information to the treatment plan
   b. Discussing treatment adjustments with the patient or a caregiver
   c. Revisions to the plan of care
   d. Reviewing treatment plans and lab results

   Rationale: Besides the above activities, communication with other health care professionals involved in the care of the patient but not employed in the same practice, would also count towards total time for care plan oversight services.

3. What is the appropriate code for a well-visit/preventive service provided to a 20-year-old established patient?
   a. 99215
   b. 99385
   c. 99395
   d. 99396

   Rationale: The preventive service codes are based on patient age and whether the patient is new or established. New patients are billed using codes 99381–99387 and established patients are billed using codes 99391–99397.

Chapter 15 Questions and Answers

1. Patients from birth to 28 days of age are considered newborns when assigning codes 99460–99486.
   a. True
   b. False

   Rationale: By definition, a patient is considered a newborn from birth to 28 days of age.

2. What codes would be used to report physician attendance of a critically ill infant less than 24 months of age being transported to the hospital?
   a. 99485–99486
   b. 99466–99467
   c. 99291–99292
   d. None of the above

   Rationale: Codes 99466–99467 are time-based codes and are billed for services of at least 30 minutes. Critical care services of less than 30 minutes should be reported with the appropriate outpatient visit or subsequent hospital care code. Codes 99291–99292 are used to report transport of patients older than 24 months of age.

3. What codes are used to report inpatient critical care services of a 3-year-old patient?
   a. 99291 and 99292
   b. 99468 and 99469
   c. 99475 and 99476
   d. 99471 and 99472

   Rationale: Neonatal and pediatric inpatient critical care codes are based on the patient's age and whether the encounter is an initial or subsequent service.

4. Subsequent *intensive* critical care codes, 99478–99480, are determined based on the patient's body weight.
   a. True
   b. False

   Rationale: Initial intensive critical care for a patient less than 28 days old is reported with code 99477. Codes 99478–99480 for subsequent intensive critical care are selected based on the patient's weight; 99478 for weight of less than 1500 grams, 99479 for weight of 1500 to 2500 grams, and 99480 for weight of 2501 to 5000 grams.

5. What code is reported when a newborn is admitted and discharged in the hospital or birthing center on the same date of service?
   a. 99460
   b. 99461
   c. 99462
   d. 99463

   Rationale: The official code description for 99463 states, "Initial hospital or birthing center care, per day, for evaluation and management of normal newborn infant admitted and discharged on the same date."

6. Adult critical care codes are reported based on the amount of time spent with the patient. What factors determine which neonatal or pediatric critical care code is appropriate?
   a. Type of visit (initial or subsequent)
   b. Time
   c. Patient age
   d. a and c

   Rationale: CPT guidelines state that neonatal and pediatric critical care services are reported per day—not on the amount of face-to-face time spent with the patient. Instead, proper code selection is based on the age of the patient, as well as whether the service is considered to be an initial or subsequent visit.

Chapter 16 Questions and Answers

1. A patient's chart indicates that 15 minutes of chronic care management services were provided for the month. What code would be reported for this service?
   a. 99490
   b. 99487
   c. 99489
   d. The service is not reportable

   Rationale: Chronic care management services of less than 20 minutes are not separately reported.

2. Care management services include both face-to-face and non-face-to-face time spent by clinical staff with the patient, caregiver, or other professionals and agencies involved in the patient's care.
   a. True
   b. False

   Rationale: See the general guidelines section in this chapter for more information on appropriate use of these codes.

3. Which of the following would be included in the care plan documentation?
   a. Expected outcomes
   b. Medication management
   c. Planned interventions
   d. All of the above

   Rationale: In addition to the above, the care plan may also include a problem list, prognosis, treatment objectives, identification of providers providing each service ordered, periodic review, and revision of the care plan as necessary.

4. Care management services may only be provided by a physician or other qualified health care professional.
   a. True
   b. False

   Rationale: These services may be performed in part by other clinical staff under direction of a physician or other qualified health care professional.

5. There are 10 required elements listed in the description for code 99483. For this patient only eight were performed. What code should be reported for the services provided?
   a. 99483-52
   b. 99483
   c. An appropriate E/M code
   d. None of the above

   Rationale: Guidance regarding 99483 from the AMA states that if all elements listed in the code description are not performed or are deemed unnecessary for the patient's condition, see the appropriate E/M code.

6. Behavioral health intervention codes 99484, 99492, and 99493, may only be reported once by the same provider in a calendar month.
   a. True
   b. False

   Rationale: These codes may only be reported once in a calendar month.

7. A patient's chart indicates that a total of 1 hour and 30 minutes of subsequent psychiatric collaborative care management services was provided for the calendar month. Which code(s) would be reported for these services?
   a. 99492 and 99494 x 1
   b. 99493
   c. 99492 and 99493
   d. 99493 and 99494 x 1

   Rationale: Subsequent psychiatric care services of less than 31 minutes are not reported separately, 31–75 minutes are reported with 99493, and 76–105 minutes are reported with 99493 and add-on code 99494. Code 99494 is reported with 99492 (initial services) or 99493 (subsequent services) for each additional increment of 30 minutes above the base time.

8. Psychiatric collaborative care management services are provided by a care team that includes a treating provider, a behavioral health care manager, and a psychiatric consultant. Which care team member reports codes 99492, 99493, and 99494 for the services provided?
   a. Behavioral health care manager
   b. Treating provider
   c. Psychiatric consultant
   d. Each provider reports their own services

   Rationale: The treating provider reports these services on behalf of the care team. In some cases, all team members may be part of the same group practice. In most situations the psychiatric consultant will be contracted directly with the treating provider to provide consultation services.

9. General behavioral health integration management services of less than 20 minutes are not reportable.
   a. True
   b. False

   Rationale: General BHI services of less than 20 minutes are not reported separately.

Chapter 17 Questions and Answers

1. Transitional care services may only be reported when a face-to-face visit by a physician or other qualified health care professional has been performed.
   a. True
   b. False

   Rationale: These codes may only be reported if at least one face-to-face visit is provided by the physician or other qualified health care professional. These codes are based on level of MDM and how soon after discharge the face-to-face service is provided, within the first seven days or within eight to 14 days after discharge.

2. When does the 30-day transitional care management period begin?
   a. The day after the patient is discharged from the inpatient setting
   b. The day the patient is discharged from the inpatient setting
   c. The day the physician performs the face-to-face visit
   d. The first Monday following discharge

   Rationale: See the general guidelines section in this chapter for more guidance on appropriate use of these codes.

3. If the physician or other qualified health care professional provides more than one face-to-face visit in a month, these services are included in the transitional care codes and are not separately reportable.
   a. True
   b. False

   Rationale: If a physician or other qualified health care professional provides more than one face-to-face visit in a month, the additional visits should be reported with the appropriate E/M code.

4. Transitional care management services require interactive contact with the patient or caregiver within how many business days of discharge?
   a. Seven
   b. Two
   c. One
   d. Five

   Rationale: CPT guidelines state that transitional care management services require a:

   - Face-to-face visit
   - Initial patient contact, and
   - Medication reconciliation within a specified period of time

   In addition, the guidelines also require "an interactive contact with the patient or caregiver, as appropriate within two business days of discharge."

5. Which of the following are acceptable methods of communication for the required interactive contact? Select all that apply.
   a. Telephone
   b. Mail
   c. Face to face
   d. E-mail

   Rationale: Per CPT guidelines, the interactive contact may be rendered face to face, over the phone or by other electronic means such as the internet or email.

Knowledge Assessments

Chapter 18 Questions and Answers

1. Which range of E/M codes should not be reported with 99497–99498 on the same date of service?
   a. 99202–99215
   b. 99304–99310
   c. 99381–99397
   d. 99475–99480

   Rationale: In addition to 99475–99480, codes 99291–99292, 99468–99469, and 99471–99472 should not be reported with the advance care planning codes.

2. The physician provides active management of the patient's problems as part of the advance care planning.
   a. True
   b. False

   Rationale: Advance care planning does not include any active management of the patient's problems. Time used to report these codes includes only the time spent in counseling and discussion of advance care directives.

Chapter 19 Questions and Answers

1. What code is reported for a Medicare patient who received 30 minutes of physician supervised care plan oversight services in the calendar month under a Medicare-approved hospice program?
   a. G0181
   b. G0182
   c. 99378
   d. The service is not reportable

   Rationale: Physician supervision of a patient receiving complex and multidisciplinary care under a Medicare approved hospice is reimbursable when 30 minutes or more are spent within a calendar month providing these services.

2. Code G0180 for physician certification for Medicare-covered, home health services can only be reported if the patient has not received any Medicare-covered, home health services for a period of at least 31 days.
   a. True
   b. False

   Rationale: Certification under a home health plan of care can only be reported when the patient has not received Medicare-covered, home health services for a period of at least 60 days.

3. Medicare does not cover preventive medicine services (99381–99429); however, the agency does cover a welcome to Medicare visit or initial preventive physical exam (IPPE). What code is used to report this visit?
   a. G0402
   b. 99387
   c. 99397
   d. G0438

   Rationale: HCPCS Level II code G0402 is used to report the IPPE for new Medicare beneficiaries, codes G0403–G0405 are used to report the global screening EKG if performed at the time of the IPPE.

4. How do providers reporting telehealth services to Medicare administrative contractors (MAC) indicate that the service was provided via telehealth real-time telecommunication systems?
   a. Report only the G code if the word telehealth is part of the code description
   b. Append modifier GT to the G code
   c. Submit using place of service (POS) code 02 or 10
   d. Both b and c

   Rationale: Beginning January 1, 2024, CMS requires the use of place of service (POS) 02 or 10 for telehealth services. POS 02 is used to report professional telehealth services when the originating site is other than the patient's home. POS 10 is used to report telehealth services when the patient is in the home.

5. Which of the following are approved distant site telehealth practitioners?
   a. Nurse practitioner
   b. Clinical psychologist
   c. Nurse midwife
   d. All of the above

   Rationale: The following list identifies approved distant site practitioners:

   - Physician
   - Physician assistant (PA)
   - Nurse practitioner (NP)
   - Clinical nurse specialist (CNS)
   - Nurse midwife
   - Clinical psychologist
   - Clinical social worker
   - Registered dietitian or nutrition professional
   - Certified registered nurse anesthetists

6. Codes G0425–G0427 and G0406–G0408 are only used to report telehealth consultations provided to Medicare beneficiaries.
   a. True
   b. False

   Rationale: G codes are only accepted by Medicare.

Knowledge Assessments

Chapter 20 Questions and Answers

1. Out of the following, which are considered part of a global surgery package?
   a. Postoperative visits
   b. Postsurgical pain management
   c. Preoperative visits
   d. All postoperative complications not requiring a return to the operating room
   e. <u>All of the above</u>

   Rationale: The CMS national definition of global surgery package includes all the items listed here as well as; intraoperative services, supplies, and miscellaneous services (i.e., dressing changes, removal of packing material, local incisional wound care, etc.). To review Medicare guidelines regarding payment for hospital observation services and observation or inpatient care services" see *Medicare Claims Processing Manual*, Pub. 100-04, chapter 12, section 30.6.8.

2. Where is Medicare's official list of postoperative days included in each surgical procedure found?
   a. *Medicare Claims Processing Manual*
   b. <u>Medicare Physician Fee Schedule Database</u>
   c. *Medicare Program Integrity Manual*
   d. National Correct Coding Initiative

   Rationale: The Medicare Physician Fee Schedule Database (MPFSDB) contains the number of days included in the postoperative period of each surgical procedure.

3. Preoperative visits for major procedures begin the day before a major procedure.
   a. <u>True</u>
   b. False

   Rationale: According to CMS guidelines preoperative visits occur after the decision for surgery has been made and begin on the day prior to a major procedure (90 global days) and begin the day of surgery for minor procedures (000 or 010 global days).

4. How many distinct components must be provided or referred to another physician, in order to bill for Medicare's initial preventive physician examination (IPPE)?
   a. Four
   b. <u>Nine</u>
   c. The number varies based on preventive services already provided to the patient
   d. 10

   Rationale: The IPPE face-to-face exam consists of the following nine distinct components:

   - Review of patient's medical and social history
   - Review the patient's potential risk factors for depression
   - Review the patient's functional ability and level of safety
   - Physical examination that includes height, weight, blood pressure, visual acuity, and BMI
   - End-of-life planning
   - Review of current prescriptions of opioids
   - Screening for potential substance use disorders
   - Education, counseling, and referral based on the results of the review and evaluation services described above
   - Education, counseling, and referral, including a brief written plan or checklist, for obtaining the appropriate screening or other Part B preventive services

5. How should providers delivering critical care services to the same patient on the same date of service representing the same specialty and group practice report their services?
   a. <u>As a single provider</u>
   b. One provider would report 99291 and the other providers would report 99292 for each additional 30 minutes of critical care time provided
   c. Each provider reports services separately
   d. None of the above

   Rationale: Medicare policy states that physicians in the same practice in the same specialty must report these claims as though they were a single physician. To review Medicare's guidance on the use of critical care services see: *Medicare Claims Processing Manual*, Pub. 100-04, chapter 12, section 30.6.12.

Glossary

25. CPT modifier, for use with CPT evaluation and management (E/M) codes, that identifies when the patient's condition requires a significant, separately identifiable E/M service(s) above and beyond other services provided or above and beyond the usual preoperative and postoperative care associated with the procedure that was performed on the same date of service. Medical record documentation must clearly support all necessary criteria required for use of the E/M service being reported, including identifying signs or symptoms of the condition for which the service was rendered. Not all payers require a separate diagnosis when billing for a procedure and E/M service on the same date of service.

57. CPT modifier, for use with CPT evaluation and management (E/M) codes, that identifies an E/M service that resulted in the initial decision to perform surgery. This modifier should be used only with procedure codes considered major surgery (90-day global period).

AAPC. National organization for coders and billers offering certification examinations based on physician-, facility-, or payer-specific guidelines or coding documentation. Upon successful completion of the selected examination, the credential for that examination is obtained.

abstractor. Person who selects and extracts specific data from the medical record and enters the information into computer files.

abuse. Medical reimbursement term that describes an incident that is inconsistent with accepted medical, business, or fiscal practices and directly or indirectly results in unnecessary costs to the Medicare program, improper reimbursement, or reimbursement for services that do not meet professionally recognized standards of care or which are medically unnecessary. Examples of abuse include excessive charges, improper billing practices, billing Medicare as primary instead of other third-party payers that are primary, and increasing charges for Medicare beneficiaries but not to other patients.

accountable care organization. Recognized legal entity under state law comprised of providers of services and suppliers with an established mechanism for shared governance who work together to coordinate care for Medicare fee-for-service beneficiaries. Section 3022 of the Affordable Care Act required CMS to develop a shared savings program to promote coordination and cooperation among providers for the purposes of improving the quality of care for Medicare fee-for-service beneficiaries and minimize costs.

Accredited Standards Committee. Organization accredited by the American National Standards Institute (ANSI) for the development of American national standards.

ACG. 1) Ambulatory care group. **2)** American College of Gastroenterologists. Professional organization for gastroenterology medical specialty.

ACH. Automated clearinghouse. Entity that processes or facilitates the processing of information received from another entity in a nonstandard format or containing nonstandard data content into standard data elements or a standard transaction, or that receives a standard transaction from another entity and processes or facilitates the processing of that information into nonstandard format or nonstandard data content for a receiving entity.

activities of daily living. Self-care activities often used to determine a patient's level of function, such as bathing, dressing, using a toilet, transferring in and out of bed or a chair, continence, eating, and walking.

acute. Sudden, severe. Documentation and reporting of an acute condition is important to establishing medical necessity.

acute care facility. Health care institution primarily engaged in providing treatment to inpatients and diagnostic and therapeutic services for medical diagnosis, treatment, and care of injured, disabled, or sick persons who are in an acute phase of illness.

add-on code. CPT code representing a procedure performed in addition to the primary procedure and designated with a + symbol in the CPT book. Add-on codes are never reported for stand-alone services but are reported secondarily in addition to the primary procedure.

adjudication. Processing and review of a submitted claim resulting in payment, partial payment, or denial. In relationship to judicial hearings, it is the process of hearing and settling a case through an objective, judicial procedure.

admission. Formal acceptance of a patient by a health care facility.

admission date. Date the patient was admitted to the health care facility for inpatient care, outpatient service, or the start of care.

against medical advice. Discharge status of patients who leave the hospital after signing a form that releases the hospital from responsibility, or those who leave the hospital premises without notifying hospital personnel.

age restriction. In health care contracting, limitation of benefits when a patient reaches a certain age.

AHA. American Hospital Association. Health care industry association that represents the concerns of institutional providers. The AHA hosts the National Uniform Billing Committee (NUBC), which has a formal consultative role under HIPAA. The AHA also publishes *Coding Clinic* for ICD-10 and HCPCS.

AHIMA. American Health Information Management Association. Association of health information management professionals offering various certification examinations for physician- and facility-based coders, clinical documentation improvement practitioners, and other technology and health informatics specialists.

allowable charge. Fee schedule amount for a medical service as determined by the physician fee schedule methodology published annually by CMS.

altering patient records. Inappropriately changing or amending patient records, usually to obtain reimbursement or because of pending audits and legal review of records.

AMA. American Medical Association. Professional organization for physicians. The AMA is the secretariat of the National Uniform Claim Committee (NUCC), which has a formal consultative role under HIPAA. The AMA also maintains the Physicians' Current Procedural Terminology (CPT) coding system.

ancillary services. Services, other than routine room and board charges, that are incidental to the hospital stay. These services include operating room; anesthesia; blood administration; pharmacy; radiology; laboratory; medical, surgical, and central supplies; physical, occupational, speech pathology, and inhalation therapies; and other diagnostic services.

any willing provider. Provider who meets the network's usual selection criteria as defined in statutes requiring a provider network.

appeal. Specific request made to a payer for reconsideration of a denial or adverse coverage or payment decision and potential restriction of benefit reimbursement.

appeal process. Steps required for appealing negative decisions related to payer denials such as denied authorization for requested services or denied charges.

arbitration. Settling of a dispute through a designated individual, group, or committee that is assigned to hear both sides of the story and has the authority to make a binding decision.

ARRA. American recovery and reinvestment act of 2009.

assessment. Process of collecting and studying information and data, such as test values, signs, and symptoms.

audit. Examination or review that establishes the extent to which performance or a process conforms to predetermined standards or criteria. An audit may target utilization, quality of care, coding, or reimbursement.

auditing and monitoring. Regular review of an organization's claim development and submission process from the point where service for a patient is initiated to the submission of a claim for payment. Monitoring involves a system of checks of and controls over, as well as a method of reporting, all areas of compliance, including regulations and audits.

auditor. Professional who evaluates a provider's utilization, quality of care, or level of reimbursement.

authentication. Characteristic of electronic signature. Under HIPAA, authentication is the product of a technology that, when it affixes a signature to a document, also includes a means of establishing that the person or entity signing the document is who he or she claims to be.

authorization. Verbal or written agreement indicating that a third-party payer will pay for services rendered by the provider as set forth in the authorization.

auxiliary personnel. Individual acting under a physician's supervision. It may be an employee, leased employee, or independent contractor of the physician (or other practitioner) or of the same entity that employs or contracts with the physician (or other practitioner).

behavior management. Education and modification techniques or methodologies aimed at helping a patient change undesirable habits or behaviors.

care plan oversight services. Physician's ongoing review and revision of a patient's care plan involving complex or multidisciplinary care modalities.

charts. Compilation of documents maintained by the provider for each patient that includes treatment/progress notes, test orders and results, correspondence from other health care providers, and other documents pertinent to the patient's care.

chief complaint. Term used in evaluation and management documentation and coding that identifies the reason or presenting problem that necessitated the patient's encounter for treatment. Typically, this is documented in the medical record using the patient's own words; for example, "My head hurts."

chronic. Persistent, continuing, or recurring.

claim. Statement of services rendered requesting payment from an insurance company or a government entity.

claim manual. Administrative guidelines used by claims processors to adjudicate claims according to company policy and procedure.

clinic. Outpatient facility that provides scheduled diagnostic, curative, rehabilitative, and educational services for walk-in (ambulatory) patients.

clinical quality measure. Tools that assist in measuring and tracking the quality of health care services rendered by eligible clinicians, eligible hospitals, and critical access hospitals (CAH). Measures use data associated with clinicians' ability to deliver high-quality care or relate to long-term goals for quality health care.

coder. Professional who translates documented, written diagnoses and procedures into numeric and alphanumeric codes.

coding guidelines. Criteria that specifies how procedure, diagnosis, or supply codes are to be translated and used in various situations. Coding guidelines are issued by the AHA, AMA, CMS, NCHVS, and various other groups. Guidelines may vary by payer, type of coding system, and intended use.

coding rules. Official rules and coding conventions used for diagnosis and procedure coding.

coding specificity. Selection of classification codes (e.g., ICD-10-CM) that provides the highest degree of accuracy and completeness based on clinical documentation. For example, a six-character ICD-10-CM code cannot be reported when the specific code requires a 7th character.

comorbid condition. Condition present that is not the primary reason for treating the patient, but one that affects the patient's care.

comorbidity. Preexisting condition that causes an increase in length of stay by at least one day in approximately 75 percent of cases. Used in DRG reimbursement.

compliance audit. Internal or external monitoring and review of activities to ensure compliance with all laws, regulations, and guidelines related to health care.

concurrent care. Medical care provided by two or more physicians on the same day. If care is medically necessary, payers usually pay both physicians. Generally, payers expect the physicians to be of different specialties and caring for different conditions or different aspects of the same condition or disease process.

constitutional. Component of evaluation and management documentation. History component review of systems used to denote general symptoms such as fever, malaise, weight change. Exam component noting vital signs and general appearance.

consultation. Advice or opinion regarding diagnosis and treatment or determination to accept transfer of care of a patient rendered by a medical professional at the request of the primary care provider.

contractor. Entity who enters into a contractual agreement with CMS to service a component of the Medicare program administration, for example, fiscal intermediaries, carriers, program safeguard coordinators.

conversion. In health care contracting, shifting a member under a group contract to an individual contract in accordance with contract terms and occurring with a change in employer benefits or when the covered person leaves the group.

conversion factor. 1) Dollar value for each relative value unit. When this dollar amount is multiplied by the total relative value units, it yields the reimbursement rate for the service. **2)** National multiplier that converts the geographically adjusted relative value units into Medicare fee schedule dollar amounts that applies to all services paid under the MPFS.

coordinated care. In health care contracting, system of health care delivery that influences utilization, quality of care, and cost of services. Managed care integrates financing and management with an employed or contracted organized provider network that delivers services to an enrolled population.

coordination of benefits. Agreement that prevents double payment for services when the member is covered by two or more sources. The agreement dictates which organization is primarily and secondarily responsible for payment.

coordination of care. Care provided concurrently with counseling that includes treatment instructions to the patient or caregiver; special accommodations for home, work, school, vacation, or other locations; coordination with other providers and agencies; and living arrangements.

copayment. Cost-sharing arrangement in which a covered person pays a specified portion of allowed charges. In relation to Medicare, the copayment designates the specific dollar amount that the patient must pay and coinsurance designates the percentage of allowed charges.

coronary care unit. Facility or service area dedicated to patients suffering from heart attack, stroke, or other serious cardiopulmonary problems.

counseling. Discussion with a patient and/or family concerning one or more of the following areas: diagnostic results, impressions, and/or recommended diagnostic studies; prognosis; risks and benefits of management (treatment) options; instructions for management (treatment) and/or follow-up; importance of compliance with chosen management (treatment) options; risk factor reduction; and patient and family education.

CPT. Current Procedural Terminology. Definitive procedural coding system developed by the American Medical Association that lists descriptive terms and identifying codes to provide a uniform language that describes medical, surgical, and diagnostic services for nationwide communication among physicians, patients, and third parties, used to report professional and outpatient services.

CPT codes. Codes maintained and copyrighted by the AMA and selected for use under HIPAA for outpatient facility and nondental professional transactions.

CPT modifier. Two-character code used to indicate that a service was altered in some way from the stated CPT or HCPCS Level II description, but not enough to change the basic definition of the service.

CQM. Clinical quality measure. Tools that assist in measuring and tracking the quality of health care services rendered by eligible clinicians, eligible hospitals, and critical access hospitals (CAH). Measures use data associated with clinicians' ability to deliver high-quality care or relate to long-term goals for quality health care.

critical care. Treatment of critically ill patients in a variety of medical emergencies that requires the constant attendance of the physician (e.g., cardiac arrest, shock, bleeding, respiratory failure, postoperative complications, critically ill neonate).

Current Procedural Terminology. Definitive procedural coding system developed by the American Medical Association that lists descriptive terms and identifying codes to provide a uniform language that describes medical, surgical, and diagnostic services for nationwide communication among physicians, patients, and third parties.

customary, prevailing, and reasonable charge. Categories used as the basis for Medicare's reimbursement rates before the resource-based relative value scale (RBRVS) was implemented. These rates were based on the lowest charge of the three categories rather than the relative values of each service, which caused wide variations in Medicare payments among physicians and specialties. "Customary" described a clinician's historical charges, "prevailing" represented the charges of other providers in the same specialty type residing in the same general locality, and "reasonable" was the lowest charge of all three categories.

date of service. Day the encounter or procedure is performed or the day a supply is issued.

diagnosis. Determination or confirmation of a condition, disease, or syndrome and its implications.

diagnostic laboratory services. Laboratory services that are required to diagnose a disease or injury, regardless of where the services are rendered. These services include certain mechanical or machine tests such as EKGs and EEGs. For Medicare purposes, these services are paid under a fee schedule.

diagnostic procedures. Procedure performed on a patient to obtain information to assess the medical condition of the patient or to identify a disease and to determine the nature and severity of an illness or injury.

diagnostic services. Examination or procedure performed on a patient to obtain information to assess the medical condition of the patient or to identify a disease and to determine the nature and severity of an illness or injury.

diagnostic x-ray services. X-ray and other related services performed for diagnostic purposes, including portable x-ray services.

direct supervision. Situation in which the physician must be present in the office suite and immediately available to provide assistance and direction throughout a given procedure. The physician is not, however, required to be present in the room when the procedure is performed.

discharge. Situation in which the patient leaves an acute care (prospective payment) hospital after receiving complete acute care treatment.

discharge date. For medical facilities, the date the patient is formally released, expires, or is transferred. In other situations, the date that medical care or treatment ended.

discharge plan. Treatment plan by the provider for continued patient care after discharge that may include home care, the services of case managers or other health care providers, or transfer to another facility.

discharge status. Disposition of the patient at discharge (e.g., left against medical advice, discharged home, transferred to an acute care hospital, expired).

discharge transfer. Discharge of a patient from one facility to another.

documentation. Physician's written or transcribed notations about a patient encounter, including a detailed operative report or written notes about a routine encounter. Source documentation must be the treating provider's own account of the encounter and may be transcribed from dictation, dictated by the physician into voice recognition software, or be hand- or typewritten. A signature or authentication accompanies each entry.

e-prescribing. Transmission of prescription or prescription-related information between the prescriber and the medication dispenser. For Medicare purposes, e-prescribing includes but is not limited to two-way transmission between the point of care and the dispenser.

E/M. Evaluation and management services. Assessment, counseling, and other services provided to a patient and reported through CPT codes.

E/M codes. Evaluation and management service codes.

EC. Eligible clinician. Term used in the Quality Payment Program (QPP) Merit-based Incentive Payment System (MIPS) track to describe medical professionals who are eligible to participate in the program.

electronic health record. Electronic version of individual patients' health-related information that has the interoperability to be created, managed, and consulted by more than one health care organization's authorized staff and clinicians and designed to streamline the clinicians' workflow processes. Information contained in an EHR includes, but is not limited to, patient demographics, process notes, problems, medications, vital signs, past medical history, immunizations, laboratory data, and radiology reports.

electronic medical record. Electronic version of individual patients' health-related information that can be created, managed, and consulted by single care organizations' authorized staff and clinicians.

eligible professional. Nonhospital based physician receiving Medicare and/or Medicaid reimbursement who is using a certified electronic health record.

emergency. Serious medical condition or symptom (including severe pain) resulting from injury, sickness, or mental illness that arises suddenly and requires immediate care and treatment, generally received within 24 hours of onset, to avoid jeopardy to the life, limb, or health of a covered person.

emergency admission. Admission in which the patient requires immediate medical or psychiatric attention because of life-threatening, severe, and potentially disabling conditions.

emergency department. Organized hospital-based facility for the provision of unscheduled episodic services to patients who present for immediate medical attention. The facility must be available 24 hours a day.

emergency outpatient. Patient admitted for diagnosis and treatment of a condition requiring immediate attention but who will not stay at that facility or be transferred to another.

emergent care. Treatment for a medical or mental health condition or symptom that arises suddenly and requires care and treatment immediately or as soon as possible.

EMR. Electronic medical record.

encoder. Computer application that assists in the assignment of a diagnosis or procedure code and may also assign reimbursement categories and values.

encounter. 1) Direct personal contact between a registered hospital outpatient (e.g., medical clinic or emergency department) and a physician (or other person authorized by state law and hospital bylaws to order or furnish services) for the diagnosis and treatment of an illness or injury. Visits with more than one health professional that take place during the same session and at a single location within the hospital are considered a single visit. **2)** Quality reporting term used to describe meetings with patients during the performance period as represented by the following: CPT Category I or Category II service or procedure code or a HCPCS Level II code located in a quality measure's denominator. Reporting of these codes counts as eligibility to meet a measure's inclusion requirements when the service occurs during the specified performance period.

end-stage renal disease. Chronic, advanced kidney disease requiring renal dialysis or a kidney transplant to prevent imminent death.

EP. Eligible professional.

episode of care. One or more health care services received during a period of relatively continuous care by a hospital or health care provider.

established patient. 1) Patient who has received professional services in a face-to-face setting within the last three years from the same physician/qualified health care professional or another physician/qualified health care professional of the exact same specialty and subspecialty who belongs to the same group practice.
2) For OPPS hospitals, patient who has been registered as an inpatient or outpatient in a hospital's provider-based clinic or emergency department within the past three years.

estimated length of stay. Average number of days of hospitalization required for a given illness or procedure, based on prior histories of patients who have been hospitalized for the same illness or procedure.

evaluation and management. Assessment, counseling, and other services provided to a patient reported through CPT codes.

evaluation and management codes. Assessment and management of a patient's health care.

examination. Comprehensive visual and tactile screening and specific testing leading to diagnosis or, as appropriate, to a referral to another practitioner.

extended care facility. Institution that provides any type of long-term care. Usually refers to a skilled nursing facility, but may be used in reference to other types of long-term institutions.

face to face. Interaction between two parties, usually provider and patient, that occurs in the physical presence of each other.

facility. Place of patient care, including inpatient and outpatient, acute or long term.

family history. Record of the health of family members, including the health status or cause of death of parents, siblings, and children, and specific diseases related to the patient's chief complaint, history of present illness, and/or review of systems.

fellow. Physician who has completed a basic residency program and is now in a formally organized and approved subspecialty program that may or may not be recognized as an approved residency program under Medicare for received GME funding.

health care provider. Entity that administers diagnostic and therapeutic services.

health history form. Document completed by the patient that contains a number of questions regarding health history; typically completed at the first patient encounter. The patient may be asked to periodically review the document at subsequent visits or as needed to ensure health history information remains current and up to date. The form should include a place for the patient to list all current prescription and over-the-counter (OTC) medications and supplements, including dosages and frequency, as well as a personal, family, and social history. All 14 body systems (constitutional, eyes, ears, nose, throat, mouth [ENT, M], respiratory, cardiovascular, gastrointestinal, genitourinary, musculoskeletal, integumentary [skin/breast], neurological, psychiatric, endocrine, hematologic/lymphatic, and allergy/immunologic) should be listed. Space should be included for any applicable insurance information, the phone number to the patient's pharmacy, and a next of kin contact.

history of present illness. Chronological account of signs and symptoms of the present condition.

HIT. Health information technology.

HITECH. Health information technology for economic and clinical health. Act that was included as part of the American Recovery and Reinvestment Act of 2009 and signed into law on February 17, 2009 for the meaningful use of health information technology. Within the Act, privacy and security measures are addressed regarding the electronic transmission of protected health information with civil and criminal enforcement of HIPAA rules defined.

home health. Palliative and therapeutic care and assistance in the activities of daily life to home bound Medicare and private plan members.

hospice. Organization that furnishes inpatient, outpatient, and home health care for the terminally ill. Hospices emphasize support and counseling services for terminally ill people and their families, pain relief, and symptom management. When the Medicare beneficiary chooses hospice benefits, all other Medicare benefits are discontinued, except physician services and treatment of conditions not related to the terminal illness.

hospital admission plan. Used to facilitate admission to the hospital and to assure prompt payment to the hospital.

HPI. History of present illness.

ICD-10. International Classification of Diseases, 10th Revision. Classification of diseases by alphanumeric code, used by the World Health Organization.

ICD-10-CM. International Classification of Diseases, 10th Revision, Clinical Modification. Clinical modification of the alphanumeric classification of diseases used by the World Health Organization, already in use in much of the world, and used for mortality reporting in the United States.

ICD-10-PCS. International Classification of Diseases, 10th Revision, Procedure Coding System. Inpatient hospital services and surgical procedures must be coded using ICD-10-PCS codes.

incident to. Services commonly provided in a physician's office or clinic that are performed by a non-physician practitioner under the direct supervision and direction of a physician who has already determined a diagnosis and documented a plan of care. For example, an evaluation and management service can be performed in the office by a mid-level provider as an "incident to" service. "Incident to" also refers to supplies that are incidental to the diagnosis or treatment of an injury or illness such as gauze or bandages.

inpatient hospitalization. Period in which a patient is housed in a single hospital usually without interruption.

intern. Medical school graduate who is in the first year of postgraduate training under the direction of a teaching physician and/or senior resident.

interpretation. Professional health care provider's review of data with a written or verbal opinion.

interval history. History documenting what has occurred in a given area since the last visit, usually associated with subsequent hospital, nursing home, rest home, and home visit services.

key portion. Part (or parts) of a service determined by the teaching physician to be the critical or key portion.

leased employee. Legal employment relationship established by a contract where an employer hires the services of an employee through another employer.

long-term care facility. Nursing home or, more specifically, a facility offering extended, nonacute care to a resident patient whose illness does not require acute care.

medical consultation. Advice or an opinion rendered by a physician at the request of the primary care provider.

medical decision making. Consideration of the differential diagnoses, the amount and/or complexity of data reviewed and considered (medical records, test results, correspondence from previous treating physicians, etc.), current diagnostic studies ordered, and treatment or management options and risk (complications of the patient's condition, the potential for complications, continued morbidity, risk of mortality, any comorbidities associated with the patient's disease process).

Glossary

medical documentation. Patient care records, including operative notes; physical, occupational, and speech-language pathology notes; progress notes; physician certification and recertifications; and emergency room records; or the patient's medical record in its entirety. When Medicare coverage cannot be determined based on the information submitted on the claim, medical documentation may be requested. The Medicare Administrative Contractor (MAC) will deny a claim for lack of medical necessity if medical documentation is not received within the stated time frame defined by the MAC (usually within 35-45 days after the date of request).

medical necessity. Medically appropriate and necessary to meet basic health needs; consistent with the diagnosis or condition and national medical practice guidelines regarding type, frequency, and duration of treatment; rendered in a cost-effective manner.

Medicare. Federally funded program authorized as part of the Social Security Act that provides for health care services for people age 65 or older, people with disabilities, and people with end-stage renal disease (ESRD).

Medicare administrative contractor. Jurisdictional entity that contracts with CMS to adjudicate professional claims under Part A and Part B, responsible for daily claims processing, utilization review, record maintenance, dissemination of information based on CMS regulations, and whether services are covered and payments are appropriate.

Medicare carrier. Organization that contracts with CMS to adjudicate professional claims under Part B, the supplemental medical insurance program. Medicare carriers are responsible for daily claims processing, utilization review, record maintenance, dissemination of information based on CMS regulations, and determining whether services are covered and payments are appropriate. This organization has been replaced by Medicare administrative contractors.

Medicare fee schedule. Fee schedule based upon physician work, expense, and malpractice designed to slow the rise in cost for services and standardize payment to physicians regardless of specialty or location of service with geographic adjustments.

Medicare Part B. Supplemental medical insurance that includes outpatient hospital care and physician and other qualified professional care. Claims from providers or suppliers other than a hospital are submitted to carriers for reimbursement. Hospital outpatient claims are submitted to their FI/MAC.

Merit-based Incentive Payment System. CMS Quality Payment Program (QPP) track that combines parts of three retired quality reporting programs—the Physician Quality Reporting System (PQRS), the Value Modifier (VM or Value-based Payment Modifier), and the Medicare EHR Incentive Program (EHR) and another CMS created performance category called Improvement Activities —into a single program. Eligible clinicians (EC) are measured on all four categories. The QPP became effective January 1, 2017.

minor procedure. Self-limited procedure, usually with an assignment of 0 or 10 follow-up days by payers. A minor procedure may be considered by many payers to be part of the global package for a primary surgical service and cannot be billed separately from the primary procedure.

MIPS. Merit-Based Incentive Payment System.

miscoding. Incorrect coding or using a code that does not apply to the procedure.

modifier. Two characters that can be appended to a HCPCS code as a means of identifying circumstances that alter or enhance the description of a service or supply.

morbidity. Diseased condition or state.

mortality. Condition of being mortal (subject to death).

new patient. Patient who is receiving face-to-face care from a provider/qualified health care professional or another physician/qualified health care professional of the exact same specialty and subspecialty who belongs to the same group practice for the first time in three years. For OPPS hospitals, a patient who has not been registered as an inpatient or outpatient, including off-campus provider based clinic or emergency department, within the past three years.

newborn admission. Infant born in the facility.

newborn intensive care unit. Special care unit for premature and seriously ill infants.

noninstitutional setting. All settings other than a hospital or skilled nursing facility.

observation patient. Patient who needs to be monitored and assessed for inpatient admission or referral to another site for care.

observation services. Services furnished on a hospital's premises, including use of a bed and periodic monitoring by a hospital's nursing or other staff, that are reasonable and necessary to evaluate an outpatient's condition or determine the need for a possible admission to the hospital as an inpatient. Such services are covered only when provided by the order of a physician or another individual authorized by state license laws and hospital staff bylaws to admit patients to the hospital or to order outpatient tests. Observation services normally do not extend beyond 23 hours.

on-call physician encounter. Physician/qualified health care professional who is on call or covering for another physician/qualified health care professional and classifies the patient's encounter as it would have been by the physician/qualified health care professional who is not available.

ONC. Office of the national coordinator for health information technology.

outpatient. Person who has not been admitted as an inpatient but who is registered on the hospital or CAH records as an outpatient and receives services (rather than supplies alone) directly from the hospital or CAH. (Code of Federal Regulations, section 410.2.)

outpatient services. Medical and other services, diagnostic or therapeutic, provided to a person who has not been admitted to the hospital as an inpatient but is registered on the hospital records as an outpatient. Outpatient services usually require a stay of less than 24 hours.

outpatient visit. Encounter in a recognized outpatient facility.

overutilization. Services rendered by providers more frequently than usual.

past history. Record of prior illnesses or conditions occurring in childhood and adulthood, such as infectious diseases, allergies, accidents, current medications, hospitalizations, and surgical/medical procedures.

patient problem. Disease, condition, illness, injury, symptom, sign, finding, complaint, or other reason for an encounter, with or without a diagnosis being established at the time of the encounter.

pediatric patient. Patient usually younger than 14 years of age.

physically present. Teaching physicians must be in the same room, or a partitioned or curtained area, as the patient and resident and/or perform a face-to-face service.

physician. Legally authorized practitioners including a doctor of medicine or osteopathy, a doctor of dental surgery or of dental medicine, a doctor of podiatric medicine, a doctor of optometry, and a chiropractor only with respect to treatment by means of manual manipulation of the spine (to correct a subluxation).

physician services. Professional services performed by physicians, including surgery, consultations, and home, office, and institutional calls.

physician work. One of three components used to develop relative value units (RVU) under the resource-based relative value scale. Physician work represents the value of the skill and time required to perform a service.

physicians at teaching hospitals. Set up by the Office of Inspector General (OIG), initiative of the National Recovery Project targeting reimbursement practices at teaching hospitals, focusing on the use of residents and the services they perform under Medicare Part B that are paid as part of Medicare Part A.

plan of treatment. Written documentation of the type of therapy services (e.g., physical, occupational, speech-language pathology, cardiac rehabilitation) to be provided to a patient and of the amount, frequency, and duration (in days, weeks, months) of the services to be provided. An active treatment plan must identify the diagnosis, the anticipated goals of the treatment, the date the plan was established, and the type of modality or procedure to be used.

practitioner. Physician or nonphysician practitioner authorized to receive payment for services or incident-to services rendered.

preexisting condition. Symptom that causes a person to seek diagnosis, care, or treatment for which medical advice or treatment was recommended or received by a physician within a certain time period before the effective date of medical insurance coverage. The preexisting condition waiting period is the time the beneficiary must wait after buying health insurance before coverage begins for a condition that existed before coverage was obtained.

present illness. Current problem, from the onset of symptoms to the time of the encounter.

presenting problem. Disease, condition, illness, injury, symptom, sign, finding, complaint, or other reason for the patient encounter.

preventive medicine service. Evaluation and management service provided as a periodic health screening and/or prophylactic service that does not typically include management of new or existing diagnoses or problems.

primary care. Basic or general health care, traditionally provided by family practice, pediatrics, and internal medicine practitioners.

primary care physician. Physician who makes an initial diagnosis and referral and retains control over the patient and utilization of services both in and outside of the plan.

primary diagnosis. Current, most significant reason for the services or procedures provided.

procedure. Diagnostic or therapeutic service provided for the care and treatment of a patient, usually conforming to a specific set of steps or instructions.

prognosis. Forecast of the probable outcome of a condition or disease and the prospects of recovery and disease residual, dependent on the nature of the disease and the patient's response to treatment.

prolonged physician services. Extended pre- or post-service care provided to a patient whose condition requires services beyond the usual.

psychiatric hospital. Specialized institution that provides, under the supervision of physicians, services for the diagnosis and treatment of mentally ill persons.

QPP. Quality Payment Program. Program that is part of the larger goal of the Centers for Medicare and Medicaid Services (CMS) to improve Medicare through a greater focus and emphasis on the quality of medical care provided to beneficiaries. The Medicare Access and CHIP Reauthorization Act of 2015 (MACRA) repealed the Sustainable Growth Rate (SGR) formula and consolidated multiple quality reporting programs into a single system called the Merit-based Incentive Payment System (MIPS), one of two tracks that makes up the Quality Payment Program. The QPP provides incentive payments to clinicians for participating in MIPS or through the second track, Advanced Alternative Payment Models (APM). The QPP's purpose is to give providers new tools and resources to help provide patients with the best possible care. Clinicians can choose how they wish to participate based on practice size, specialty, location, or patient population. Clinicians who opt to participate in an Advanced APM through Medicare Part B may earn an incentive payment for participating in an innovative payment model. However, if clinicians choose to participate in traditional Medicare Part B, they will participate in MIPS where they are eligible to earn a performance-based payment adjustment. The QPP became effective on January 1, 2017.

qualified health care professional. Educated, licensed or certified, and regulated professional operating under a specified scope of practice to provide patient services that are separate and distinct from other clinical staff. Services may be billed independently or under the facility's services.

referral. Approval from the primary care physician to see a specialist or receive certain services. May be required for coverage purposes before a patient receives care from anyone except the primary physician.

referred outpatient. Person sent to a special diagnostic facility or to a hospital service department for the diagnostic tests or procedures.

rehabilitation hospital. Institution that serves inpatients of whom the vast majority require intensive rehabilitative services for the treatment of certain conditions (e.g., stroke, amputation, brain or spinal cord injuries, and neurological disorders).

resident. Individual participating in an approved graduate medical education (GME) program or a physician who is not in an approved GME program but who is authorized to practice only in a hospital setting including interns and fellows but not medical students.

rural health clinic. Clinic in an area where there is a shortage of health services staffed by a nurse practitioner, physician assistant, or certified nurse midwife under physician direction that provides routine diagnostic services, including clinical laboratory services, drugs, and biologicals, and that has prompt access to additional diagnostic services from facilities meeting federal requirements.

second opinion. Medical opinion obtained from another health care professional, relevant to clinical evaluation, before the performance of a medical service or surgical procedure. Includes patient education regarding treatment alternatives and/or to determine medical necessity.

secondary care. Services provided by medical specialists, such as cardiologists, urologists, and dermatologists who generally do not have first contact with patients.

self-referral. Patient who was not referred by a physician or other health care practitioner, but who chose that facility or provider on his or her own.

severity of illness. Relative levels of loss of function and mortality that may be experienced by patients with a particular disease.

short-stay patients. Inpatients admitted for 48 hours or less, or outpatients who stay 24 hours or less.

signature. Physician's signature acknowledges that he/she has performed or supervised the service or procedure and that the transcription has been read and corrections made before signing. Signed or initialed laboratory and x-ray results show auditors that the physician has reviewed the information.

skilled nursing facility. Institution or a distinct part of an institution that is primarily engaged in providing skilled nursing care and related services for residents who require medical or nursing care; or rehabilitation services for the rehabilitation of injured, disabled, or sick persons.

SOAP. Subjective, objective, assessment, plan. When documenting patients' visits, the SOAP approach has been used historically as it standardizes physician documentation and easily adapts to history, exam, and medical decision-making. The steps are defined as follows: **1)** Subjective: The information the patient tells the physician. **2)** Objective: The physician's observed, objective overview, including the patient's vital signs and the findings of the physical exam and any diagnostic tests. **3)** Assessment: A list the physician prepares in response to the patient's condition, including the problem, diagnoses, and reasons leading the physician to the diagnoses. **4)** Plan: The physician's workup or treatment planned for each problem in the assessment.

social history. Review of pertinent past and current activities of the patient including marital status, employment or occupation, use of drugs, alcohol and tobacco, educational background, sexual history, and other related social factors such as travel, avocations, and hobbies.

swing bed. Bed used for acute or long-term care, depending on the patient's need and the hospital's level of occupancy. Swing beds typically are available in small and rural hospitals. A swing-bed patient may be admitted and discharged from acute care and readmitted to a swing bed to receive skilled or intermediate levels of care. At times, the patient may remain in the same bed while changes occur in his or her care, charges, and payment.

teaching physician. Physician, other than another resident, who involves residents in the care of his or her patients.

telehealth service. Care by a provider with the patient at a remote site, usually rural, utilizing electronic communication to evaluate, monitor, and treat a patient.

tertiary care facility. Hospital providing specialty care to patients referred from other hospitals because of the severity of their injuries or illnesses.

treatment plan. Plan of care established by the provider outlining specific deficits and planned treatment that may be submitted to the case manager when seeking certification for a plan member.

type A emergency department. Emergency department licensed and advertised to be available to provide emergent care 24 hours a day, seven days a week. Type A emergency departments must meet both the CPT book definition of an emergency department and the EMTALA definition of a dedicated emergency department.

type B emergency department. Emergency department licensed and advertised to provide emergent care less than 24 hours a day, seven days a week. Type B emergency departments must meet the EMTALA definition of a dedicated emergency department.

UCR. Usual, customary, and reasonable. Fees charged for medical services that are considered normal, common, and in line with the prevailing fees in a given geographical area. May also be referred to as "customary, prevailing, and reasonable" charges.

upcoding. Practice of billing a code that represents a higher reimbursement than the code for the procedure actually performed.

Appendix A. Physician E/M Code Self-Audit Forms

Note: For 2025, the forms contained in this appendix will also be available as a downloadable PDF. To access the forms, use the following URL and password: www.optumcoding.com/support/product-updates/ Password: **EM25**

Evaluation and Management Services Worksheet

The following worksheet may be used to collect the necessary data when auditing a medical record for office and other outpatient services (99202-99205 and 99212-99215).

Note: For definitions and details regarding each MDM element, refer to chapters 3 to 11 of this publication.

Example 1: Office and Other Outpatient Services Audit Worksheet

Record Number			DOS billed	
Attending		Signed ❑ Yes ❑ No	DOS Rendered	
E/M Billed	**E/M Documented**	**E/M Mod Billed**	**E/M Mod Doc**	
Incident to:				
When a yes is answered for **all** of the following, the service may be billed as incident to under Medicare guidelines.			**Yes**	**No**
Is the NPP an employee of the practice?			❑	❑
If this is a new patient, did the physician participate in the patient's care?			❑	❑
Was direct personal supervision by the physician provided for in-office encounters?			❑	❑
Does the physician have an active part in the ongoing care of the patient?			❑	❑
History	Was a medically appropriate history documented?		Yes ❑	No ❑
Examination	Was a medically appropriate exam documented?		Yes ❑	No ❑

Medical Decision Making		
Number and Complexity of Problems Addressed	**Amount and/or Complexity of Data to be Reviewed and Analyzed** ***Each unique test, order, or document contributes to the combination of 2 or combination of 3 in Category 1 below.***	**Risk of Complications and/or Morbidity or Mortality of Patient Management**
Minimal ❏ 1 self-limited or minor problem	❏ **Minimal or none**	❏ **Minimal risk of morbidity from additional diagnostic testing or treatment**
Low ❏ 2 or more self-limited or minor problems; **or** ❏ 1 stable chronic illness; **or** ❏ 1 acute, uncomplicated illness or injury **or** ❏ 1 stable, acute illness **or** ❏ 1 acute, uncomplicated illness or injury requiring hospital inpatient or observation level of care	❏ **Limited** *(Must meet the requirements of at least 1 of the 2 categories)* ❏ **Category 1: Tests and documents** Any combination of 2 from the following: • Review of prior external note(s) from each unique source* • Review of the result(s) of each unique test* • Ordering of each unique test* **or** ❏ **Category 2: Assessment requiring an independent historian(s)**	❏ **Low risk of morbidity from additional diagnostic testing or treatment**
Moderate ❏ 1 or more chronic illnesses with exacerbation, progression, or side effects of treatment; **or** ❏ 2 or more stable chronic illnesses; **or** ❏ 1 undiagnosed new problem with uncertain prognosis; **or** ❏ 1 acute illness with systemic symptoms; **or** ❏ 1 acute, complicated injury	❏ **Moderate** *(Must meet the requirements of at least 1 out of 3 categories)* ❏ **Category 1: Tests, documents, or independent historian(s).** Any combination of **3** from the following: • Review of prior external note(s) from each unique source* • Review of the result(s) of each unique test* • Ordering of each unique test* • Assessment requiring an independent historian(s) **or** ❏ **Category 2: Independent interpretation of tests** • Independent interpretation of a test performed by another physician/other qualified health care professional (not separately reported) **or** ❏ **Category 3: Discussion of management or test interpretation** • Discussion of management or test interpretation with external physician/other qualified health care professional/appropriate source (not separately reported)	❏ **Moderate risk of morbidity from additional diagnostic testing or treatment** *Examples only:* • Prescription drug management • Decision regarding minor surgery with identified patient or procedure risk factors • Decision regarding elective major surgery without identified patient or procedure risk factors • Diagnosis or treatment significantly limited by social determinants of health
High ❏ 1 or more chronic illnesses with severe exacerbation, progression, or side effects of treatment; **or** ❏ 1 acute or chronic illness or injury that poses a threat to life or bodily function	**Extensive** *(Must meet the requirements of at least 2 out of 3 categories)* ❏ **Category 1: Tests, documents, or independent historian(s)** Any combination of 3 from the following: • Review of prior external note(s) from each unique source*; • Review of the result(s) of each unique test*; • Ordering of each unique test*; • Assessment requiring an independent historian(s) **or** ❏ **Category 2: Independent interpretation of tests** • Independent interpretation of a test performed by another physician/other qualified health care professional (not separately reported) **or** ❏ **Category 3: Discussion of management or test interpretation** • Discussion of management or test interpretation with external physician/other qualified health care professional/appropriate source (not separately reported)	❏ **High risk of morbidity from additional diagnostic testing or treatment** *Examples only:* • Drug therapy requiring intensive monitoring for toxicity • Decision regarding elective major surgery with identified patient or procedure risk factors • Decision regarding emergency major surgery • Decision regarding hospitalization or escalation of hospital-level care • Decision not to resuscitate or to de-escalate care because of poor prognosis • Decision regarding parenteral controlled substances

* Note: Test panels such as 80047 are counted as a single laboratory test. The differentiation between single or multiple unique tests is defined in accordance with the CPT code set.

Evaluation and Management Services Worksheet

The following worksheet may be used to collect the necessary data when auditing a medical record for hospital inpatient or observation E/M services (99221-99223, 99231-99233, 99234-99236, and 99238-99239).

Note: For definitions and details regarding each MDM element, refer to Chapter 2 and Chapter 5 of this publication. For definitions and details regarding incident-to and shared services, refer to Chapter 5 of this publication.

Example 2: Hospital Care Services Audit Worksheet

Record Number		DOS billed	
Attending	Signed ❑ Yes ❑ No	DOS Rendered	
E/M Billed	**E/M Documented**	**E/M Mod Billed**	**E/M Mod Doc**

Shared Services:			
For a service to be considered shared, **all** of the following questions must have an answer of yes.		❑	❑
Are the NPP and physician employed by the same practice?		❑	❑
Are the clinically relevant portions of the E/M service documented by the physician?		❑	❑
Is there documentation from the physician for this encounter?		❑	❑
Is the physician documentation tied to the NPP's documentation?		❑	❑
History	Was a medically appropriate history documented?	Yes ❑	No ❑
Examination	Was a medically appropriate exam documented?	Yes ❑	No ❑

Physician E/M Self-Audit Formss

Medical Decision Making		
Number and Complexity of Problems Addressed	**Amount and/or Complexity of Data to be Reviewed and Analyzed** *Each unique test, order, or document contributes to the combination of 2 or combination of 3 in Category 1 below.*	**Risk of Complications and/or Morbidity or Mortality of Patient Management**
Minimal ❑ 1 self-limited or minor problem	❑ **Minimal or none**	❑ **Minimal risk of morbidity from additional diagnostic testing or treatment**
Low ❑ 2 or more self-limited or minor problems; **or** ❑ 1 stable chronic illness; **or** ❑ 1 acute, uncomplicated illness or injury **or** ❑ 1 stable, acute illness **or** ❑ 1 acute, uncomplicated illness or injury requiring hospital inpatient or observation level of care	❑ **Limited** *(Must meet the requirements of at least 1 of the 2 categories)* ❑ **Category 1: Tests and documents** Any combination of 2 from the following: • Review of prior external note(s) from each unique source* • Review of the result(s) of each unique test* • Ordering of each unique test* **or** ❑ **Category 2: Assessment requiring an independent historian(s)**	❑ **Low risk of morbidity from additional diagnostic testing or treatment**
Moderate ❑ 1 or more chronic illnesses with exacerbation, progression, or side effects of treatment; **or** ❑ 2 or more stable chronic illnesses; **or** ❑ 1 undiagnosed new problem with uncertain prognosis; **or** ❑ 1 acute illness with systemic symptoms; **or** ❑ 1 acute, complicated injury	❑ **Moderate** *(Must meet the requirements of at least 1 out of 3 categories)* ❑ **Category 1: Tests, documents, or independent historian(s).** Any combination of **3** from the following: • Review of prior external note(s) from each unique source* • Review of the result(s) of each unique test* • Ordering of each unique test* • Assessment requiring an independent historian(s) **or** ❑ **Category 2: Independent interpretation of tests** • Independent interpretation of a test performed by another physician/other qualified health care professional (not separately reported) **or** ❑ **Category 3: Discussion of management or test interpretation** • Discussion of management or test interpretation with external physician/other qualified health care professional/appropriate source (not separately reported)	❑ **Moderate risk of morbidity from additional diagnostic testing or treatment** *Examples only:* • Prescription drug management • Decision regarding minor surgery with identified patient or procedure risk factors • Decision regarding elective major surgery without identified patient or procedure risk factors • Diagnosis or treatment significantly limited by social determinants of health
High ❑ 1 or more chronic illnesses with severe exacerbation, progression, or side effects of treatment; **or** ❑ 1 acute or chronic illness or injury that poses a threat to life or bodily function	**Extensive** *(Must meet the requirements of at least 2 out of 3 categories)* ❑ **Category 1: Tests, documents, or independent historian(s)** Any combination of 3 from the following: • Review of prior external note(s) from each unique source*; • Review of the result(s) of each unique test*; • Ordering of each unique test*; • Assessment requiring an independent historian(s) **or** ❑ **Category 2: Independent interpretation of tests** • Independent interpretation of a test performed by another physician/other qualified health care professional (not separately reported) **or** ❑ **Category 3: Discussion of management or test interpretation** • Discussion of management or test interpretation with external physician/other qualified health care professional/appropriate source (not separately reported)	❑ **High risk of morbidity from additional diagnostic testing or treatment** *Examples only:* • Drug therapy requiring intensive monitoring for toxicity • Decision regarding elective major surgery with identified patient or procedure risk factors • Decision regarding emergency major surgery • Decision regarding hospitalization or escalation of hospital-level care • Decision not to resuscitate or to de-escalate care because of poor prognosis • Decision regarding parenteral controlled substances

* Note: Test panels such as 80047 are counted as a single laboratory test. The differentiation between single or multiple unique tests is defined in accordance with the CPT code set.

Evaluation and Management Services Worksheet

The following worksheet may be used to collect the necessary data when auditing a medical record for consultation (99242-99245 and 99252-99255).

Note: For definitions and details regarding each MDM element, refer to Chapter 2 and Chapter 5 of this publication. For definitions and details regarding incident-to and shared services, refer to Chapter 5 of this publication.

Example 3: Consultation Services Audit Worksheet

Record Number			DOS billed	
Attending		Signed ❑ Yes ❑ No	DOS Rendered	
E/M Billed	**E/M Documented**		**E/M Mod Billed**	**E/M Mod Doc**

Incident to:			
When a yes is answered for **all** of the following, the service may be billed as incident to under Medicare guidelines.		**Yes**	**No**
Is the NPP an employee of the practice?		❑	❑
If this is a new patient, did the physician participate in the patient's care?		❑	❑
Was direct personal supervision by the physician provided for in-office encounters?		❑	❑
Does the physician have an active part in the ongoing care of the patient?		❑	❑
Shared Services:			
For a service to be considered shared, **all** of the following questions must have an answer of yes.		❑	❑
Are the NPP and physician employed by the same practice?		❑	❑
Are the clinically relevant portions of the E/M service documented by the physician?		❑	❑
Is there documentation from the physician for this encounter?		❑	❑
Is the physician documentation tied to the NPP's documentation?		❑	❑
History	Was a medically appropriate history documented?	Yes ❑	No ❑
Examination	Was a medically appropriate exam documented?	Yes ❑	No ❑

Physician E/M Self-Audit Formss

Medical Decision Making		
Number and Complexity of Problems Addressed	**Amount and/or Complexity of Data to be Reviewed and Analyzed** ***Each unique test, order, or document contributes to the combination of 2 or combination of 3 in Category 1 below.***	**Risk of Complications and/or Morbidity or Mortality of Patient Management**
Minimal ❑ 1 self-limited or minor problem	❑ **Minimal or none**	❑ **Minimal risk of morbidity from additional diagnostic testing or treatment**
Low ❑ 2 or more self-limited or minor problems; **or** ❑ 1 stable chronic illness; **or** ❑ 1 acute, uncomplicated illness or injury **or** ❑ 1 stable, acute illness **or** ❑ 1 acute, uncomplicated illness or injury requiring hospital inpatient or observation level of care	❑ **Limited** *(Must meet the requirements of at least 1 of the 2 categories)* ❑ **Category 1: Tests and documents** Any combination of 2 from the following: • Review of prior external note(s) from each unique source* • Review of the result(s) of each unique test* • Ordering of each unique test* **or** ❑ **Category 2: Assessment requiring an independent historian(s)**	❑ **Low risk of morbidity from additional diagnostic testing or treatment**
Moderate ❑ 1 or more chronic illnesses with exacerbation, progression, or side effects of treatment; **or** ❑ 2 or more stable chronic illnesses; **or** ❑ 1 undiagnosed new problem with uncertain prognosis; **or** ❑ 1 acute illness with systemic symptoms; **or** ❑ 1 acute, complicated injury	❑ **Moderate** *(Must meet the requirements of at least 1 out of 3 categories)* ❑ **Category 1: Tests, documents, or independent historian(s).** Any combination of **3** from the following: • Review of prior external note(s) from each unique source* • Review of the result(s) of each unique test* • Ordering of each unique test* • Assessment requiring an independent historian(s) **or** ❑ **Category 2: Independent interpretation of tests** • Independent interpretation of a test performed by another physician/other qualified health care professional (not separately reported) **or** ❑ **Category 3: Discussion of management or test interpretation** • Discussion of management or test interpretation with external physician/other qualified health care professional/appropriate source (not separately reported)	❑ **Moderate risk of morbidity from additional diagnostic testing or treatment** *Examples only:* • Prescription drug management • Decision regarding minor surgery with identified patient or procedure risk factors • Decision regarding elective major surgery without identified patient or procedure risk factors • Diagnosis or treatment significantly limited by social determinants of health
High ❑ 1 or more chronic illnesses with severe exacerbation, progression, or side effects of treatment; **or** ❑ 1 acute or chronic illness or injury that poses a threat to life or bodily function	**Extensive** *(Must meet the requirements of at least 2 out of 3 categories)* ❑ **Category 1: Tests, documents, or independent historian(s)** Any combination of 3 from the following: • Review of prior external note(s) from each unique source*; • Review of the result(s) of each unique test*; • Ordering of each unique test*; • Assessment requiring an independent historian(s) **or** ❑ **Category 2: Independent interpretation of tests** • Independent interpretation of a test performed by another physician/other qualified health care professional (not separately reported) **or** ❑ **Category 3: Discussion of management or test interpretation** • Discussion of management or test interpretation with external physician/other qualified health care professional/appropriate source (not separately reported)	❑ **High risk of morbidity from additional diagnostic testing or treatment** *Examples only:* • Drug therapy requiring intensive monitoring for toxicity • Decision regarding elective major surgery with identified patient or procedure risk factors • Decision regarding emergency major surgery • Decision regarding hospitalization or escalation of hospital-level care • Decision not to resuscitate or to de-escalate care because of poor prognosis • Decision regarding parenteral controlled substances

* Note: Test panels such as 80047 are counted as a single laboratory test. The differentiation between single or multiple unique tests is defined in accordance with the CPT code set.

Evaluation and Management Services Worksheet

The following worksheet may be used to collect the necessary data when auditing a medical record for emergency department services (99281-99285).

Note: For definitions and details regarding each MDM element, refer to Chapter 2 and Chapter 5 of this publication. For definitions and details regarding incident-to and shared services, refer to Chapter 5 of this publication.

Example 4: Emergency Department Services Audit Worksheet

Record Number			DOS billed		
Attending		Signed ❑ Yes ❑ No	DOS Rendered		
E/M Billed	**E/M Documented**		**E/M Mod Billed**	**E/M Mod Doc**	
Shared Services:					
For a service to be considered shared, **all** of the following questions must have an answer of yes.				❑	❑
Are the NPP and physician employed by the same practice?				❑	❑
Are the clinically relevant portions of the E/M service documented by the physician?				❑	❑
Is there documentation from the physician for this encounter?				❑	❑
Is the physician documentation tied to the NPP's documentation?				❑	❑
History	Was a medically appropriate history documented?			Yes ❑	No ❑
Examination	Was a medically appropriate exam documented?			Yes ❑	No ❑

Physician E/M Self-Audit Formss

Medical Decision Making		
Number and Complexity of Problems Addressed	**Amount and/or Complexity of Data to be Reviewed and Analyzed** ***Each unique test, order, or document contributes to the combination of 2 or combination of 3 in Category 1 below.***	**Risk of Complications and/or Morbidity or Mortality of Patient Management**
Minimal ❑ 1 self-limited or minor problem	❑ **Minimal or none**	❑ **Minimal risk of morbidity from additional diagnostic testing or treatment**
Low ❑ 2 or more self-limited or minor problems; **or** ❑ 1 stable chronic illness; **or** ❑ 1 acute, uncomplicated illness or injury **or** ❑ 1 stable, acute illness **or** ❑ 1 acute, uncomplicated illness or injury requiring hospital inpatient or observation level of care	❑ **Limited** *(Must meet the requirements of at least 1 of the 2 categories)* ❑ **Category 1: Tests and documents** Any combination of 2 from the following: • Review of prior external note(s) from each unique source* • Review of the result(s) of each unique test* • Ordering of each unique test* **or** ❑ **Category 2: Assessment requiring an independent historian(s)**	❑ **Low risk of morbidity from additional diagnostic testing or treatment**
Moderate ❑ 1 or more chronic illnesses with exacerbation, progression, or side effects of treatment; **or** ❑ 2 or more stable chronic illnesses; **or** ❑ 1 undiagnosed new problem with uncertain prognosis; **or** ❑ 1 acute illness with systemic symptoms; **or** ❑ 1 acute, complicated injury	❑ **Moderate** *(Must meet the requirements of at least 1 out of 3 categories)* ❑ **Category 1: Tests, documents, or independent historian(s).** Any combination of **3** from the following: • Review of prior external note(s) from each unique source* • Review of the result(s) of each unique test* • Ordering of each unique test* • Assessment requiring an independent historian(s) **or** ❑ **Category 2: Independent interpretation of tests** • Independent interpretation of a test performed by another physician/other qualified health care professional (not separately reported) **or** ❑ **Category 3: Discussion of management or test interpretation** • Discussion of management or test interpretation with external physician/other qualified health care professional/appropriate source (not separately reported)	❑ **Moderate risk of morbidity from additional diagnostic testing or treatment** *Examples only:* • Prescription drug management • Decision regarding minor surgery with identified patient or procedure risk factors • Decision regarding elective major surgery without identified patient or procedure risk factors • Diagnosis or treatment significantly limited by social determinants of health
High ❑ 1 or more chronic illnesses with severe exacerbation, progression, or side effects of treatment; **or** ❑ 1 acute or chronic illness or injury that poses a threat to life or bodily function	**Extensive** *(Must meet the requirements of at least 2 out of 3 categories)* ❑ **Category 1: Tests, documents, or independent historian(s)** Any combination of 3 from the following: • Review of prior external note(s) from each unique source*; • Review of the result(s) of each unique test*; • Ordering of each unique test*; • Assessment requiring an independent historian(s) **or** ❑ **Category 2: Independent interpretation of tests** • Independent interpretation of a test performed by another physician/other qualified health care professional (not separately reported) **or** ❑ **Category 3: Discussion of management or test interpretation** • Discussion of management or test interpretation with external physician/other qualified health care professional/appropriate source (not separately reported)	❑ **High risk of morbidity from additional diagnostic testing or treatment** *Examples only:* • Drug therapy requiring intensive monitoring for toxicity • Decision regarding elective major surgery with identified patient or procedure risk factors • Decision regarding emergency major surgery • Decision regarding hospitalization or escalation of hospital-level care • Decision not to resuscitate or to de-escalate care because of poor prognosis • Decision regarding parenteral controlled substances

* Note: Test panels such as 80047 are counted as a single laboratory test. The differentiation between single or multiple unique tests is defined in accordance with the CPT code set.

Evaluation and Management Services Worksheet

The following worksheet may be used to collect the necessary data when auditing a medical record for nursing facility services (99304-99310 and 99315-99316).

Note: For definitions and details regarding each MDM element, refer to Chapter 2 and Chapter 5 of this publication. For definitions and details regarding incident-to and shared services, refer to Chapter 5 of this publication.

Example 5: Nursing Facility Services Audit Worksheet

Record Number			DOS billed	
Attending		Signed ❑ Yes ❑ No	DOS Rendered	
E/M Billed	**E/M Documented**		**E/M Mod Billed**	**E/M Mod Doc**
Shared Services:				
For a service to be considered shared, **all** of the following questions must have an answer of yes.			❑	❑
Are the NPP and physician employed by the same practice?			❑	❑
Are the clinically relevant portions of the E/M service documented by the physician?			❑	❑
Is there documentation from the physician for this encounter?			❑	❑
Is the physician documentation tied to the NPP's documentation?			❑	❑
History	Was a medically appropriate history documented?		Yes ❑	No ❑
Examination	Was a medically appropriate exam documented?		Yes ❑	No ❑

Physician E/M Self-Audit Formss

Medical Decision Making		
Number and Complexity of Problems Addressed	**Amount and/or Complexity of Data to be Reviewed and Analyzed** ***Each unique test, order, or document contributes to the combination of 2 or combination of 3 in Category 1 below.***	**Risk of Complications and/or Morbidity or Mortality of Patient Management**
Minimal ❑ 1 self-limited or minor problem	❑ **Minimal or none**	❑ **Minimal risk of morbidity from additional diagnostic testing or treatment**
Low ❑ 2 or more self-limited or minor problems; **or** ❑ 1 stable chronic illness; **or** ❑ 1 acute, uncomplicated illness or injury **or** ❑ 1 stable, acute illness **or** ❑ 1 acute, uncomplicated illness or injury requiring hospital inpatient or observation level of care	❑ **Limited** *(Must meet the requirements of at least 1 of the 2 categories)* ❑ **Category 1: Tests and documents** Any combination of 2 from the following: • Review of prior external note(s) from each unique source* • Review of the result(s) of each unique test* • Ordering of each unique test* **or** ❑ **Category 2: Assessment requiring an independent historian(s)**	❑ **Low risk of morbidity from additional diagnostic testing or treatment**
Moderate ❑ 1 or more chronic illnesses with exacerbation, progression, or side effects of treatment; **or** ❑ 2 or more stable chronic illnesses; **or** ❑ 1 undiagnosed new problem with uncertain prognosis; **or** ❑ 1 acute illness with systemic symptoms; **or** ❑ 1 acute, complicated injury	❑ **Moderate** *(Must meet the requirements of at least 1 out of 3 categories)* ❑ **Category 1: Tests, documents, or independent historian(s).** Any combination of **3** from the following: • Review of prior external note(s) from each unique source* • Review of the result(s) of each unique test* • Ordering of each unique test* • Assessment requiring an independent historian(s) **or** ❑ **Category 2: Independent interpretation of tests** • Independent interpretation of a test performed by another physician/other qualified health care professional (not separately reported) **or** ❑ **Category 3: Discussion of management or test interpretation** • Discussion of management or test interpretation with external physician/other qualified health care professional/appropriate source (not separately reported)	❑ **Moderate risk of morbidity from additional diagnostic testing or treatment** *Examples only:* • Prescription drug management • Decision regarding minor surgery with identified patient or procedure risk factors • Decision regarding elective major surgery without identified patient or procedure risk factors • Diagnosis or treatment significantly limited by social determinants of health
High ❑ 1 or more chronic illnesses with severe exacerbation, progression, or side effects of treatment; **or** ❑ 1 acute or chronic illness or injury that poses a threat to life or bodily function	**Extensive** *(Must meet the requirements of at least 2 out of 3 categories)* ❑ **Category 1: Tests, documents, or independent historian(s)** Any combination of 3 from the following: • Review of prior external note(s) from each unique source*; • Review of the result(s) of each unique test*; • Ordering of each unique test*; • Assessment requiring an independent historian(s) **or** ❑ **Category 2: Independent interpretation of tests** • Independent interpretation of a test performed by another physician/other qualified health care professional (not separately reported) **or** ❑ **Category 3: Discussion of management or test interpretation** • Discussion of management or test interpretation with external physician/other qualified health care professional/appropriate source (not separately reported)	❑ **High risk of morbidity from additional diagnostic testing or treatment** *Examples only:* • Drug therapy requiring intensive monitoring for toxicity • Decision regarding elective major surgery with identified patient or procedure risk factors • Decision regarding emergency major surgery • Decision regarding hospitalization or escalation of hospital-level care • Decision not to resuscitate or to de-escalate care because of poor prognosis • Decision regarding parenteral controlled substances

* Note: Test panels such as 80047 are counted as a single laboratory test. The differentiation between single or multiple unique tests is defined in accordance with the CPT code set.

Evaluation and Management Services Worksheet

The following worksheet may be used to collect the necessary data when auditing a medical record for home or residence services (99341-99345 and 99347-99350).

Note: For definitions and details regarding each MDM element, refer to Chapter 2 and Chapter 5 of this publication. For definitions and details regarding incident-to and shared services, refer to Chapter 5 of this publication.

Example 6: Home and Residence Services Audit Worksheet

Record Number		DOS billed	
Attending	Signed ❑ Yes ❑ No	DOS Rendered	
E/M Billed	**E/M Documented**	**E/M Mod Billed**	**E/M Mod Doc**

Incident to:		
When a yes is answered for **all** of the following, the service may be billed as incident to under Medicare guidelines.	**Yes**	**No**
Is the NPP an employee of the practice?	❑	❑
If this is a new patient, did the physician participate in the patient's care?	❑	❑
Was direct personal supervision by the physician provided for in-office encounters?	❑	❑
Does the physician have an active part in the ongoing care of the patient?	❑	❑

History	Was a medically appropriate history documented?	Yes ❑	No ❑
Examination	Was a medically appropriate exam documented?	Yes ❑	No ❑

Physician E/M Self-Audit Formss

Medical Decision Making		
Number and Complexity of Problems Addressed	**Amount and/or Complexity of Data to be Reviewed and Analyzed** ***Each unique test, order, or document contributes to the combination of 2 or combination of 3 in Category 1 below.***	**Risk of Complications and/or Morbidity or Mortality of Patient Management**
Minimal ❑ 1 self-limited or minor problem	❑ **Minimal or none**	❑ **Minimal risk of morbidity from additional diagnostic testing or treatment**
Low ❑ 2 or more self-limited or minor problems; **or** ❑ 1 stable chronic illness; **or** ❑ 1 acute, uncomplicated illness or injury **or** ❑ 1 stable, acute illness **or** ❑ 1 acute, uncomplicated illness or injury requiring hospital inpatient or observation level of care	❑ **Limited** *(Must meet the requirements of at least 1 of the 2 categories)* ❑ **Category 1: Tests and documents** Any combination of 2 from the following: • Review of prior external note(s) from each unique source* • Review of the result(s) of each unique test* • Ordering of each unique test* **or** ❑ **Category 2: Assessment requiring an independent historian(s)**	❑ **Low risk of morbidity from additional diagnostic testing or treatment**
Moderate ❑ 1 or more chronic illnesses with exacerbation, progression, or side effects of treatment; **or** ❑ 2 or more stable chronic illnesses; **or** ❑ 1 undiagnosed new problem with uncertain prognosis; **or** ❑ 1 acute illness with systemic symptoms; **or** ❑ 1 acute, complicated injury	❑ **Moderate** *(Must meet the requirements of at least 1 out of 3 categories)* ❑ **Category 1: Tests, documents, or independent historian(s).** Any combination of **3** from the following: • Review of prior external note(s) from each unique source* • Review of the result(s) of each unique test* • Ordering of each unique test* • Assessment requiring an independent historian(s) **or** ❑ **Category 2: Independent interpretation of tests** • Independent interpretation of a test performed by another physician/other qualified health care professional (not separately reported) **or** ❑ **Category 3: Discussion of management or test interpretation** • Discussion of management or test interpretation with external physician/other qualified health care professional/appropriate source (not separately reported)	❑ **Moderate risk of morbidity from additional diagnostic testing or treatment** *Examples only:* • Prescription drug management • Decision regarding minor surgery with identified patient or procedure risk factors • Decision regarding elective major surgery without identified patient or procedure risk factors • Diagnosis or treatment significantly limited by social determinants of health
High ❑ 1 or more chronic illnesses with severe exacerbation, progression, or side effects of treatment; **or** ❑ 1 acute or chronic illness or injury that poses a threat to life or bodily function	**Extensive** *(Must meet the requirements of at least 2 out of 3 categories)* ❑ **Category 1: Tests, documents, or independent historian(s)** Any combination of 3 from the following: • Review of prior external note(s) from each unique source*; • Review of the result(s) of each unique test*; • Ordering of each unique test*; • Assessment requiring an independent historian(s) **or** ❑ **Category 2: Independent interpretation of tests** • Independent interpretation of a test performed by another physician/other qualified health care professional (not separately reported) **or** ❑ **Category 3: Discussion of management or test interpretation** • Discussion of management or test interpretation with external physician/other qualified health care professional/appropriate source (not separately reported)	❑ **High risk of morbidity from additional diagnostic testing or treatment** *Examples only:* • Drug therapy requiring intensive monitoring for toxicity • Decision regarding elective major surgery with identified patient or procedure risk factors • Decision regarding emergency major surgery • Decision regarding hospitalization or escalation of hospital-level care • Decision not to resuscitate or to de-escalate care because of poor prognosis • Decision regarding parenteral controlled substances

* Note: Test panels such as 80047 are counted as a single laboratory test. The differentiation between single or multiple unique tests is defined in accordance with the CPT code set.

Appendix B. Evaluation and Management (E/M) Services Guidelines

E/M Guidelines Overview

The E/M guidelines have sections that are common to all E/M categories and sections that are category specific. Most of the categories and many of the subcategories of service have special guidelines or instructions unique to that category or subcategory. Where these are indicated, eg, "Hospital Inpatient and Observation Care," special instructions are presented before the listing of the specific E/M services codes. It is important to review the instructions for each category or subcategory. These guidelines are to be used by the reporting physician or other qualified health care professional to select the appropriate level of service. These guidelines do not establish documentation requirements or standards of care. The main purpose of documentation is to support care of the patient by current and future health care team(s). These guidelines are for services that require a face-to-face encounter with the patient and/or family/caregiver. (For 99211 and 99281, the face-to-face services may be performed by clinical staff.)

▶In the **Evaluation and Management** section (98000-98016, 99202-99499), there are many code categories. Each category may have specific guidelines, or the codes may include specific details. These E/M guidelines are written for the following categories:

- Office or Other Outpatient Services
- Telemedicine Services
- Hospital Inpatient and Observation Care Services
- Consultations
- Emergency Department Services
- Nursing Facility Services
- Home or Residence Services
- Prolonged Service With or Without Direct Patient Contact on the Date of an Evaluation and Management Service◀

Classification of Evaluation and Management (E/M) Services

The E/M section is divided into broad categories, such as office visits, hospital inpatient or observation care visits, and consultations. Most of the categories are further divided into two or more subcategories of E/M services. For example, there are two subcategories of office visits (new patient and established patient) and there are two subcategories of hospital inpatient and observation care visits (initial and subsequent). The subcategories of E/M services are further classified into levels of E/M services that are identified by specific codes.

The basic format of codes with levels of E/M services based on medical decision making (MDM) or time is the same. First, a unique code number is listed. Second, the place and/or type of service is specified (eg, office or other outpatient visit). Third, the content of the service is defined. Fourth, time is specified. (A detailed discussion of time is provided in the Guidelines for Selecting Level of Service Based on Time.)

The place of service and service type are defined by the location where the face-to-face encounter with the patient and/or family/caregiver occurs. For example, service provided to a nursing facility resident brought to the office is reported with an office or other outpatient code.

New and Established Patients

Solely for the purposes of distinguishing between new and established patients, **professional services** are those face-to-face services rendered by physicians and other qualified health care professionals who may report evaluation and management services. A new patient is one whohas not received any professional services from the physician or other qualified health care professional or another physician or other qualified health care professional of the **exact** same specialty **and subspecialty** who belongs to the same group practice, within the past three years.

An established patient is one who has received professional services from the physician or other qualified health care professional or another physician or other qualified health care professional of the **exact** same specialty **and subspecialty** who belongs to the same group practice, within the past three years. See Decision Tree for New vs Established Patients.

In the instance where a physician or other qualified health care professional is on call for or covering for another physician or other qualified health care professional, the patient's encounter will be classified as it would have been by the physician or other qualified health care professional who is not available. When advanced practice nurses and physician assistants are working with physicians, they are considered as working in the **exact** same specialty **and subspecialty** as the physician.

▶ ◀ = Contains new or revised text

No distinction is made between new and established patients in the emergency department. E/M services in the emergency department category may be reported for any new or established patient who presents for treatment in the emergency department.

The Decision Tree for New vs Established Patients is provided to aid in determining whether to report the E/M service provided as a new or an established patient encounter.

Decision Tree for New vs Established Patients

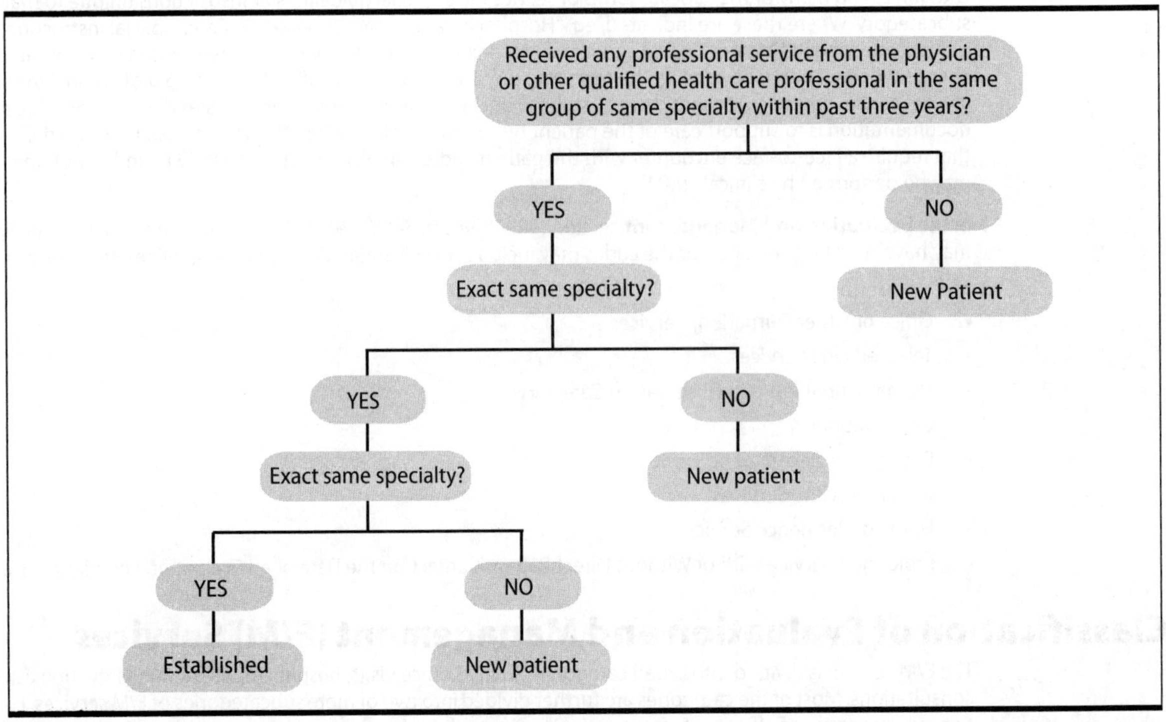

Initial and Subsequent Services

Some categories apply to both new and established patients (eg, hospital inpatient or observation care). These categories differentiate services by whether the service is the initial service or a subsequent service. For the purpose of distinguishing between initial or subsequent visits, professional services are those face-to-face services rendered by physicians and other qualified health care professionals who may report evaluation and management services. An initial service is when the patient has not received any professional services from the physician or other qualified health care professional or another physician or other qualified health care professional of the exact same specialty and subspecialty who belongs to the same group practice, during the inpatient, observation, or nursing facility admission and stay.

A subsequent service is when the patient has received professional service(s) from the physician or other qualified health care professional or another physician or other qualified health care professional of the exact same specialty and subspecialty who belongs to the same group practice, during the admission and stay.

In the instance when a physician or other qualified health care professional is on call for or covering for another physician or other qualified health care professional, the patient's encounter will be classified as it would have been by the physician or other qualified health care professional who is not available. When advanced practice nurses and physician assistants are working with physicians, they are considered as working in the exact same specialty and subspecialty as the physician.

For reporting hospital inpatient or observation care services, a stay that includes a transition from observation to inpatient is a single stay. For reporting nursing facility services, a stay that includes transition(s) between skilled nursing facility and nursing facility level of care is the same stay.

E/M Services Guidelines

Split or Shared Visits

Physician(s) and other qualified health care professional(s) (QHP[s]) may act as a team in providing care for the patient, working together during a single E/M service. The split or shared visits guidelines are applied to determine which professional may report the service. If the physician or other QHP performs a substantive portion of the encounter, the physician or other QHP may report the service. If code selection is based on total time on the date of the encounter, the service is reported by the professional who spent the majority of the face-to-face or non-face-to-face time performing the service. For the purpose of reporting E/M services within the context of team-based care, performance of a substantive part of the MDM requires that the physician(s) or other QHP(s) made or approved the management plan for the ***number and complexity of problems addressed at the encounter*** and takes responsibility for that plan with its inherent ***risk of complications and/or morbidity or mortality of patient management***. By doing so, a physician or other QHP has performed two of the three elements used in the selection of the code level based on MDM. If ***the amount and/or complexity of data to be reviewed and analyzed*** is used by the physician or other QHP to determine the reported code level, assessing an independent historian's narrative and the ordering or review of tests or documents do not have to be personally performed by the physician or other QHP, because the relevant items would be considered in formulating the management plan. Independent interpretation of tests and discussion of management plan or test interpretation must be personally performed by the physician or other QHP if these are used to determine the reported code level by the physician or other QHP.

Multiple Evaluation and Management Services on the Same Date

The following guidelines apply to services that a patient may receive for hospital inpatient care, observation care, or nursing facility care. For instructions regarding transitions to these settings from the office or outpatient, home or residence, or emergency department setting, see guidelines for **Hospital Inpatient and Observation Care Services or Nursing Facility Services**.

A patient may receive E/M services in more than one setting on a calendar date. A patient may also have more than one visit in the same setting on a calendar date. The guidelines for multiple E/M services on the same date address circumstances in which the patient has received multiple visits or services from the same physician or other QHP or another physician or other QHP of the exact same specialty and subspecialty who belongs to the same group practice.

Coding Tip

Instructions for Use of the CPT Codebook

When advanced practice nurses and physician assistants are working with physicians, they are considered as working in the exact same specialty and subspecialty as the physician. A "physician or other qualified health care professional" is an individual who is qualified by education, training, licensure/regulation (when applicable), and facility privileging (when applicable) who performs a professional service within his or her scope of practice and independently reports that professional service. These professionals are distinct from "clinical staff." A clinical staff member is a person who works under the supervision of a physician or other qualified health care professional, and who is allowed by law, regulation and facility policy to perform or assist in the performance of a specific professional service but does not individually report that professional service. Other policies may also affect who may report specific services.

CPT Coding Guidelines, Introduction, Instructions for Use of the CPT Codebook

Per day: The hospital inpatient and observation care services and the nursing facility services are "per day" services. When multiple visits occur over the course of a single calendar date in the same setting, a single service is reported. When using MDM for code level selection, use the aggregated MDM over the course of the calendar date. When using time for code level selection, sum the time over the course of the day using the guidelines for reporting time.

Multiple encounters in different settings or facilities: A patient may be seen and treated in different facilities (eg, a hospital-to-hospital transfer). When more than one primary E/M service is reported and time is used to select the code level for either service, only the time spent providing that individual service may be allocated to the code level selected for reporting that service. No time may be counted twice when reporting more than one E/M service. Prolonged services are also based on the same allocation and their relationship to the primary service. The designation of the facility may be defined by licensure or regulation. Transfer from a hospital bed to a nursing facility bed in a hospital with nursing facility beds is considered as two services in two facilities because there is a discharge from one type of designation to another. An intra-facility transfer for a different level of care (eg, from a routine unit to a critical care unit) does not constitute a new stay, nor does it constitute a transfer to a different facility.

Emergency department (ED) and services in other settings (same or different facilities): Time spent in an ED by a physician or other QHP who provides subsequent E/M services may be included in calculating total time on the date of the encounter when ED services are not reported and another E/M service is reported (eg, hospital inpatient and observation care services).

Discharge services and services in other facilities: Each service may be reported separately as long as any time spent on the discharge service is not counted towards the total time of a subsequent service in which code level selection for the subsequent service is based on time. This includes any hospital inpatient or observation care services (including admission and discharge services) time (99234, 99235, 99236) because these services may be selected based on MDM or time. When these services are reported with another E/M service on the same calendar date, time related to the hospital inpatient or observation care service (including admission and discharge services) may not be used for code selection of the subsequent service.

Discharge services and services in the same facility: If the patient is discharged and readmitted to the same facility on the same calendar date, report a subsequent care service instead of a discharge or initial service. For the purpose of E/M reporting, this is a single stay.

Discharge services and services in a different facility: If the patient is admitted to another facility, for the purpose of E/M reporting this is considered a different stay. Discharge and initial services may be reported as long as time spent on the discharge service is not counted towards the total time of the subsequent service reported when code level selection is based on time.

Critical care services (including neonatal intensive care services and pediatric and neonatal critical care): Reporting guidelines for intensive and critical care services that are performed on the same calendar date as another E/M service are described in the service specific section guidelines.

Transitions between office or other outpatient, home or residence, or emergency department and hospital inpatient or observation or nursing facility: See the guidelines for **Hospital Inpatient and Observation Care Services** or **Nursing Facility Services**. If the patient is seen in two settings and only one service is reported, the total time on the date of the encounter or the aggregated MDM is used for determining the level of the single reported service. If prolonged services are reported, use the prolonged services code that is appropriate for the primary service reported, regardless of where the patient was located when the prolonged services time threshold was met. The choice of the primary service is at the discretion of the reporting physician or other QHP.

Services Reported Separately

Any specifically identifiable procedure or service (ie, identified with a specific CPT code) performed on the date of E/M services may be reported separately.

The ordering and actual performance and/or interpretation of diagnostic tests/studies during a patient encounter are not included in determining the levels of E/M services when the professional interpretation of those tests/studies is reported separately by the physician or other qualified health care professional reporting the E/M service. Tests that do not require separate interpretation (eg, tests that are results only) and are analyzed as part of MDM do not count as an independent interpretation, but may be counted as ordered or reviewed for selecting an MDM level. The performance of diagnostic tests/studies for which specific CPT codes are available may be reported separately, in addition to the appropriate E/M code. The interpretation of the results of diagnostic tests/studies (ie, professional component) with preparation of a separate distinctly identifiable signed written report may also be reported separately, using the appropriate CPT code and, if required, with modifier 26 appended.

The physician or other qualified health care professional may need to indicate that on the day a procedure or service identified by a CPT code was performed, the patient's condition required a significant separately identifiable E/M service. The E/M service may be caused or prompted by the symptoms or condition for which the procedure and/or service was provided. This circumstance may be reported by adding modifier 25 to the appropriate level of E/M service. As such, different diagnoses are not required for reporting of the procedure and the E/M services on the same date.

History and/or Examination

E/M codes that have levels of services include a medically appropriate history and/or physical examination, when performed. The nature and extent of the history and/or physical examination are determined by the treating physician or other qualified health care professional reporting the service. The care team may collect information, and the patient or caregiver may supply information directly (eg, by electronic health record [EHR] portal or questionnaire) that is reviewed by the reporting physician or other qualified health care professional. The extent of history and physical examination is not an element in selection of the level of these E/M service codes.

Levels of E/M Services

Select the appropriate level of E/M services based on the following:

1. The level of the MDM as defined for each service, **or**
2. The total time for E/M services performed on the date of the encounter.

Within each category or subcategory of E/M service based on MDM or time, there are three to five levels of E/M services available for reporting purposes. Levels of E/M services are **not** interchangeable among the different categories or subcategories of service. For example, the first level of E/M services in the subcategory of office visit, new patient, does not have the same definition as the first level of E/M services in the subcategory of office visit, established patient. Each level of E/M services may be used by all physicians or other qualified health care professionals.

Guidelines for Selecting Level of Service Based on Medical Decision Making

Four types of MDM are recognized: straightforward, low, moderate, and high. The concept of the level of MDM does not apply to 99211, 99281.

MDM includes establishing diagnoses, assessing the status of a condition, and/or selecting a management option. MDM is defined by three elements. The elements are:

- ***The number and complexity of problem(s) that are addressed during the encounter.***
- ***The amount and/or complexity of data to be reviewed and analyzed.*** These data include medical records, tests, and/or other information that must be obtained, ordered, reviewed, and analyzed for the encounter. This includes information obtained from multiple sources or interprofessional communications that are not reported separately and interpretation of tests that are not reported separately. Ordering a test is included in the category of test result(s) and the review of the test result is part of the encounter and not a subsequent encounter. Ordering a test may include those considered but not selected after shared decision making. For example, a patient may request diagnostic imaging that is not necessary for their condition and discussion of the lack of benefit may be required. Alternatively, a test may normally be performed, but due to the risk for a specific patient it is not ordered. These considerations must be documented. Data are divided into three categories:
  - Tests, documents, orders, or independent historian(s). (Each unique test, order, or document is counted to meet a threshold number.)
  - Independent interpretation of tests (not separately reported).
  - Discussion of management or test interpretation with external physician or other qualified health care professional or appropriate source (not separately reported).
- ***The risk of complications and/or morbidity or mortality of patient management***. This includes decisions made at the encounter associated with diagnostic procedure(s) and treatment(s). This includes the possible management options selected and those considered but not selected after shared decision making with the patient and/or family. For example, a decision about hospitalization includes consideration of alternative levels of care. Examples may include a psychiatric patient with a sufficient degree of support in the outpatient setting or the decision to not hospitalize a patient with advanced dementia with an acute condition that would generally warrant inpatient care, but for whom the goal is palliative treatment.

Shared decision making involves eliciting patient and/or family preferences, patient and/or family education, and explaining risks and benefits of management options.

MDM may be impacted by role and management responsibility.

When the physician or other qualified health care professional is reporting a separate CPT code that includes interpretation and/or report, the interpretation and/or report is not counted toward the MDM when selecting a level of E/M services. When the physician or other qualified health care professional is reporting a separate service for discussion of management with a physician or another qualified health care professional, the discussion is not counted toward the MDM when selecting a level of E/M services.

The Levels of Medical Decision Making (MDM) table (Table 1) is a guide to assist in selecting the level of MDM for reporting an E/M services code. The table includes the four levels of MDM (ie, straightforward, low, moderate, high) and the three elements of MDM (ie, number and complexity of problems addressed at the encounter, amount and/or complexity of data reviewed and analyzed, and risk of complications and/or morbidity or mortality of patient management). To qualify for a particular level of MDM, two of the three elements for that level of MDM must be met or exceeded.

Examples in the table may be more or less applicable to specific settings of care. For example, the decision to hospitalize applies to the outpatient or nursing facility encounters, whereas the decision to escalate hospital level of care (eg, transfer to ICU) applies to the hospitalized or observation care patient. See also the introductory guidelines of each code family section.

The elements listed in Table 1, Levels of Medical Decision Making, are defined in the guidelines for number and complexity of problems addressed at the encounter, amount and/or complexity of data to be reviewed and analyzed, and risk of complications and/or morbidity or mortality of patient management.

Table 1: Levels of Medical Decision Making (MDM)

Level of MDM (Based on 2 out of 3 Elements of MDM)	Number and Complexity of Problems Addressed at the Encounter	Amount and/or Complexity of Data to Be Reviewed and Analyzed **Each unique test, order, or document contributes to the combination of 2 or combination of 3 in Category 1 below.*	Risk of Complications and/or Morbidity or Mortality of Patient Management
Straightforward	**Minimal** • **1** self-limited or minor problem	**Minimal or none**	**Minimal risk of morbidity from additional diagnostic testing or treatment**
Low	**Low** • **2** or more self-limited or minor problems; **or** • **1** stable, chronic illness; **or** • **1** acute, uncomplicated illness or injury; **or** • **1** stable, acute illness; **or** • **1** acute, uncomplicated illness or injury requiring hospital inpatient or observation level of care	**Limited** *(Must meet the requirements of at least 1 out of 2 categories)* **Category 1: Tests and documents** • Any combination of 2 from the following: – Review of prior external note(s) from each unique source*; – Review of the result(s) of each unique test*; – Ordering of each unique test* **or** **Category 2: Assessment requiring an independent historian(s)** *(For the categories of independent interpretation of tests and discussion of management or test interpretation, see moderate or high)*	**Low risk of morbidity from additional diagnostic testing or treatment**
Moderate	**Moderate** • **1** or more chronic illnesses with exacerbation, progression, or side effects of treatment; **or** • **2** or more stable, chronic illnesses; **or** • **1** undiagnosed new problem with uncertain prognosis; **or** • **1** acute illness with systemic symptoms; **or** • **1** acute, complicated injury	**Moderate** *(Must meet the requirements of at least 1 out of 3 categories)* **Category 1: Tests, documents, or independent historian(s)** • Any combination of 3 from the following: – Review of prior external note(s) from each unique source*; – Review of the result(s) of each unique test*; – Ordering of each unique test*; – Assessment requiring an independent historian(s) **or** **Category 2: Independent interpretation of tests** • Independent interpretation of a test performed by another physician/other qualified health care professional (not separately reported); **or** **Category 3: Discussion of management or test interpretation** • Discussion of management or test interpretation with external physician/other qualified health care professional/appropriate source (not separately reported)	**Moderate risk of morbidity from additional diagnostic testing or treatment** *Examples only:* • Prescription drug management • Decision regarding minor surgery with identified patient or procedure risk factors • Decision regarding elective major surgery without identified patient or procedure risk factors • Diagnosis or treatment significantly limited by social determinants of health
High	**High** • **1** or more chronic illnesses with severe exacerbation, progression, or side effects of treatment; **or** • **1** acute or chronic illness or injury that poses a threat to life or bodily function	**Extensive** *(Must meet the requirements of at least 2 out of 3 categories)* **Category 1: Tests, documents, or independent historian(s)** • Any combination of 3 from the following: – Review of prior external note(s) from each unique source*; – Review of the result(s) of each unique test*; – Ordering of each unique test*; – Assessment requiring an independent historian(s) **or** **Category 2: Independent interpretation of tests** • Independent interpretation of a test performed by another physician/other qualified health care professional (not separately reported); **or** **Category 3: Discussion of management or test interpretation** • Discussion of management or test interpretation with external physician/other qualified health care professional/appropriate source (not separately reported)	**High risk of morbidity from additional diagnostic testing or treatment** *Examples only:* • Drug therapy requiring intensive monitoring for toxicity • Decision regarding elective major surgery with identified patient or procedure risk factors • Decision regarding emergency major surgery • Decision regarding hospitalization or escalation of hospital-level care • Decision not to resuscitate or to de-escalate care because of poor prognosis • Decision regarding parenteral controlled substances

Number and Complexity of Problems Addressed at the Encounter

One element used in selecting the level of service is the number and complexity of the problems that are addressed at the encounter. Multiple new or established conditions may be addressed at the same time and may affect MDM. Symptoms may cluster around a specific diagnosis and each symptom is not necessarily a unique condition. Comorbidities and underlying diseases, in and of themselves, are not considered in selecting a level of E/M services **unless** they are addressed, and their presence increases the amount and/or complexity of data to be reviewed and analyzed or the risk of complications and/or morbidity or mortality of patient management. The final diagnosis for a condition does not, in and of itself, determine the complexity or risk, as extensive evaluation may be required to reach the conclusion that the signs or symptoms do not represent a highly morbid condition. Therefore, presenting symptoms that are likely to represent a highly morbid condition may "drive" MDM even when the ultimate diagnosis is not highly morbid. The evaluation and/or treatment should be consistent with the likely nature of the condition. Multiple problems of a lower severity may, in the aggregate, create higher risk due to interaction.

The term "risk" as used in the definition of this element relates to risk from the condition. While condition risk and management risk may often correlate, the risk from the condition is distinct from the risk of the management.

Problem: A problem is a disease, condition, illness, injury, symptom, sign, finding, complaint, or other matter addressed at the encounter, with or without a diagnosis being established at the time of the encounter.

Problem addressed: A problem is addressed or managed when it is evaluated or treated at the encounter by the physician or other qualified health care professional reporting the service. This includes consideration of further testing or treatment that may not be elected by virtue of risk/benefit analysis or patient/parent/guardian/surrogate choice. Notation in the patient's medical record that another professional is managing the problem without additional assessment or care coordination documented does not qualify as being addressed or managed by the physician or other qualified health care professional reporting the service. Referral without evaluation (by history, examination, or diagnostic study[ies]) or consideration of treatment does not qualify as being addressed or managed by the physician or other qualified health care professional reporting the service. For hospital inpatient and observation care services, the problem addressed is the problem status on the date of the encounter, which may be significantly different than on admission. It is the problem being managed or co-managed by the reporting physician or other qualified health care professional and may not be the cause of admission or continued stay.

Minimal problem: A problem that may not require the presence of the physician or other qualified health care professional, but the service is provided under the physician's or other qualified health care professional's supervision (see 99211, 99281).

Self-limited or minor problem: A problem that runs a definite and prescribed course, is transient in nature, and is not likely to permanently alter health status.

Stable, chronic illness: A problem with an expected duration of at least one year or until the death of the patient. For the purpose of defining chronicity, conditions are treated as chronic whether or not stage or severity changes (eg, uncontrolled diabetes and controlled diabetes are a single chronic condition). "Stable" for the purposes of categorizing MDM is defined by the specific treatment goals for an individual patient. A patient who is not at his or her treatment goal is not stable, even if the condition has not changed and there is no short-term threat to life or function. For example, a patient with persistently poorly controlled blood pressure for whom better control is a goal is not stable, even if the pressures are not changing and the patient is asymptomatic. The risk of morbidity **without** treatment is significant.

Acute, uncomplicated illness or injury: A recent or new short-term problem with low risk of morbidity for which treatment is considered. There is little to no risk of mortality with treatment, and full recovery without functional impairment is expected. A problem that is normally self-limited or minor but is not resolving consistent with a definite and prescribed course is an acute, uncomplicated illness.

Acute, uncomplicated illness or injury requiring hospital inpatient or observation level care: A recent or new short-term problem with low risk of morbidity for which treatment is required. There is little to no risk of mortality with treatment, and full recovery without functional impairment is expected. The treatment required is delivered in a hospital inpatient or observation level setting.

Stable, acute illness: A problem that is new or recent for which treatment has been initiated. The patient is improved and, while resolution may not be complete, is stable with respect to this condition.

Chronic illness with exacerbation, progression, or side effects of treatment: A chronic illness that is acutely worsening, poorly controlled, or progressing with an intent to control progression and requiring additional supportive care or requiring attention to treatment for side effects.

Undiagnosed new problem with uncertain prognosis: A problem in the differential diagnosis that represents a condition likely to result in a high risk of morbidity without treatment.

Acute illness with systemic symptoms: An illness that causes systemic symptoms and has a high risk of morbidity without treatment. For systemic general symptoms, such as fever, body aches, or fatigue in a minor illness that may be treated to alleviate symptoms, see the definitions for ***self-limited or minor problem*** or ***acute, uncomplicated illness or injury.*** Systemic symptoms may not be general but may be single system.

Acute, complicated injury: An injury which requires treatment that includes evaluation of body systems that are not directly part of the injured organ, the injury is extensive, or the treatment options are multiple and/or associated with risk of morbidity.

Chronic illness with severe exacerbation, progression, or side effects of treatment: The severe exacerbation or progression of a chronic illness or severe side effects of treatment that have significant risk of morbidity and may require escalation in level of care.

Acute or chronic illness or injury that poses a threat to life or bodily function: An acute illness with systemic symptoms, an acute complicated injury, or a chronic illness or injury with exacerbation and/or progression or side effects of treatment, that poses a threat to life or bodily function in the near term without treatment. Some symptoms may represent a condition that is significantly probable and poses a potential threat to life or bodily function. These may be included in this category when the evaluation and treatment are consistent with this degree of potential severity.

Amount and/or Complexity of Data to Be Reviewed and Analyzed

One element used in selecting the level of services is the amount and/or complexity of data to be reviewed or analyzed at an encounter.

Analyzed: The process of using the data as part of the MDM. The data element itself may not be subject to analysis (eg, glucose), but it is instead included in the thought processes for diagnosis, evaluation, or treatment. Tests ordered are presumed to be analyzed when the results are reported. Therefore, when they are ordered during an encounter, they are counted in that encounter. Tests that are ordered outside of an encounter may be counted in the encounter in which they are analyzed. In the case of a recurring order, each new result may be counted in the encounter in which it is analyzed. For example, an encounter that includes an order for monthly prothrombin times would count for one prothrombin time ordered and reviewed. Additional future results, if analyzed in a subsequent encounter, may be counted as a single test in that subsequent encounter. Any service for which the professional component is separately reported by the physician or other qualified health care professional reporting the E/M services is not counted as a data element ordered, reviewed, analyzed, or independently interpreted for the purposes of determining the level of MDM.

Test: Tests are imaging, laboratory, psychometric, or physiologic data. A clinical laboratory panel (eg, basic metabolic panel [80047]) is a single test. The differentiation between single or multiple tests is defined in accordance with the CPT code set. For the purpose of data reviewed and analyzed, pulse oximetry is not a test.

Unique: A unique test is defined by the CPT code set. When multiple results of the same unique test (eg, serial blood glucose values) are compared during an E/M service, count it as one unique test. Tests that have overlapping elements are not unique, even if they are identified with distinct CPT codes. For example, a CBC with differential would incorporate the set of hemoglobin, CBC without differential, and platelet count. A unique source is defined as a physician or other qualified health care professional in a distinct group or different specialty or subspecialty, or a unique entity. Review of all materials from any unique source counts as one element toward MDM.

Combination of data elements: A combination of different data elements, for example, a combination of notes reviewed, tests ordered, tests reviewed, or independent historian, allows these elements to be summed. It does not require each item type or category to be represented. A unique test ordered, plus a note reviewed and an independent historian would be a combination of three elements.

External: External records, communications and/or test results are from an external physician, other qualified health care professional, facility, or health care organization.

External physician or other qualified health care professional: An external physician or other qualified health care professional who is not in the same group practice or is of a different specialty or subspecialty. This includes licensed professionals who are practicing independently. The individual may also be a facility or organizational provider such as from a hospital, nursing facility, or home health care agency.

Discussion: Discussion requires an interactive exchange. The exchange must be direct and not through intermediaries (eg, clinical staff or trainees). Sending chart notes or written exchanges that are within progress notes does not qualify as an interactive exchange. The discussion does not need to be on the date of the encounter, but it is counted only once and only when it is used in the decision making of the encounter. It may be asynchronous (ie, does not need to be in person), but it must be initiated and completed within a short time period (eg, within a day or two).

Independent historian(s): An individual (eg, parent, guardian, surrogate, spouse, witness) who provides a history in addition to a history provided by the patient who is unable to provide a complete or reliable history (eg, due to developmental stage, dementia, or psychosis) or because a confirmatory history is judged to be necessary. In the case where there may be conflict or poor communication between multiple historians and more than one historian is needed, the independent historian requirement is met. It does not include translation services. The independent history does not need to be obtained in person but does need to be obtained directly from the historian providing the independent information.

Independent interpretation: The interpretation of a test for which there is a CPT code, and an interpretation or report is customary. This does not apply when the physician or other qualified health care professional who reports the E/M service is reporting or has previously reported the test. A form of interpretation should be documented but need not conform to the usual standards of a complete report for the test. A test that is ordered and independently interpreted may count both as a test ordered and interpreted.

Appropriate source: For the purpose of the **discussion of management** data element (see Table 1, Levels of Medical Decision Making), an appropriate source includes professionals who are not health care professionals but may be involved in the management of the patient (eg, lawyer, parole officer, case manager, teacher). It does not include discussion with family or informal caregivers. For the purpose of ***documents reviewed,*** documents from an appropriate source may be counted.

Risk of Complications and/or Morbidity or Mortality of Patient Management

One element used in selecting the level of service is the risk of complications and/or morbidity or mortality of patient management at an encounter. This is distinct from the risk of the condition itself.

Risk: The probability and/or consequences of an event. The assessment of the level of risk is affected by the nature of the event under consideration. For example, a low probability of death may be high risk, whereas a high chance of a minor, self-limited adverse effect of treatment may be low risk. Definitions of risk are based upon the usual behavior and thought processes of a physician or other qualified health care professional in the same specialty. Trained clinicians apply common language usage meanings to terms such as *high, medium, low,* or *minimal* risk and do not require quantification for these definitions (though quantification may be provided when evidence-based medicine has established probabilities). For the purpose of MDM, level of risk is based upon consequences of the problem(s) addressed at the encounter when appropriately treated. Risk also includes MDM related to the need to initiate or forego further testing, treatment, and/or hospitalization. The risk of patient management criteria applies to the patient management decisions made by the reporting physician or other qualified health care professional as part of the reported encounter.

Morbidity: A state of illness or functional impairment that is expected to be of substantial duration during which function is limited, quality of life is impaired, or there is organ damage that may not be transient despite treatment.

Social determinants of health: Economic and social conditions that influence the health of people and communities. Examples may include food or housing insecurity.

Surgery (minor or major, elective, emergency, procedure or patient risk):

Surgery—Minor or Major: The classification of surgery into minor or major is based on the common meaning of such terms when used by trained clinicians, similar to the use of the term "risk." These terms are not defined by a surgical package classification.

Surgery—Elective or Emergency: Elective procedures and emergent or urgent procedures describe the timing of a procedure when the timing is related to the patient's condition. An elective procedure is typically planned in advance (eg, scheduled for weeks later), while an emergent procedure is typically performed immediately or with minimal delay to allow for patient stabilization. Both elective and emergent procedures may be minor or major procedures.

Surgery—Risk Factors, Patient or Procedure: Risk factors are those that are relevant to the patient and procedure. Evidence-based risk calculators may be used, but are not required, in assessing patient and procedure risk.

Drug therapy requiring intensive monitoring for toxicity: A drug that requires intensive monitoring is a therapeutic agent that has the potential to cause serious morbidity or death. The monitoring is performed for assessment of these adverse effects and not primarily for assessment of therapeutic efficacy. The monitoring should be that which is generally accepted practice for the agent but may be patient-specific in some cases. Intensive monitoring may be long-term or short-term. Long-term intensive monitoring is not performed less than quarterly. The monitoring may be performed with a laboratory test, a physiologic test, or imaging. Monitoring by history or examination does not qualify. The monitoring affects the level of MDM in an encounter in which it is considered in the management of the patient. An example may be monitoring for cytopenia in the use of an antineoplastic agent between dose cycles. Examples of monitoring that do not qualify include monitoring glucose levels during insulin therapy, as the primary reason is the therapeutic effect (unless severe hypoglycemia is a current, significant concern); or annual electrolytes and renal function for a patient on a diuretic, as the frequency does not meet the threshold.

Parenteral controlled substances: The level of risk is based on the usual behavior and thought processes of a physician or other qualified health care professional in the same specialty and subspecialty and not simply based on the presence of an order for parenteral controlled substances.

Guidelines for Selecting Level of Service Based on Time

Certain categories of time-based E/M codes that do not have levels of services based on MDM (eg, Critical Care Services) in the E/M section use time differently. It is important to review the instructions for each category.

Time is **not** a descriptive component for the emergency department levels of E/M services because emergency department services are typically provided on a variable intensity basis, often involving multiple encounters with several patients over an extended period of time.

When time is used for reporting E/M services codes, the time defined in the service descriptors is used for selecting the appropriate level of services. The E/M services for which these guidelines apply require a face-to-face encounter with the physician or other qualified health care professional and the patient and/or family/caregiver. For office or other outpatient services, if the physician's or other qualified health care professional's time is spent in the supervision of clinical staff who perform the face-to-face services of the encounter, use 99211.

For coding purposes, time for these services is the total time on the date of the encounter. It includes both the face-to-face time with the patient and/or family/caregiver and non-face-to-face time personally spent by the physician and/or other qualified health care professional(s) on the day of the encounter (includes time in activities that require the physician or other qualified health care professional and does not include time in activities normally performed by clinical staff). It includes time regardless of the location of the physician or other qualified health care professional (eg, whether on or off the inpatient unit or in or out of the outpatient office). It does not include any time spent in the performance of other separately reported service(s).

Each service that may be reported using time for code level selection has a required time threshold. The concept of attaining a mid-point between levels does not apply. A full 15 minutes is required to report any unit of prolonged services codes 99417, 99418.

Physician(s) and other qualified health care professional(s) may each provide a portion of the face-to-face and non-face-to-face work related to the service. When time is being used to select the appropriate level of services for which time-based reporting is allowed, the time personally spent by the physician(s) and other qualified health care professional(s) assessing and managing the patient and/or counseling, educating, communicating results to the patient/family/caregiver on the date of the encounter is summed to define total time. Only distinct time should be summed (ie, when two or more individuals jointly meet with or discuss the patient, only the time of one individual should be counted).

When prolonged time occurs, the appropriate prolonged services code may be reported. The total time on the date of the encounter spent caring for the patient should be documented in the medical record when it is used as the basis for code selection.

Physician or other qualified health care professional time includes the following activities, when performed:

- preparing to see the patient (eg, review of tests)
- obtaining and/or reviewing separately obtained history
- performing a medically appropriate examination and/or evaluation
- counseling and educating the patient/family/caregiver
- ordering medications, tests, or procedures
- referring and communicating with other health care professionals (when not separately reported)
- documenting clinical information in the electronic or other health record
- independently interpreting results (not separately reported) and communicating results to the patient/family/caregiver
- care coordination (not separately reported)

Do not count time spent on the following:

- the performance of other services that are reported separately
- travel
- teaching that is general and not limited to discussion that is required for the management of a specific patient

For split or shared visits, see the split or shared visits guidelines.

Unlisted Service

An E/M service may be provided that is not listed in this section of the CPT codebook. When reporting such a service, the appropriate unlisted code may be used to indicate the service, identifying it by "Special Report," as discussed in the following paragraph. The "Unlisted Services" and accompanying codes for the E/M section are as follows:

99429 **Unlisted preventive** medicine service
99499 **Unlisted evaluation and management** service

Special Report

An unlisted service or one that is unusual, variable, or new may require a special report demonstrating the medical appropriateness of the service. Pertinent information should include an adequate definition or description of the nature, extent, and need for the procedure and the time, effort, and equipment necessary to provide the service. Additional items that may be included are complexity of symptoms, final diagnosis, pertinent physical findings, diagnostic and therapeutic procedures, concurrent problems, and follow-up care.

Index